FOURTH EDITION

BIOLOGICAL PERFORMANCE of MATERIALS

Fundamentals of Biocompatibility

FOURTH EDITION

BIOLOGICAL PERFORMANCE of MATERIALS

Fundamentals of Biocompatibility

Jonathan Black

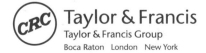

Taylor & Francis
Taylor & Francis Group
Boca Raton   London   New York

A CRC title, part of the Taylor & Francis imprint, a member of the
Taylor & Francis Group, the academic division of T&F Informa plc.

Published in 2006 by
CRC Press
Taylor & Francis Group
6000 Broken Sound Parkway NW, Suite 300
Boca Raton, FL 33487-2742

1005283051

International Standard Book Number-10: 0-8493-3959-6 (Hardcover)
International Standard Book Number-13: 978-0-8493-3959-2 (Hardcover)
Library of Congress Card Number 2005051081

Library of Congress Cataloging-in-Publication Data

Black, Jonathan, 1939-
  Biological performance of materials : fundamentals of biocompatibility / Jonathan Black.-- 4th ed.
    p. cm.
  Includes bibliographical references and index.
  ISBN 0-8493-3959-6 (alk. paper)
  1. Biomedical materials. 2. Biomedical materials--Testing. 3. Biocompatibility. I. Title.

R857.M3B59 2006
617.9'5'028--dc22   2005051081

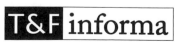

Taylor & Francis Group
is the Academic Division of T&F Informa plc.

Visit the Taylor & Francis Web site at
http://www.taylorandfrancis.com

and the CRC Press Web site at
http://www.crcpress.com

Preface

Biocompatibility of materials increasingly occupies the consciousness of engineers dealing with medical and biological problems. The engineer has long been accustomed to dealing with materials, limits on design. These limits, such as yield stress, endurance limit, and rupture life, are reflected in design margins tailored to the criticality of the specific application. In situations involving biological interactions as a portion of the design problem, the additional materials limit of biocompatibility must be considered.

Failure of compatibility (that is, incompatibility) is proving to be the ultimate limit to the engineering solution of many biomedical problems. As a result, it is necessary to incorporate a thorough grounding in the aspects of biocompatibility — or, as I prefer to term it more generally, biological performance of materials — into the training of bioengineers.

When this book was first conceived, in the early 1970s, no suitable textbooks dealing with broad aspects of biomedical materials or, as the field rapidly came to be called, biomaterials, were available. Today, as this field has matured into biomaterials science and engineering (BSE), many edited collections and topical monographs are available for students and workers at many different levels. However, none seems to suit the neophyte: the former are invariably written by a panel of experts and thus tend to be uneven in attempting to be comprehensive and the latter are the work of a single investigator or research group focusing on relatively narrow and parochial interests. Both of these types of books have a place and many are extremely valuable to the advanced worker, but they all fail to meet the needs of the student or the professional without a background in the field. Thus, it appears that the current work is still needed; it focuses primarily on principles of biological performance at a relatively fundamental level: interactions between living and nonliving materials whose consideration sets BSE apart as a distinct field of investigation and knowledge.

Biological Performance of Materials: Fundamentals of Biocompatibility was originally intended for use as an undergraduate text for a one-term, junior–senior-level bioengineering course on biological performance. I and others have used it in this role. However, with the assignment of selected articles as reading and study sources, it has also proven useful as the central text in undergraduate survey courses on biomaterials and on artificial organs. With additional reading material from the scientific and clinical literature and from materials science texts, it has also been used as the focus of a first-year graduate course in biomaterials for students with engineering (but not biological or medical) backgrounds and, conversely, as a supplementary text for courses on implants for nursing students with little or no engineering training. Finally, engineers working in medical device development and evaluation in industrial as well as governmental settings have found it a useful reference book. The scarcity of reference to actual materials and specific applications has apparently made this diversity of use possible; this revision attempts to maintain the versatility of the work. Primary training in materials science and biology is useful, but not totally essential, because this book is intended for use in conjunction with undergraduate texts in materials science and biology, as needed, so as to accommodate variations in individual degrees of preparation.

We begin with an examination of the concept of "biocompatibility" and arguments for the broader concept of biological performance. Two major sections are devoted to the effect of biological systems on materials ("biodegradation" = material response) and of materials on biological systems ("biocompatibility" = host response), respectively. Selected additional readings are provided at the end of each chapter.

The reader will note an emphasis on methods for determination of biological performance, throughout and especially in Chapter 17 and Chapter 18. This reflects the centrality of material and host response in the clinical performance of medical devices and surgical implants as well as the continued need to select new and modified materials for specific applications. These questions become even more challenging and complex as increasing numbers of viable and nonviable untraditional materials come under consideration for clinical use. The practicing engineer will find this book a useful source of references, test methods, and approaches to the problem of establishing biological performance of materials. Generic materials properties are tabulated in Interpart 1; Interpart 2 is an example of diagnostic approaches to detection of clinical issues associated with biomaterials in animal models and in patients. The final four chapters deal with design, qualification, standardization, and regulation of implant materials and will be of special assistance to the professional. In response to comments on earlier editions, an extensive glossary is also included.

Due to the fundamental nature of this examination, I have elected in this revision to retain many earlier examples and studies, providing updated material and more current references only when needed. The reader is advised to make use of the online resources of the National Library of Medicine (PubMed*) to provide additional, more recent, and more specialized information.

I wish to thank the many undergraduate and graduate students and colleagues whose ideas, questions, and discussions have contributed significantly to the scope and content of this work. Special thanks are due to G.K. Smith and J.L. Woodman for their seminal contributions to Chapter 14 and Chapter 15. An appeal for corrections and suggestions was issued to readers of two listserves (BIOMAT-L and BIOMCH-L) and considerable useful feedback was received.

---

* http://www.ncbi.nlm.nih.gov/entrez/query.fcgi?db=PubMed.

In the preface to the second edition (1992), I suggested that inappropriate host response to implants and premature device failure secondary to materials degradation continue to impose unwanted limits on engineering solutions to biological and medical problems. This is still the case today. It can only be hoped that ideas and information contained in this revised work will contribute to the further' improvement of biomaterials in their application to the alleviation of human disability, disorder, and disease.

Jonathan Black

Abstract

Biological Performance of Materials: Fundamentals of Biocompatibility presents an organized approach to examining and understanding the interactions between materials used in medical devices and implants and living organisms. After an introductory section addressing definitions and aspects of biological environments, the work is divided into three principal sections. These deal with material response to biological systems, host response to biomaterials, and test methods for determining biological response *in vitro* as well as in animal models and clinical settings. Interparts provide summaries of physical properties of commonly used metallic, polymeric, and ceramic biomaterials as well as a guide to understanding clinical performance of implanted biomaterials. In addition to numerous references to the literature, each chapter includes an additional bibliography; an extensive glossary completes the work. Now in its fourth edition, this work draws on Black's more than 35 years experience as a teacher, researcher, and consultant in biomaterials science and engineering.

The Author

Jonathan Black is professor emeritus of bioengineering at Clemson University in Clemson, South Carolina. He holds degrees in physics (Cornell University), engineering science (Pennsylvania State University), and metallurgy (biomaterials) (University of Pennsylvania). Before his appointment as the first occupant of the Hunter Chair of Bioengineering at Clemson in 1988, he was a member of the Department of Orthopaedic Surgery at the University of Pennsylvania for 17 years with a secondary appointment in the Department of Bioengineering. From 1992 to 1995, he was a senior visiting fellow in the IRC for biomaterials at Queen Mary and Westfield College (London), with support from an SERC fellowship.

Black has been active in research and teaching in several areas of biomaterials, with special reference to the biological performance of metallic implants and to the needs of orthopaedic clinical practice. He is the author of many articles and several textbooks, including *Biological Performance of Materials* (1981, 1992, 1999, 2005), *Orthopaedic Biomaterials in Research and Practice* (1988), and, with G. Hastings, *Handbook of Biomaterial Properties* (1998). He has a long-term interest in implant retrieval and analysis and is the author of a major 1992–1993 study of the field for the USFDA.

Black has been involved in professional activities in biomaterials for more than 30 years and is a charter fellow of biomaterials science and engineering (FBSE). He is a charter member and past president of the Society for Biomaterials (U.S.) and has been a frequent presenter and session chair at the Gordon Research Conferences on Biomaterials and an organizer of the triennial Biointeractions conference series in the United Kingdom. He has served on a number of advisory and editorial boards and was an assistant editor of the *Journal of Biomedical Materials Research* from 1978 to 1995. Black is an associate member of the American Academy of Orthopaedic Surgeons and recipient of the presidential gold medal from the British Orthopaedic Association.

In 1992, Black established and served as principal of IMN Biomaterials, a professional consultancy in biomaterials and orthopaedic engineering. He concentrated his efforts in this area after retirement from Clemson in 1993 and closed this enterprise at the end of 1998. He continues to chair the Scientific Advisory Board for Stryker Orthopaedics.

Contents

Part III Host Response: Biological Effects of Implants

Part I

General Considerations

1

Biocompatibility: Definitions and Issues

1.1 Introduction

The issue of biocompatibility arises from recognition of the profound differences between living tissues and nonliving materials. In an historical and a practical perspective, a wide range of interactive behavior occurs between tissues and materials. In any of these interactions, beneficial and adverse effects may be observed. Thus, materials considered foods and beverages can be nutritious or non-nutritious. From another viewpoint, they can be considered toxic or nontoxic. Such judgments are relative to use or abuse rather than to an absolute scale. Although it is a central nervous system depressor, alcohol has a positive virtue as a disinhibiting stimulant and social drug in small doses. Internally, large doses are toxic, and still larger doses are lethal. However, even in toxic doses, alcohol is a useful external antiseptic.

It is desirable to extend this sort of relativism of dose and type of use to examination of the interactions between biomaterials and living systems. Biomaterials are materials of natural or man-made origin that are used to direct, supplement, or replace the functions of living tissues. When these materials evoke a minimal biological response, they have come to be termed biocompatible. As it is typically used, the term biocompatible is inappropriate and defective of content. Compatibility is strictly the quality of harmonious interaction. Thus, the label biocompatible suggests that the material described displays universally "good" or harmonious behavior in contact with tissue and body fluids. It is an absolute term without any referent.

Furthermore, the traditional ideas of biocompatibility refer essentially to the effect of the material on the biological system. Effects of biological processes on materials are rarely included in the meaning, unless the results of material changes elicit a change in biological response. The effects of the biological system on the material are usually lumped in the term biodegradation, which implies "bad" behavior — again without a referent. However, in the case of a deeply implanted suture, biodegradation may be a sought-after result.

One can protest that this is a semantic discussion without content. On the contrary, I think that the terminology used and the assumptions inherent in that terminology tend to condition the approach taken in experiment and analysis. Thus, the most common approach to establishing the biocompatibility of a material is still to establish the absence of deleterious effects associated with its use in biological applications. Once such tests are completed, the material is regarded as qualified. I believe that the absolute nature of the language employed has led to the use of absolute, and thus inappropriate, criteria.

The real issues in the use of materials in medical and surgical devices are not any more absolute than is the choice of a material for any other engineering application. The choice of materials for construction of a device or machine is made early in the design process. The properties of the candidate materials, particularly those properties that bear on the intended function of the complete assembly, then interact strongly with the design. The ultimate test of the appropriateness of the choice of materials is the performance of the completed device in its intended application. In this performance, the interaction between design choices (shape, size, linkage, etc.) and materials properties (strength, density, composition, etc.) can be seen. Chapter 21 deals with some of these points more fully.

The real issue of biocompatibility is not whether there are adverse biological reactions to a material, but whether that material performs satisfactorily (that is, in the intended fashion) in the intended biomedical application and thus can be considered a successful biomaterial. This goal should lead directly to a traditional engineering design process of considering the advantages and disadvantages inherent in the selection of a particular material for a design in a specific application. Among the factors considered must be the interaction of the material with the biological processes in its intended site of operation.

One of the consequences of this relative approach to material performance in contact with living tissues must also be the rejection of the idea that any material in any selected application can be categorically safe or unsafe. In dealing with food additives, it is possible to draw up a list of materials that are "generally regarded as safe" (GRAS).* This results from the situation in which each dye, sweetener, flavoring agent, etc. is serving the same function, no matter what the apparent application, and is consistently used in a low but relatively uniform amount or "dose." Food is always ingested and never implanted, and all food is subjected to the same succession of physiological degradation, storage, and excretion processes. By contrast, a material used successfully in one medical device, and thus considered a biomaterial, may then be used in a different form in a different location with another intended response, with an unsatisfactory result. Thus, it should be no surprise that there is no GRAS list for biomaterials.**

---

* This register or list is maintained by the US-FDA's Center for Food Safety and Applied Nutrition (CFSAN) and, as of May 2005, contained 158 completed entries. See: http:// www.cfsan.fda.gov/~rdb/opa-gras.html.
** However, see Section 20.4.1 for an attempt to create such a list.

1.2   Biological Performance

I adopted the term biological performance as a descriptor of materials in order to replace the historical or classical idea of biocompatibility. Biological performance and two closely related terms are defined as follows:

Biological performance: the interaction between materials and living systems

The two aspects of this performance are:

Host response: the local and systemic response, other than the intended therapeutic response, of living systems to the material

Material response: the response of the material to living systems

The generality of these terms is obvious. Their definitions have no inherent value judgments, and they do not suggest absolute qualities.

However, these terms are not sufficient for a full discussion. I have stressed the need for consideration of interactions between materials and living systems on a relative, rather than an absolute, basis. This suggests the need for a system of grading or ranking based upon the results of tests. Additional terms are needed to implement such a concept. The first three definitions are therefore supplemented with several others:

Reference (or control) material: a material that, by standard test, has been determined to elicit a reproducible, quantifiable host or material response*

Level of host (or material) response: the nature of the host (or material) response in a standard test with respect to the response obtained with a reference material

A standard test, as referred to in these two definitions, is simply any well-defined, repeatable test. The requirements for such tests are discussed in Chapter 17 and Chapter18.

Finally, I suggest that the use of the term biocompatibility be retained for historical reasons, but with a narrow and careful redefinition:

Biocompatible (-ility): biological performance in a specific application that is judged suitable to that situation

---

* Note that this definition carries no implication of "good" or "bad" behavior on the part of the reference material. A reference material might be a material with minimal host response (a negative reference) or an extreme host response (a positive reference). Reference materials may or may not be selected from those conventionally used for implant fabrication. The use of a material as a reference material does not qualify it as a biomaterial.

So, at the end of the consideration, when host and material responses are known and the particular device application is examined, a final value judgment can then be made that leads to the acceptance or rejection of the material for that application. Such a selection and a resulting record of adequate performance do not "qualify" a material. Rather, they increase the confidence in the use of the material as a biomaterial in that particular application and point to possible successful use in similar applications.

This last point is extremely important. The final arbiter of biocompatibility, as defined here, can only be satisfactory clinical performance, insofar as material properties affect the outcome of the treatment. Thus, if a biomaterial has been in use for a long time, it makes no sense to go back to the materials science laboratory, the tissue culture laboratory, and the animal colony in an attempt to determine its biocompatibility. The experiment has already been performed during human clinical use; what is required is careful observation to determine and interpret the outcome. This point is discussed at length in Chapter 22.

1.3   Consensus Definitions

A major attempt has been made to reach consensus concerning some definitions related to biocompatibility. A working consensus conference, sponsored by the European Society for Biomaterials, was held in 1986 to discuss these matters in an international setting (Williams 1987). Of the 13 terms that gained consensus definitions; the following are relevant to this discussion:

Biomaterial: a nonviable material used in a medical device, intended to interact with biological systems

Host response: the reaction of a living system to the presence of a material

Biocompatibility: the ability of a material to perform with an appropriate host response in a specific situation

Although they are terse, these are not bad definitions. They preserve the idea of interaction and of relative, rather than absolute, attributes. They are limited definitions in that they specifically exclude living tissues from the spectrum of biomaterials. In addition to exhibiting active physiological processes, tissues are materials with definable physical structure and properties; thus, their exclusion seems unwarranted and unwise. It is unfortunate that the conferees chose to deprecate the terms biological performance and material response because I consider them to embody concepts that lend clarity to the discussion of biocompatibility.

The success of this conference and, in particular, the widespread acceptance of biocompatibility as a relative rather than an absolute attribute of biomaterials led to the convening in 1991 of a second consensus conference, again in Chester, U.K., under the same sponsorship (Williams et al. 1992). After intensive discussion, five additional terms related to biomaterials and biological performance were agreed to by consensus:

Biomaterial: a material intended to interface with biological systems to evaluate, treat, augment, or replace any tissue, organ, or function of the body

Bioactive material: a biomaterial designed to elicit or modulate biological activity

Bone bonding: the establishment, by physicochemical processes, of continuity between implant and bone matrix

Biodegradation: the breakdown of a material mediated by a biological system

Inherent thrombogenicity: thrombus formation controlled by the material surface

The definition of biomaterials clearly matured in the interval between these two conferences. The concept of bioactivity will be discussed in the next section in the context of interactivity. Biodegradation now was given a special meaning: not merely the passive response of a material to the physicochemical conditions found in living systems, but also involving actual cellular effects on the pericellular environment (see Section 2.3). Finally, the compound term inherent thrombogenicity represents the first small, solid achievement in defining the very complex interactions between blood and biomaterials (see Chapter 9 for further discussion).

However, words become part of language by the repetition of their use or they are abandoned, in the same way that paths broken through the wild may or may not become superhighways. Thus, it remains to be seen how these and other terms discussed here will be conventionally understood and used in the scientific literature.*

1.4 Discussion

The use of the definitions discussed here has gradually redirected the study of interactions between biological systems and materials. It has moved from efforts to obtain qualification and blanket assurances of safety to description and grading of biological performance based upon the careful development

---

* See the Glossary for additional consensus definitions.

of standard tests and the characterization of reproducible response relative to reference materials. This is a central idea that will guide considerations throughout this work.

I feel strongly that absolute qualification of an artificial or processed material in biological applications is not possible now or in the foreseeable future. It is necessary to establish minimum requirements for performance at various stages of materials development. Strategies for setting such levels are discussed in Chapter 21.

It has been suggested that no foreign material is biocompatible (old meaning) and that the best that can be expected is that the results of its use are "physiologically tolerable." This is a somewhat negative view that overlooks the essentially benign responses elicited by many materials in living systems. However, such a suggestion should attract attention to another important point. Living systems differ most from machines in respect to the constant flux and change of their components — that is, in their physiology. Biological performance, particularly host response, ought not to be defined in terms of tissue structure and pathology but primarily in terms of local, organ, and systemic physiology. Deviations from usual physiological conditions may lead to changes in the structure and function of living tissues.

The key to understanding host response and, to a lesser degree, material response, is knowledge of the participation of the material in the physiology of the host. Extrapolation of results obtained in tissue culture and animal models rests significantly on knowledge of how normal and abnormal physiological processes in these systems differ from those in humans, in health and in disease. Thus, in addition to concentrating on making relative rather than absolute determinations, care will also be taken to attend to physiology (normal and abnormal) and its interspecies variations.

Osborn (1979) attempted to take such physiological considerations into account by classifying all biomaterials as biotolerant, bioinert, or bioactive, conveying respectively the sense of negative (but tolerable) local host response, absence of local host response, and positive (desired) local host response. Slutskii and Vetra (1996) revived Osborn's approach by defining a term, reactogenicity, as the intrinsic property (or combination of properties) of a biomaterial that produces a certain tissue reaction. This approach essentially converts Osborn's categories into a continuous scale — presumably running from normal to some degree of inflammation (see Chapter 8) — because Slutskii prefers to restrict reactogenicity to the description of the intrinsic properties of "biocompatible," that is, successful biomaterials. Both of these treatments mirror an earlier approach by Steinemann (1975), in which he explicitly classified metallic implant materials, by reference to the nature of the local encapsulization response, as toxic, scar tissue, or vital. Steinemann's approach is of particular interest in that he tried, somewhat unsuccessfully, to correlate these categories with an intrinsic material property, polarization resistance (see Section 4.6), thus presaging Slutskii and Vetra.

Collectively, these approaches provide little illumination because they fail to look beyond the immediate biomaterial–tissue interface to the larger requirements of specific clinical applications. However, it is possible to extend these ideas, taking into account the development of the field of biomaterials and eliminating the undesirable use of the prefix bio- (as used by Osborn). Examining the historical development of biomaterials, I have identified four phases (or types) of biomaterials, based upon changing concepts of host response:

- Phase 1. Inert (biomaterials): implantable materials that elicit little or no host response
- Phase 2. Interactive (biomaterials): implantable materials designed to elicit specific, beneficial responses, such as ingrowth, adhesion, etc.
- Phase 3. Viable (biomaterials)*: implantable materials, incorporating or attracting live cells at implantation, that are treated by the host as normal tissue matrices and are actively resorbed and/or remodeled
- Phase 4. Replant (biomaterials)*: implantable materials consisting of native tissue cultured *in vitro* from cells obtained previously from the specific implant patient

It is now recognized that searches for type 1** materials are as pointless as the historical pursuit of the Philosopher's Stone — the talisman that would turn any base material into gold. Many biomaterials in present clinical use, such as porous structures and bioactive coatings, as well as ones in development are properly called type 2 materials. Type 3 materials are the subject of active research and commercial interest, with initial examples in limited clinical use (see Warnke et al. 2004). Advances in control and manipulation of the genetic code in mammals suggest that no intellectual barrier exists to prevent the broad future realization of type 4 materials at the tissue and organ levels. In fact, a true type 4 material (implantable, live tissue with the identical genetic code and immunological determinants of the recipient patient) represents the ultimate fulfillment of the original search for biocompatibility: implantable materials demonstrating harmonious interaction.

Medical practice today utilizes great numbers of artificial devices and implants. As long ago as 1988, by some estimates (Moss et al. 1991), as many as one in 22 Americans had at least one implant and the proportion clearly continues to increase. For any one application, a wide variety of

---

* In the 15 years since I conceived these definitions, the field has advanced rapidly. Thus, I now implicitly include the implantation of DNA, as plasmids or in transfected cells, in the definition of phase 3 and 4 biomaterials and similarly broaden the phase 4 definition to read "*in vitro* or *in vivo*."

** I have generally used the term *phase* to discuss the historical development and *type* to address the actual biomaterials.

similar designs exist with different degrees of efficacy. In contrast to this profusion of design, materials suitable as biomaterials continue to be scarce. Perhaps no more than a few dozen of the millions of available metal, polymer, and ceramic compositions have proven useful in medical devices and implants.

The limiting factor in the use of materials as biomaterials continues to be achieving appropriate biological performance. Better understanding of biological performance and the factors affecting it will lead to a variety of useful new materials options. This in turn will lead to substantial expansion of the role that artificial devices can play in the prevention and treatment of human disability and disease. At the end of this progression, when the technology for preparation of type 4 materials is readily, widely, and affordably available, artificial devices will be called upon to serve only as "bridges" to replantation and the field of biomaterials will emerge in its rightful place as one of the healing arts.

1.5   The Discipline of Biomaterials*

The concluding comments in the preceding section presuppose that a field of study or an intellectual discipline — biomaterials — exists. Such a field exists when a definition that includes all valid aspects and excludes all other aspects is recognized. I define the field of biomaterials thus:

> Biomaterials: the organized study of the materials properties of the tissues and organs of living organisms; the development and characterization of pharmacologically inert materials to measure, restore, and improve function in such organisms; and the interaction between viable and nonviable materials

This definition can be seen in graphic form in Figure 1.1. The bases for the field, its foundation disciplines, are the traditional intellectual fields of engineering, medicine, and the physical and biological sciences. The body of the field is the materials science approach to manufactured (artificial) and natural (or native) biomaterials (including tissues). The apex or distinguishing feature of the field is the study of biological performance of materials as defined by their host and material responses. This last area is unique to the discipline of biomaterials and leads to a further definition:

> Biomaterials science: the study and knowledge of the interaction between living and nonliving materials

---

* Parts of this section were previously published, in different form, in Black et al. (1992).

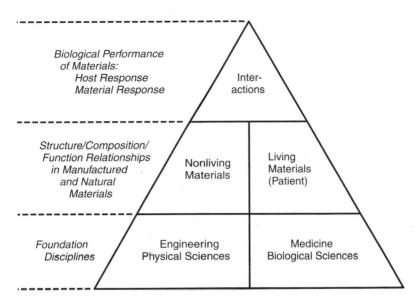

FIGURE 1.1
The structure of the discipline of biomaterials.

A complementary definition is:

> Biomaterials engineering: the application of the principles of biomaterials science and its foundation sciences to the solution of practical problems of human health, disability, and disease

Taking into account the definitions of biomaterials as objects and as a field of study, I advance three propositions about the nature of the intellectual field of biomaterials:

> Biomaterials is a materials science: the central issue is the dependence of physical properties on composition and structure.
>
> Biomaterials is an interdisciplinary science: its unique feature is consideration of the interactions between living and nonliving materials.
>
> Biomaterials is a medical science: its ultimate goal is the improvement of human health and quality of life.

Biomaterials science and engineering are evolving fields of study, investigation, and development. However, their meets and bounds are now understood well enough to assert safely that they are parts of an established discipline, the field of biomaterials.

1.6   Afterword: Paradigmatic Shift

As the field of biomaterials began to be organized as a field of research and an academic discipline in the early 1970s,* a recognizable paradigm emerged that dominated the efforts in the field (Figure 1.2). In this analysis, the central issue was seen as the interaction between implant and patient at the interface: the effect of the patient on the implant ("biodegradation" = material response) and the converse effect of the implant on the patient ("biocompatibility" = [local] host response). The principal foci of investigation of material response were fracture, wear, corrosion, and dissolution, with lesser interests in transport, storage, and excretion of degradation products. Host response was viewed primarily in a local or interface context, with emphasis on ingrowth, inflammation, fibrosis (encapsulation), and, when in chronic contact with blood, coagulation and hemolysis.

As the field began to mature and interest moved away from the apparently impossible and fruitless search for inert (type 1) materials to active pursuit and design of bioactive (type 2: interactive) materials, some trends could be noted:

- Biological models began to focus less on animals and patients and more on cells and molecules.

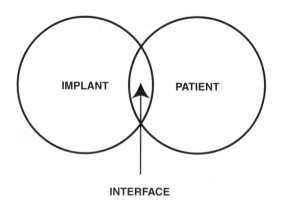

INTERFACE

Material Degradation

(fracture; wear; corrosion

[transport, storage, excretion])

Local Host Response

(ingrowth; inflammation;

fibrosis; coagulation/hemolysis

[remote; systemic])

FIGURE 1.2
The old biomaterials paradigm.

---

* A key milestone was the organization of the Society for Biomaterials (SFB) in 1973.

- Investigations and design of materials began to emphasize three-dimensional structures over two-dimensional interfaces.

- Effects of material-living systems' interactions were increasingly examined in terms of systemic biology as well as local biological response.

- Initial efforts at replacement of absent, damaged, or diseased parts of the human body broadened into concern for diagnosis, repair, and regeneration.

- Overall, the field moved from a more applied engineering approach of providing pragmatic solutions to clinical problems to a concern for more science-based fundamental understanding of clinical problems and of potential routes to their solution.

These shifts in emphasis are contained in the modern reference to the field as "biomaterials science and engineering," rather than as "biomaterials," and are reflected in a new paradigm (Figure 1.3). Here, *material* is replaced by *matrix* and *patient* by *cell*, and a third factor, *signal*, is added. Each of these factors interacts with the other two: the cells are affected by their matrix and by bound and free signals; the signals are modified by cellular activity and by association with matrix while the matrix can be remodeled by cells, based upon its native structure and upon interaction with signaling molecules. The emphasis is now larger than merely a study of the interface between body and biomaterial, as in the old paradigm; now it is on interactions and their local, systemic, and remote consequences.

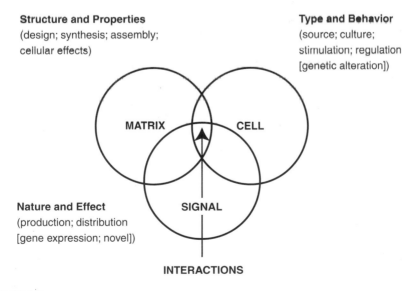

Structure and Properties
(design; synthesis; assembly;
cellular effects)

Type and Behavior
(source; culture;
stimulation; regulation
[genetic alteration])

MATRIX CELL

Nature and Effect
(production; distribution
[gene expression; novel])

SIGNAL

INTERACTIONS

FIGURE 1.3
The emerging new biomaterials paradigm.

The foci of interest have also shifted:

- Matrix: here interest still closely resembles traditional materials scientists' concerns for the relationships between structure and properties; however, rather than mere selection and adaptation of materials, the activities tend to involve prospective design, synthesis, and assembly and investigation of cellular effects on the resulting material.

- Cells: replacing earlier attention centered on the biological response (of tissues) at the interface, the studies now address the cells, which can interact with the matrix as well as local and systemic signals. The focus is on cell source, *in vitro* culture, stimulation, and regulation, as well as the possibility of transient or permanent genetic alteration.

- Signals: the final member of the triad is a class of molecules of biological and synthetic origins that can affect cellular behavior, especially insofar as cell–matrix interactions are concerned. Here, the focus of interest is on characterization, production, and distribution of known and novel molecular sequences and molecules and on the possibility of their production *in situ* through genetic expression.

An obvious early exemplar of this new or modern paradigm is the type 3 or biohybrid biomaterial: a matrix capable of being remodeled by implanted or attracted cells, cells cultured *in vitro* or recruited upon implantation, and signals to regulate cell–matrix and construct–host interactions. This paradigm makes it clear that the newly emerging bioengineering fields of genetic, cellular, and tissue engineering are, in fact, not new but simply logical extensions of the historic and maturing field of biomaterials science and engineering.

Thus, as a basic science field, as an engineering field allied to clinical medicine, and as a class of materials, biomaterials continues to grow and diversify. The new paradigm questions our earlier assertions of knowledge and suggests that biomaterials science and engineering will continue to be an exciting and viable field for the foreseeable future.

References

Black, J., Shalaby, S.W. and LaBerge, M., Biomaterials education: an academic viewpoint, *J. Appl. Biomater.*, 3, 231, 1992.

Moss, A.J. et al., Use of selected medical device implants in the United States, 1988, *Advance Data No. 191*, February 26, 1991, Centers for Disease Control, National Center for Health Statistics, Washington, D.C.

Osborn, J.F., Biomaterials and their use in implants, *Schw. Mschr. Zahnheilk.*, 89, 1138, 1979.

Slutskii, L.I. and Vetra, J.J., Letter to the editor: biocompatibility and reactogenicity of materials: a semantic and logical analysis of definitions and their practical significance, *Cells Mater.*, 6, 137, 1996.

Steinemann, S., [Corrosion, compatibility, and mechanical properties of metallic implants] (Ger.), *Fortschr. Kiefer Gesichtschir.*, 19, 50, 1975, discussed in Steinemann, S., Introduction, in Winter, G.D., Leray, J.L., de Groot, K.(Eds), *Evaluation of Biomaterials*, John Wiley & Sons, Chichester, U.K., 1, 1980.

Warnke, P.H. et al., Growth and transplantation of a custom vascularised bone graft in a man, *Lancet*, 364, 766, 2004.

Williams, D.F. (Ed.), *Definitions in Biomaterials: Proceedings of a Consensus Conference of the European Society for Biomaterials*, Chester, England, March 3–5, 1986. Elsevier, Amsterdam, 1987.

Williams, D.F., Black, J. and Doherty, P.J., Second consensus conference on definitions in biomaterials, in Doherty, P.J. et al. (Eds.), *Biomaterial–Tissue Interfaces. Advances in Biomaterials* Vol. 10, Elsevier, Amsterdam, 525, 1992.

Bibliography

Bush, R.B., Biomaterials: an introduction for librarians, *Sci. Technol. Lib.*, 15(4), 3, 1996.

Feldman, D.S. et al., A biocompatibility hierarchy: justification for biomaterial enhanced regeneration, in Wise, D.L., Trantolo, D.J., Altobelli, D.E. et al. (Eds.), *Encyclopedic Handbook of Biomaterials and Bioengineering, Part A: Materials*, Vol. 1, Marcel Dekker, New York, 223, 1995.

Peppas, N.A. and Langer, R., New challenges in biomaterials, *Science*, 264, 25 March 1994, 1715.

2

Introduction to the Biological Environment

2.1 General Considerations

The central idea developed in the previous chapter is that biological performance should be defined in terms of interaction between materials and their operational setting, the biological environment. This is not qualitatively different from the normal consideration given to the material aspects of performance and durability during any engineering design process. However, two relative quantitative aspects set biological performance apart and create the need for an independent study of material and host responses:

- High demand: the biological environment, especially internal to living systems, is a remarkably aggressive one, resembling tropical marine conditions. It is a milieu of high chemical activity combined with a highly variable spectrum of combined mechanical stresses.

- Invariant conditions: despite its aggressive aspects, the biological environment displays an extraordinary quality of constancy in physical conditions and composition. Complex control systems exist to maintain that constancy; thus, deviations from established conditions attendant to the presence of materials may be expected to incite restoring responses.

The latter portions of this work deal with many aspects of this peculiar environment during examination of typical material and host responses. At this point, it is advisable to examine general points that will serve as guides for discussion.

2.2 Comparison of External and Internal Conditions

The aggressive aspects of the biological environment may be understood if the differences between conditions external and internal to living systems are examined. Externally, the familiar aspects of the physical world can be found. Most materials are inorganic and are partially or fully oxidized. Although physical processes are interrelated, there is an absence of active environmental control systems. Time constants for change are long, determined by processes of chemical reaction and diffusion, and driven by sources that supply energy primarily through radiation, conduction, and convection. A wide variety of atomic species are present. Structure and chemical content vary greatly and little evidence of compositional or structural optimization can be found.

By contrast, the internal environment arises from a system in which materials (molecules and tissues) are largely organic and are partially or fully reduced. Most changes are mediated by active, energy-requiring control systems. In many cases, multiple parallel systems with different time constants and extensive intersystem interactions control a single transformation or process. Time constants are orders of magnitude shorter than for most inorganic reactions due to mediation by specialized organic catalysts (enzymes) and the derivation of energy from chemical sources through coupled reactions. Although a great variety of chemical content and structure exists, arrangements and combinations of a few elements — primarily carbon, oxygen, hydrogen, and nitrogen — comprise the vast majority of this complexity. Elements that are present are generally utilized and structures display a parsimonious efficiency, providing an overall impression of design optimization.

Whatever one's views on the origin and development of biological systems, one must be impressed by the complexity of these systems and their economy of action. They obtain their objectives by excluding, through accident, design, or active process, materials that are unnecessary or harmful to the function of their individual processes. These phenomena act to exclude all materials other than healthy, autologous (belonging to the same organism) tissue. Furthermore, the systems interact locally as well as on a regional and global (whole organism) scale. Thus, a constant aspect of the biological environment is that the introduction of a foreign material will elicit a host response, which may have local, systemic, and remote aspects.

2.3   Problems in Definition of the Biological Environment

Until now, I have referred to "a" biological environment. However, a variety of sets of conditions is associated with life processes, and it is difficult to define the actual environment in which a material or device is called upon to function. More will be said about this later. The difficulty arises from a lack of detailed knowledge of *in vivo* conditions and the local variations that can occur in the face of overall maintenance of conditions, termed homeostasis, necessary for life. Also, there is ambiguity in defining the region that is coupled with an implant. Implants in isolated locations can interact with the rest of the system through diffusion of ions and fluids, circulation of blood, and drainage of the lymphatics. Even the definition of absolute volumes of material in communication with an implant is difficult. As Chapter 15 will show, the volume of water in which an implant is immersed in the human body may be taken as 10^{-15}, 8.4, or 1000 l, depending upon the details of consideration.

A last general point has to do with the maintenance of homeostasis. In a particular location, temperature, pH, pO_2, equivalent electrical potential, hydrostatic and osmotic pressure, and tissue/fluid composition are closely controlled. However, the observation of such active control should not lead to unwarranted conclusions concerning its adaptability. The control systems most in evidence are those that control for the usual situation and small deviations. Superimposed upon these are "emergency" protection systems, such as coagulation, inflammation, and nonspecific immune response. These initiate programmed deviations that attempt to restore normal conditions locally, as long as systemic integrity is maintained. Taking a control systems viewpoint, one can foresee challenges that can overwhelm the restorative capabilities of local and systemic control. Only challenges that occur within the "design" spectrum of the system can be expected to elicit satisfactory responses, except by chance. Thus, when viewing host response, it is wise to recognize the limited environmental variations that occur in the absence of outside intrusion. It is also prudent to consider the qualitative and quantitative differences between chance intrusion and deliberate functional implantation of biomaterials.

Materials must be tested *in vitro* before implantation, even in animals. It is desirable to attempt, in large or small part, to replicate the operating environment that the material may encounter after implantation. Here it is useful to distinguish among four classes of exposure environments:

- Physiological: chemical (inorganic) and thermal conditions controlled to normative mammalian values for the intended application
- Biophysiological: physiological conditions with the addition of appropriate types and concentrations of initially nondenatured (active) cell products (serum proteins, enzymes, etc.)
- Biological: biophysiological conditions with the addition of appropriate viable, active cells
- Pericellular (circumcellular): a special case of "biological": the conditions in the immediate vicinity of appropriate, viable, active cells

I term these "classes" of environments because the exact value of parameters within each depends upon the specific details of the location within tissue or organ and, in the case of materials (rather than device) testing, upon the design details and functional goals of the device.

In vitro testing is usually carried out under physiological or biophysiological conditions only. The problems associated with *in vitro* testing and its comparison to *in vivo* conditions will be discussed further in Chapter 17 and Chapter 18. In this chapter, "biological environment" is taken to mean, most generally, the combination of conditions that an implanted material will encounter acutely and chronically in actual service: the combination of biological and pericellular conditions, as well as the instantaneous requirements placed upon the design and function of the device in which it is incorporated. The combination of these intrinsic and extrinsic environmental effects with the overall patient requirements during the proposed period of implantation produces what is properly termed the implant life history: the total combination of requirements that the biomaterial must meet to be successful in a specific application.

2.4   Elements of the Biological Environment

The human body is generally considered in terms of a standard or reference configuration: this is the 70-kg man.* This standard has the macroscopic parameters given in Table 2.1. Wide individual variations from these parameters exist. Age, type and level of activity, disease state, national origin, and genetic factors will also affect the absolute values. Furthermore, the values given here, as in the following tables in this chapter, are mean normative values for a male Anglo–Saxon individual aged in his mid-30s. They represent an average expectation and do not account for any variations within physiological limits. It is common to describe such variations under the overall term "biological variation." The physicochemical and mechanical conditions encountered in the body can also be defined (Table 2.2).

When the effects of release of material from the implant into the body are considered, it is necessary to know the starting or nominal inorganic chemical composition of the body. Although the concentrations of major elements have been known for some time, those of trace elements, present in very low concentrations, are just beginning to be appreciated fully. Table 2.3 presents nominal or reference mean values; see Chapter 15 for a more detailed discussion.

Taken together, these parameters define the intrinsic physicochemical and mechanical parameters appropriate to generic biological environments. Exact dimensional and functional details of a particular anatomical site may be required when designing tests for particular materials or devices. In another area, more detailed information is desirable. Blood is a delicate and pervasive

* It is usual practice to speak of the standard man rather than the standard human. Recent comments in the lay literature concerning the focus of federal funding for biomedical research have drawn attention, once again, to important differences between men and women. Thus, the values in Table 2.1 should be taken as guidelines; other sources, such as Lentner (1981), should be addressed for values applicable to gender-specific applications for northern hemisphere Anglo–Saxon subjects.

TABLE 2.1

Macroscopic Parameters of the Reference Human[a]

Weight: 70 kg	Height (medium frame): 1.80 m
Surface area: 1.88 m²	Volume: 0.065 m³
Composition:	Density:
Water: 60% (42 l)	Fat: 0.9 g/cm³
Solid: 40% (28 kg)	Whole body: 1.07 g/cm³
Distribution of tissue types (as percentages of body weight)	
Muscle:	43
Bone:	30
Internal organs:	
Heart:	0.4
Liver:	2
Kidneys (2):	0.5
Spleen:	0.2
Lungs:	1.6
Brain:	2.3
Viscera:	5.6
Skin:	7
Blood:	7.2 (5 l)
Basal metabolic rate: 37/kcal.m²/h	

[a]Values given for a male individual in his mid-30s.

Source: Lentner, C. (Ed.), *Geigy Scientific Tables*, Ciba–Geigy, Basle, 1981.

tissue. It is essential to understand its makeup and normal values, especially for applications involving blood contact on a chronic basis. Information describing the composition and cellular distribution of blood is given in Table 2.4.

It is difficult to obtain engineering properties of biological materials for use in design processes. With a group of contributors, Black and Hastings (1998) took a major step by attempting to collate reliable properties of normal human tissues and fluids. However, effects of age and disease processes on engineering properties of tissues are still not well reported. Reference should be made to contemporary literature or individual experimental studies may need to be undertaken to obtain design data for specific applications.

Beginning with the information given in Table 2.1 to Table 2.4 and from other sources, it is possible to develop a picture of the thermal, mechanical, and chemical environment that an implant will encounter when it is implanted in a specific anatomical site. Some of the material responses during implant service life will be described in Chapter 3 to Chapter 7 of this work. This defined environment may be changed acutely and chronically by the presence of an implant.* Chapter 8 to Chapter 15 deal with some

---

* Although it is possible to define four types of "biological" environments, it should be appreciated that the fourth — the pericellular environment — is the least known and understood. On this scale of consideration, it is clear that cellular events produce dynamic and continuing changes (Konttinen et al. 2005). These are difficult to measure and to replicate *in vitro*. In the general case, there can probably be no substitute for *in vivo* studies in intact animals to examine host–material interactions at this level.

TABLE 2.2

Physicochemical and Mechanical Conditions in Humans

	Value	Location
pH	1.0	Gastric contents
	4.5–6.0	Urine
	6.8	Intracellular
	7.0	Interstitial
	7.15–7.35	Blood
pO_2 (mmHg)	2–40	Interstitial
	12	Intramedullary
	40	Venous
	100	Arterial
	160	Atmospheric
pCO_2 (mmHg)	40	Alveolar
	2	Atmospheric
Temperature (°C)	37	Normal core
	20–42.5	Deviations in disease
	28	Normal skin
	0–45	Skin at extremities

Mechanical	Stress (MPa)	Tissues
	0–0.4	Cancellous bone
	0.08–0.1	Across aortic valve (ventricular diastole)
	0.12–0.16	Across mitral valve (ventricular systole)
	0–4	Cortical bone
	4	Muscle (peak stress)
	40	Tendon (peak stress)
	80	Ligament (peak stress)

Stress Cycles (per year)	Activity
3×10^5	Peristalsis
3×10^6	Swallowing
$0.5–4 \times 10^7$	Heart contraction
$0.1–1 \times 10^6$	Finger joint motion
$1–2 \times 10^6$	Walking

variations in the biological environment that arise, locally and systemically, as a result of implantation — that is, the host response.

2.5   Implant Life History

The thermal, mechanical, and chemical parameters described in previous sections are sufficient to predict, in general, the acute or instantaneous biological environment encountered by an implant. These acute values differ little from patient to patient; differences have only small effects on acute host and material responses. Phenotypic and genotypic biological differences that

TABLE 2.3

Inorganic Composition of the Human Body

		Total Body Burden	Conc. (aver.)
Basic	Oxygen	43,000 g	61.4%
elements[a]	Carbon	16,000 g	22.9%
	Hydrogen	7,000 g	10.0%
	Nitrogen	1,800 g	2.6%
	Total	67,800 g	96.9%
Physiological	Calcium	1000 g	1.43%
elements[a]	Phosphorus	780 g	1.11%
	Potassium	140 g	0.20%
	Sulfur	140 g	0.20%
	Sodium	100 g	0.14%
	Chlorine	95 g	0.14%
	Total	2255 g	3.22%
Trace	Magnesium	19 g	271 ppm
elements[a]	Iron	4.2 g	61.4 ppm
	Zinc	2.3 g	33 ppm
	Iodine	130 mg	1.9 ppm
	Copper	72 mg	1.0 ppm
	Aluminum	61 mg	0.9 ppm
	Vanadium	18 mg	260 ppb
	Selenium	<13 mg	<190 ppb
	Manganese	12 mg	170 ppb
	Nickel	10 mg	140 ppb
	Molybdenum	<9.5 mg	<136 ppb
	Titanium	9 mg	130 ppb
	Chromium	<6.6 mg	<94 ppb
	Cobalt	<1.5 mg	<21 ppb
	Total	<25.84 g	<0.37%

[a] Total of body burdens exceeds 70,000 g and 100% due to variety of primary sources and experimental error in individual values.

Source: Data from Lentner, C. (Ed.), *Geigy Scientific Tables*, Ciba–Geigy, Basle, 1981.

affect chronic host response to materials do exist. These may only be discernible by clinical testing of a specific patient; analyses of body fluids and tissues are probably inadequate for a full understanding of individual differences. It is unfortunate that technology for determination of the functional behavior of implants and implant–patient interactions is weak compared with that available to biological scientists for the study of natural organs *in situ*.

Beyond these obvious similarities and possible individual biological differences, the demands and expectations of individuals vary considerably. A total hip replacement prosthesis for a 40-year-old head of a family presents

TABLE 2.4

Components and Composition of Human Blood

Blood			
Packed cell volume	**38.5%**		
Serum volume	**61.5%**		
Serum composition (mean values)			
Cations	mEq/l	Anions	mEq/l
Sodium	142	Chlorine	101
Potassium	4	Bicarbonate	27
Calcium	5	Phosphate	2
Magnesium	2	Sulfate	1
Total	153	Organic acids	6
		Proteins	16
		Total	153

Other elements		
Iron	0.75–1.75	mg/l (ppm)
Nickel	1.0–5.0	µg/l (ppb)
Titanium	3.3	µg/l
Aluminum	2.0	µg/l
Copper	0.8–1.4	µg/l
Chromium	0.3	µg/l
Manganese	0.4–1.0	µg/l
Vanadium	<0.2	µg/l
Cobalt	0.15	µg/l

Serum proteins	
Total	65–80 g/l
Distribution (%):	
Albumin	61.5
Globulins (total)	34.5
α	8.2
β	10.3
δ	12.6
Fibrinogen	4.0

Cellular Distribution Type	Blood Concentration	Typical Dimension (µm)
Erythrocyte	4–$5.6 \times 10^6/\mu l$	8–9
Platelet	1.5–$3 \times 10^5/\mu l$	2–4
Leukocyte	2.8–$11.2 \times 10^3/\mu l$	—

Leukocyte Distribution Type	(%)	Typical Dimension (µm)
Neutrophils	59	10–15
Eosinophils	2.4	10–15
Basophils	0.6	10–15
Monocytes	6.5	12–20
Lymphocytes	31	7–18

Sources: Data from Lentner, C. (Ed.), *Geigy Scientific Tables*, Ciba–Geigy, Basle, 1981, and author's research.

TABLE 2.5

Implant Life History

Implant: anterior cruciate ligament replacement
Type: permanent
Patient indications:
Post-traumatic replacement, age: 35–48
(est. mean life expectancy: 40 years)

    pH   = 7 ± 0.3
    pO_2 = <40 mmHg
    pCO_2 = <40 mmHg
    25°C ≤ T ≤ 37°C

Mechanical conditions[a]
  Strain (range of maximum): 5–10%
  Loads: (moderate activity level, including recreational jogging)

Activity	Peak Load (N)	Cycles/Year	Total Cycles
Stairs:			
Ascending	67	4.2×10^4	1.7×10^6
Descending	133	3.5×10^4	1.4×10^6
Ramp walking:			
Ascending	107	3.7×10^3	1.5×10^5
Descending	485	3.7×10^3	1.5×10^5
Sitting and rising	173	7.6×10^4	3.0×10^6
Undifferentiated	<210	9.1×10^5	3.6×10^7
Level walking	210	2.5×10^6	1.0×10^8
Jogging	630	6.4×10^5	2.6×10^7
Jolting	700	1.8×10^3	7.3×10^5
Totals		4.2×10^6	2.9×10^8

[a] Adapted from Table III in Chen, E.H. and Black, J., *J. Biomed. Mater. Res.*, 14, 567, 1980.

a quite different engineering problem from such a device for an 80-year-old nursing home resident. Accounting for these functional differences completes the description of the service environment; the full picture thus formed is termed, as previously defined, the implant life history.

Implant life histories vary considerably from application to application and, of necessity, involve a high degree of engineering estimation. Within given target (patient) groups, the choice and intensity of work and leisure activities will vary widely (e.g., Schmalzried et al. 2000). As a result, implant life histories can only be regarded as predictive guides in the development, evaluation, and study of implantable biomaterials.

Table 2.5 gives an example of an implant life history, in this case for a permanent anterior cruciate ligament replacement. The supposed patient presents an example of an individual with moderate demands: presumably a full-time worker with evening and/or weekend physical recreational interests. If this individual were disabled in some manner or employed in a setting with unusual physical demands, such as mining or construction, or took part in other more demanding physical activities, such as wind surfing, mountain climbing, or parachute jumping, these facts should be noted and the physical consequences accounted for, in terms of different estimated peak loads and numbers of repetitions.

Asymmetry may also be a factor. Whether it is intrinsic or acquired, "handedness" is a possible source of laterality in physical properties of tissues, such as bone (Dane et al. 2001), subject to dynamic remodeling (see Chapter 10). Less controversial and more obvious are the visible effects of repetitive asymmetric physical activities, such as certain sports (soft- and hard-ball pitching, golf, archery, etc.) or work tasks (using a sledge hammer, painting, etc.). In some individual cases, laterality in tissue properties or material response (Joshi et al. 2001) is observed without any obvious source.

Within a particular application, the selection of particular materials and designs incorporating them has come to be termed demand matching. Demand matching cannot account for changes in a patient's life postimplantation, but it can be used to guide selection of technologies preimplantation. In the best of all possible words, one would try to design the longest lived, most durable materials that evoked optimum responses. However, present concerns about the cost of medical care and the way in which biomaterials and biomedical devices contribute to these costs result in cost containment, or more properly cost minimization, as a stimulus for "good enough" provided devices (and their constituent biomaterials) — that is, that will meet the patient's needs and expectations without excessive cost.

There is no general agreement on what patient features contribute to demand and how these features should be balanced in deriving a predictive formula. Demand matching tends to be individualized for the medical practitioner and to depend upon subjective as well as objective measures. Of the objective measures available, age (as measured by life expectancy) and gender (as a predictor of body weight and activity level) are the most widely accepted.

The mean U.S. life expectancy as a function of age is shown graphically in Figure 2.1 (NCHS 2002). Life expectancy now declines nearly linearly from early childhood (~6 months of age) to around age 50. Thereafter, however, the curve has a positive upward bend. Thus, mean life expectancy at age 60 is 21.6 years and, by age 70, it has declined by only 7.2 years to 14.4 years. Table 2.6 shows the clear effect of gender and national origin on life expectancy. It should be remembered that these data are averages.* Therefore, although mean life expectancy of U.S. residents at 75 is 11.3 years, only 24 of every 1000 that turn 75 will die before their next birthday.

In an example of demand matching (Black 1997), I have discussed selection of alternate bearing technologies in implants for total hip replacement arthroplasty; patient age at surgery, as well as other, less well defined demand components, has been taken into account.

---

* It is interesting to note that U.S. life expectancy at birth continues to increase, although it rose by more than 50% (49.2 to 76.9 years) during the 20th century. Thus, although Figure 2.1 and Table 2.6 reflect data only to age 100, U.S. life insurance underwriters have recently begun to use tables that extend to 110 years of life.

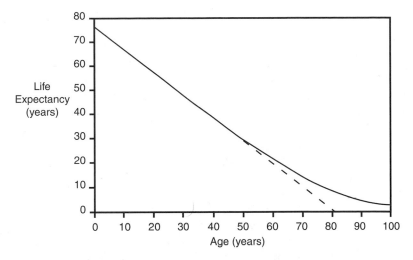

FIGURE 2.1

Average U.S. life expectancy 2000 mean (average of male and female, all national origins). (National Center for Health Statistics (NCHS), *National Vital Statistics Reports*, 51(3), 29, 2002.)

TABLE 2.6

U.S. Life Expectancy (Years)[a]

Age	Total Persons	All Races		White		Black	
		Male	Female	Male	Female	Male	Female
0	76.9	74.1	79.5	74.8	80.0	68.2	74.9
20	57.8	55.2	60.3	55.7	60.7	49.9	56.3
35	43.6	41.3	45.8	41.7	46.1	36.6	42.1
50	30.0	27.9	31.8	28.2	32.0	24.2	28.9
65	17.9	16.3	19.2	16.3	19.2	14.2	17.4
70	14.4	13.0	15.5	13.0	15.5	11.7	14.1
75	11.3	10.1	12.1	10.3	12.1	9.4	11.2
80	8.6	7.6	9.1	7.6	9.1	7.3	8.6
85	6.3	5.6	6.7	5.5	6.6	5.7	6.5
90	4.7	4.1	4.8	4.0	4.7	4.5	4.8
100	2.6	2.4	2.7	2.2	2.4	2.9	2.7

[a] Year 2000.

Source: National Center for Health Statistics (NCHS), *National Vital Statistics Reports*, 51(3), 29, 2002.

2.6   Preimplantation Handling Effects

One tends to think of the biological environment as that into which the implant passes after manufacture and storage. This assumption overlooks two intermediate processes common to all implant applications. In the first place, the implant may become contaminated, accidentally or as a side effect of planned processing and handling during manufacture, storage, and insertion. It is usually assumed that the implant surface is a pure, clean one with the composition of the bulk material. The truth may be far different. Organic films introduced during manufacture or by inadvertent handling may persist. Oxidation or other attack may occur during preoperative storage. Materials may be picked up from packaging used for storage or during sterilization. Contaminants may be transferred from surgical instruments.

For this reason, experimental studies of biological performance should include surface characterization of actual implant specimens selected from the full group fabricated in a particular study in the condition just before surgical insertion. Furthermore, care should be taken when materials are incorporated into devices for clinical trials and use, to see that the surface conditions are the same as those found during earlier developmental studies.

Second, all implants must be cleaned and sterilized before use; the manufacturer may supply some in sterile, double-wrapped packages, but others must be sterilized in the laboratory or hospital before use. The common forms of sterilization used in implant practice are:

- Cold solution
- Dry heat
- Moist heat (steam)
- Gas
- Gas plasma
- Gamma irradiation

Some typical sterilization parameters for each of these common methods are listed in Table 2.7. The particular method and parameters used must be suited to the individual implant type to provide maximum safety with minimum cost and implant degradation. Newer methods include electron beam irradiation and radio frequency plasma gas sterilization (Chau et al. 1996; Feldman and Hui 1997), which have the virtue of cleaning implant surfaces as well as sterilizing them.

The process of sterilization, if overlooked, may affect perception of the material and the host response. It is possible for some sterilization processes, such as irradiation, to change material properties, particularly of polymers,

TABLE 2.7

Methods and Typical Parameters of Sterilization

Method	Temperature	Time	Notes
Cold solution	RT	1–3 h	Commercial solutions; usually include formaldehyde or gluteraldehyde
Dry heat	160–175°C (max.)	0.5–2 h	Time/temperature vary inversely
Moist heat	120–130°C (max.)	2–15 min	Time/temperature vary inversely
Gas	RT — 55°C	1–24 h	Gas is usually ethylene oxide, 400–1200 mg/l; 48-h degassing required
Plasma discharge	45–55°C	1–2 h	RF discharge (var. frequencies) in <0.5 torr gas; hydrogen peroxide or peracetic acid most common
Irradiation	RT	2–24 h	^{60}Co gamma irradiation, 10–40 kGy dose; time/dose rate vary inversely

immediately (Nuutinen et al. 2002) and/or during subsequent preimplantation storage (Edidin et al. 2002). This might be interpreted, in error, as a material response effect if it is detected after implantation, or it might produce changes in host response secondary to the changes in the materials' properties (Stanford et al. 1994). It is also possible for traces of liquid or gaseous sterilants to be carried into the implant site, thus modifying the host response. Finally, sterilization of an unclean implant may render it sterile but not clean or pyrogen free (Gorbet and Sefton 2005), thus affecting the host response (see Section 8.2.2). Therefore, in any examination of material and host responses to implanted materials, it is necessary to pay close attention to actual surface conditions and sterilization effects as a prologue to exposure to the biological environment.

References

Black, J., Prospects for alternate bearing surfaces in total replacement arthroplasty of the hip, in *Performance of the Wear-Couple BIOLOX Forte in Hip Arthroplasty*, Puhl, W. (Ed.), Enke Verlag, Stuttgart, 1997, 2.

Black, J. and Hastings, G.W. (Eds.), *Handbook of Biomaterial Properties*, Part 1, Chapman & Hall, London, 1998.

Chau, T.T. et al., Microwave plasmas for low-temperature dry sterilization, *Biomaterials*, 17, 1273, 1996.

Chen, E.H. and Black, J., Materials design analysis of the prosthetic anterior cruciate ligament, *J. Biomed. Mater. Res.*, 14, 567, 1980.

Dane, S. et al., Differences between right- and left-femoral bone mineral densities in right- and left-handed men and women, *Int. J. Neurosci.*, 111(3–4), 187, 2001.

Edidin, A.A. et al., Accelerated aging studies of UHMWPE. I. Effect of resin, processing, and radiation environment on resistance to mechanical degradation, *J. Biomed. Mater. Res.*, 61(2), 312, 2002.

Feldman, L.A. and Hui, H.K., Compatibility of medical devices and materials with low-temperature hydrogen peroxide gas plasma, *Med. Dev. Diagn. Ind.*, 19(12), 57, 1997.

Gorbet, M.B. and Sefton, M.V., Endotoxin: The uninvited guest, *Biomaterials*, 26, 6811, 2005.

Joshi, A., Ilchmann, T. and Markovic, L., Socket wear in bilateral simultaneous total hip arthroplasty, *J. Arthrop.*, 16(1), 117, 2001.

Konttinen, Y.T. et al., The microenvironment around total hip replacement prostheses, *Clin. Orthop. Rel. Res.*, 430, 28, 2005.

Lentner, C. (Ed.), *Geigy Scientific Tables,* Ciba–Geigy, Basle, 1981.

National Center for Health Statistics (NCHS), *National Vital Statistics Reports*, 51(3), 29, 2002.

Nuutinen, J.P. et al., Effect of gamma, ethylene oxide, electron beam, and plasma sterilization on the behavior of SR-PLLA fibers *in vitro, J. Biomater. Sci. Polym. Ed.*, 13(12), 1325, 2002.

Schmalzried, T.P. et al., Wear is a function of use, not time, *Clin. Orthop. Rel. Res.*, 381, 36, 2000.

Stanford, C.M., Keller, J.C. and Solursh, M., Bone cell expression on titanium surfaces is altered by sterilization treatments, *J. Dent. Res.*, 73(5), 1061, 1994.

Bibliography

Altman, P.L. and Dittmer, D.S. (Eds.), *Biological Handbooks: Blood and Other Body Fluids,* 1961; *Biology Data Book,* 1964. Federation of American Societies for Experimental Biology (FASEB), Bethesda, MD.

Åstrand, P.-O. et al., *Textbook of Work Physiology: Physiological Bases of Exercise*, 4th ed., Human Kinetics Pub., Champaign, IL, 2003.

Baier, R.E. et al., Radiofrequency gas plasma (glow discharge) disinfection of dental operative instruments, including handpieces, *J. Oral Implantol.*, 18(3), 236, 1992.

Block, S.S. (Ed.), *Disinfection, Sterilization and Preservation*, 5th ed., Lippincott, Williams & Wilkins, Philadelphia, 2000.

Cooney, D.O., *Biomedical Engineering Principles*, Marcel Dekker, New York, 1976.

Ganong, W.F., *Review of Medical Physiology,* 21st ed., McGraw–Hill, New York, 2003.

Gaughran, E.R.L. and Kereluk, K. (Eds.), *Sterilization of Medical Products*, Johnson & Johnson, New Brunswick, NJ, 1977.

Kurtz, S.M. et al., Advances in the processing, sterilization, and crosslinking of ultra-high molecular weight polyethylene for total joint arthroplasty, *Biomaterials*, 20, 1659, 1999.

LeVeau, B. (Ed.), *Williams and Lissner: Biomechanics of Human Motion,* 2nd ed., W.B. Saunders, Philadelphia, 1977.

Matthews, I.P., Gibson, C. and Samuel A.H., Sterilization of implantable devices, *Clin. Mater.*, 15, 191, 1994.

Nair, P.D., Currently practiced sterilization methods — some inadvertent consequences, *J. Biomater. Appl.*, 10, 121, 1955.

Nordin, M., Frankel, V.H. and Frankel, V.H., *Basic Biomechanics of the Skeletal System,* 3rd ed. Lippincott Williams & Wilkins, Philadelphia, 2001.

Northrip, J.W., *Introduction to Biomechanic Analysis of Sport,* 2nd ed., Wm. C. Brown, Dubuque, IA, 1979.

Snyder, W.S. (Ed.), *Report of the Task Group on Reference Man*, International Commission on Radiological Protection, No. 23, Pergamon, Oxford, 1975.

Staff, Plastics Design Library (Eds.), *The Effect of Sterilization Methods on Plastics and Elastomers*. W.A. Morris, Inc. (for Plastics Design Library), Norwich, NY, 1994.

Wise, D.L. et al. (Eds.), *Encyclopedic Handbook of Biomaterials and Bioengineering, Part B: Applications*. (Vols. 1, 2), Marcel Dekker, New York, 1995.

Part II

Material Response: Function and Degradation of Materials *In Vivo*

3

Swelling and Leaching

3.1 Introduction

The simplest form of interaction between implant materials and the biological environment is the transfer of material across the material–tissue interface in the absence of reaction. If the substance — ions or fluid — moves from the tissue into the biomaterial, the result in a fully dense material will be swelling due to conservation of volume. Even in the absence of fluid uptake, the biomaterial may absorb some component or solute from the surrounding fluid phase. If the fluid moves into the tissue, or if one component of the biomaterial dissolves in the fluid phase of the tissue, the resulting material porosity is said to be due to leaching. Both of these effects have profound influences on the behavior of materials despite the absence of externally applied mechanical stresses and obvious shape changes. Swelling and leaching result from the process of diffusion. Before considering the effects on materials' properties, the fundamentals of diffusion and the diffusion models appropriate to each situation will be examined.

3.2 Fick's Laws of Diffusion

The fundamental relationship that governs diffusion in isotropic materials is

$$F = -D\frac{\partial C}{\partial x} \tag{3.1}$$

where
F = rate of transfer per unit area of cross section
D = diffusion constant
x = coordinate normal to cross section
C = concentration of diffusing material

Equation 3.1 is called Fick's first law; diffusion that obeys this relationship is termed Fickian or type I diffusion. In this simple case, the diffusion constant, D, depends only upon the material diffusing (the solute) and the matrix through which it moves. Thus, D is independent of concentration, position, and time. However, D does depend upon the type of diffusion process taking place, which includes surface, grain boundary, and volume diffusion. This dependence is given by

$$D = D_o e^{[-Q/KT]} \tag{3.2}$$

with dimensions of cm^2 sec^{-1},
where

Q = energy of activation of the diffusion process
$\quad$ ($Q_{volume} > Q_{grain\ boundary} > Q_{surface}$ [4:3:2 or 4:2:1])
D_o = intrinsic diffusion constant (D_o [surface] >
$\quad$ D_o [grain boundary] > D_o [volume])

Thus, it is easy to see that, within a given material system (a substance diffusing through a biomaterial) $D_{surface} > D_{grain\ boundary} > D_{volume}$ and surface diffusion is favored at typical biological temperatures.

When Equation 3.1 is applied to the problem of one-directional flow in an infinite medium, a differential equation of this form can be obtained:

$$\frac{\partial C}{\partial t} = D \frac{\partial^2 C}{\partial x^2} \tag{3.3}$$

Equation 3.3 is usually called Fick's second law. The application of Equation 3.1 and Equation 3.3 to different geometries, and to the initial and boundary conditions, of specific situations is sufficient to determine the distribution and mass transfer rate of diffusing materials in all cases.

3.3   Absorption

The simplest case that results in swelling is that of diffusion from a fluid with a fixed concentration, in the presence of perfect mixing, into an infinite medium. This is the case for the early period of absorption in any geometric arrangement; when the diffusing material is mostly near the surface, geometric factors have little effect. The arrangement, initial conditions, and change of concentration in the solid (biomaterial) phase with time are shown in Figure 3.1.

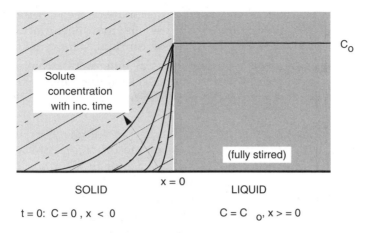

FIGURE 3.1
Absorption from a liquid into a solid biomaterial.

The exact solution for the concentration at a given point as a function of time is

$$C = C_o \left(\frac{x}{2(Dt)} \right)^{\frac{1}{2}}$$ (3.4)

where
C_o = external concentration
x = distance perpendicular to interface

$$\text{erfc}(a) = \left[\frac{2}{\sqrt{\pi}} \right] \int_a^\infty e^{-y^2} dy$$ (3.5)

The function erfc(a) is related to the error function erf(a) and will be found tabulated in texts on diffusion and heat transfer.

Integration of Equation 3.4 over distance for two values of time leads to the following relationship for the total mass transfer, M_t, across the boundary:

$$M_t = 2C_o \left[\frac{Dt}{\pi} \right]^{\frac{1}{2}}$$ (3.6)

The following conclusions follow directly from Equation 3.4 and Equation 3.6:

- The distance of penetration of any given concentration ("the diffusion front") increases in proportion to the square root of time.

- The time required for any point to reach a given concentration is proportional to the square of the distance from the surface and is inversely proportional to the diffusion constant.
- The total amount of diffusing material entering the biomaterial through a unit area of interface increases as the square root of time and is proportional to the diffusion constant.

The situation shown in Figure 3.1 is correct for volume or grain boundary diffusion, with appropriate values for the diffusion constant, when the liquid phase is well mixed, as in the case of fluid or solute uptake from arterial blood. If the liquid phase is not well mixed, as in the case of interstitial fluid surrounding a soft tissue implant site, then the situation is more complex. The simplest case occurs when a stagnation layer exists at the solid surface: this may be modeled as a third phase with a "resistance" to diffusion, often expressed by reducing the fluid phase concentration by a multiplier, k, which is less than unity. Thus, the adjusted concentration, C_o', is given by:

$$C_o' = k\, C_o \tag{3.7}$$

A second complication arises when the solid phase is able to absorb water (or another solvent) as well as the solute under study. This produces a steadily thickening solvated surface layer in which the solute can diffuse more readily than in the unsolvated solid. This has the effect of increasing the $1/2$ power exponent in Equation 3.4 and Equation 3.6 to values closer to one (and similarly of altering the preceding conclusions). Such a process is termed non-Fickian or type II diffusion.

3.4 Examples of Undesirable Absorption

One special case will be examined: diffusional pickup by a sphere in a medium of constant concentration. The application is the problem of the "variant" heart valve poppet. The poppet-type of heart valve consists of a polymeric sphere (the "poppet") usually fabricated from a silicone elastomer, a metal constraining cage, and valve seat with a fabric sewing ring (Figure 3.2). This was an early and usually successful design for human aortic valve replacement; however, for a small percentage of patients, the ball jammed in the cage or, in some cases, the ball actually escaped. Discoloration of such recovered balls, termed "variant," suggested that some material had been absorbed, leading to swelling.

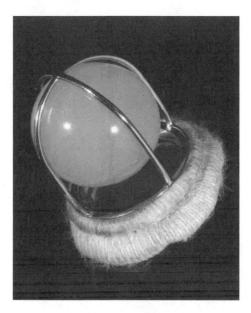

FIGURE 3.2
Starr–Edwards "poppet" type aortic heart valve. Note polyester fabric sewing ring, metal (co-base alloy) cage, and seat and silicone ball ("poppet"). (Courtesy R. Baier.)

The mathematical solution for this case is reached by transforming Equation 3.3 into spherical coordinates and solving for the appropriate boundary conditions. One finds that M_t is proportional to Dt/a^2, where a is the radius of the sphere. That is,

$$\frac{M_t}{M_\infty} = k\left(\frac{Dt}{a^2}\right) \qquad (3.8)$$

where
   M_∞ = maximum amount of material absorbed
   k = constant

The solution suggests that simple absorption should produce a weight gain that is linear with time. Data obtained by Carmen and Kahn (1968) from a study of ten variant poppets are given in Table 3.1. A linear regression (r = 0.91) yields a linear rate of weight gain of 0.27% per month in good functional agreement with our calculation. This rate presumably equals kD/a^2 from Equation 3.8.

The absorption of materials from blood can have a variety of consequences. McHenry et al. (1970) studied poppets retrieved from five patients with clinical symptoms of aortic valve malfunction and reported discoloration (yellowing), fatty smell, and strut (cage) grooves. These poppets, which were

TABLE 3.1

Weight Gain by "Variant" Poppets

Weight Gain (%)	Period of Implantation (weeks)
0.1	1
0.1	2
0.9	11
2.1	18
4.15	34
3.4	39
2.5	48
3.1	52
3.3	52
5.5	80

Source: Adapted from Carmen, R. and Kahn, P., *J. Biomed. Mater. Res.*, 2, 457, 1968.

implanted for longer times than those studied by Carmen and Kahn (1968), contained up to 16% simple and complex lipids by weight. The simple lipids (1.5 to 2% by weight) were composed of 60 to 65% cholesterol esters, 15 to 20% triglycerides, 5% fatty acids, and 10% cholesterol. The material absorbed (in these two reports) is a portion of the "fatty" component of blood serum, usually called lipid on a collective basis. It can be presumed that the shape and physical property changes observed were a result of lipid absorption. Lipids are present in other body fluids and may be absorbed by implants that are not in the blood flow.

Swanson et al. (1973) reported on a study of 49 silicone elastomer finger joint prostheses that were retrieved, for various reasons, after implantation for up to 36 months in patients. All implants were examined for lipid content by chloroform extraction, the resulting weight change was determined, and a direct analysis of the extractant fluid was performed. Of these implants, 12 had fractured in use. A summary of the findings is given in Table 3.2. The question was raised as to whether lipid absorption had any relationship to the fracture in service. The authors concluded that there is no relationship between time of implantation, or lipid content, and risk of fracture.

It is surprising in the light of the Carmen and Kahn study that no relationship was seen between lipid content and time. However, two points must be made:

- The boundary conditions for an implant within the tissue capsule in a finger joint are quite different from those present in flowing blood; C_o, C_s, and mass transfer are all different in this case. Thus, the previous solution not predicting the results is not surprising.
- The maximum weight gain reported in Table 3.2 is 0.515%. This is the value that would be expected after less than 2 months if one used

TABLE 3.2

Lipid Content of Retrieved Finger Joint Prostheses

Implantation Duration (months)	Intact Implants		Fractured Implants			
	No.	Cumulative Lipids (wt.%)[a]	No.	Cumulative Lipids (wt.%)	No.	Estimated Lipids (wt.%)[b]
12	15	0.475 ± 0.05	8	0.515 ± 0.2	8	0.515
24	24	0.461 ± 0.04	10	0.447 ± 0.2	2	0.175
36	37	0.469 ± 0.03	12	0.443 ± 0.1	2	0.423

[a] Cumulative: 24 month group includes data from 12 months; 36 month group includes data from 24 months.

[b] Estimated: 24 months = estimated lipid (wt.%) for implants failing between 12 and 24 months; 36 months = estimated lipid (wt.%) for implants failing between 24 and 36 months.

Source: Adapted from Swanson, A.B. et al., *Orthop. Clin. N. Am.*, 4(4), 1097, 1973.

the rate computed from Table 3.1 and is one-tenth of the maximum value reported for the heart valve poppets. Therefore, an alternate explanation for the failure to observe a linear increase in weight with time might be that the equilibrium level is far lower in the finger joint and is reached before 12 months, the earliest summary date given in Table 3.2.

Examination of the data in Table 3.2, with an attempt to estimate mean lipid values of the failed implants within 12-month intervals, suggests another possible conclusion concerning the relationship between lipid content and device fracture. It is possible that there are two populations of failed implants: those that take up lipid with abnormal rapidity (represented by the failures in the first 12-month period) and those that take it up quite slowly (represented by the later failures). In the first case, one might invoke weakening due to swelling, perhaps secondary to reaction between lipids and the implant (Pfleiderer et al. 1995); in the second, decreased tear resistance associated with the absence of a plasticizing effect might be suggested. (See Chapter 6 for a more complete discussion of these phenomena.)

The effects of absorption in these series can be summarized as change in color, change in volume (swelling), and possible change in mechanical properties (as evidenced by the presence of strut grooves). Mechanical property changes secondary to absorption, in the general case, can include reduction in modulus of elasticity, increase in internal viscosity, increase in ductility (or possible decrease in the presence of reaction with the absorbed species), change in the coefficient of friction, and reduction of wear resistance.

3.5 Osmotic Equilibrium

Problems arise even in the absence of obvious property changes. The increase in volume due to absorption results in the application of a negative internal hydrostatic stress to the material. This effect can be understood through the following calculation. If a material is immersed in a solution so that the solute is soluble in the liquid phase (solvent) and the solid phase (material), there will be an initial interfacial pressure:

$$\Pi = MRT \tag{3.9}$$

where
M = molarity of solute in liquid phase
R = gas constant = 8.31×10^7 erg $°K^{-1}$ mol^{-1}
T = absolute temperature

This is van't Hoff's law and the pressure, Π, is called the osmotic pressure. It is an expression of the fact that the activity of the solute in the liquid phase is greater than that in the solid phase.

Driven by the osmotic pressure, the solid phase will absorb solute. When this happens, the solid phase expands as if subject to a negative hydrostatic pressure. This pressure, P, is called the swelling pressure and

$$P = \Pi - p \tag{3.10}$$

where p = hydrostatic restoring force of the swollen material. That is, as the material swells, an elastic restoring force is generated through the strain of the material that counteracts the osmotic pressure. As the material swells, this restoring force rises, the activity of the solute in the solid phase rises, and the swelling pressure approaches zero as equilibrium conditions are obtained. Obviously, changes of solute concentration in the liquid phase disturb this equilibrium and can produce further expansion or contraction of the solid phase.

Advantage is taken of this phenomenon in the production of hydrophilic gels for biomedical applications such as contact lenses. These materials have low elastic moduli and high affinity for water. Because water has a molarity of 55.6, high osmotic pressure coupled with low negative hydrostatic restoring forces permit the fabrication of compositions with an equilibrium water content approaching 98%; volume expansions may exceed 5000% (Refojo 1976). Even more modest swelling affects mechanical properties; see Section 6.3.2.

3.6 Leaching

The simplest case that results in leaching is that of removal of diffusing material from the surface at a constant rate. This is approximately the case of elution by moving blood; it is closely parallel to the *in vitro* situation of evaporation from a surface. The arrangement, initial conditions, and change of concentration of the solute in the solid (biomaterial) phase with time are shown in Figure 3.3.

In most real situations, an additional condition is present. If the fluid medium is in motion but not fully stirred (as shown), some rate of transfer must be assumed. The simplest case is to take this rate as proportional to the surface concentration at any moment. In particular, this rate is taken to be linearly dependent upon the difference between a surface concentration, C_s, and bulk concentration, C_o. Thus, the boundary condition is:

$$-D\frac{\partial C}{\partial x} = \alpha\left(C_o - C_s\right) \quad \text{at } x = 0 \qquad (3.11)$$

If $h = \alpha/D$, Equation 3.10 leads to the following solution:

$$\frac{C - C_s}{C_o - C_s} = \text{erfc}\left(\frac{x}{2\sqrt{Dt}}\right)\left(-e^{\left[hx + h^2 Dt\right]}\right)\text{erfc}\left(\frac{x}{2\sqrt{Dt}} + h\sqrt{Dt}\right) \qquad (3.12)$$

For a particular value of h, M_t is proportional to $(Dt)^{1/2}$. Other conditions, such as concentration-dependent diffusion constants, surface and bulk reactions, etc., can affect the former of these relationships.

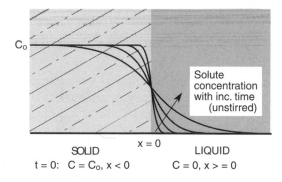

FIGURE 3.3
Leaching from a solid biomaterial into a liquid.

3.7   Example of Planned Leaching: Drug Release

When drugs are administered by intramuscular injection, their release into other compartments of the body is governed by diffusion. The effect of this may be seen in Figure 3.4. On the left-hand portion of this figure, the saw-toothed trace shows the effective drug concentration, at some point distant from the point of administration, resulting from three divided doses. After the first dose, the concentration at that point rises through the suboptimal into the optimal therapeutic range, then begins to decline rapidly due to the combined effects of storage in other tissues, metabolic degradation, and excretion. The declining dashed line segment shows the continued concentration decline that would occur if the second (and third) doses were not administered. Unfortunately, the selected temporal spacing of the doses, for their size, was too short: the concentration after the third dose is sufficient to produce toxic side effects. The relationship between drug concentration in the target tissue or organ and its effect is shown on the right side of Figure 3.4; this relationship is referred to as a "dose–response" curve, sometimes called a Bertrand curve.

The curvilinear dashed line in the left-hand portion of Figure 3.4 represents an optimum strategy: the drug concentration rises smoothly and rapidly to an optimal level and then is maintained at constant. With care, such an effect can be obtained by continuous intravenous injection. However, it is possible to utilize diffusional effects to produce a device that can produce the same results.

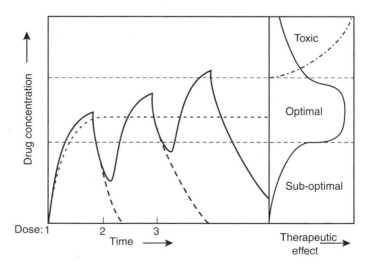

FIGURE 3.4
Drug release strategies. (Adapted from Chien, Y.W., *Med. Prog. Technol.*, 15, 21, 1989.)

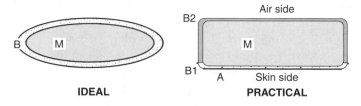

FIGURE 3.5
Sustained (reservoir) drug release device.

Figure 3.5 schematically depicts (left side) an ideal implantable drug release device that would accomplish this goal. It consists of two design elements: a barrier membrane (B) and a drug reservoir or matrix (M). The drug is dissolved as a solute in the filler or may be present simply as an imiscible dispersed, but diffusable, phase. If the intrinsic diffusion properties for the drug in question are such that the conditions

$$D_B << D_M, D_{tissue} \tag{3.13}$$

can be maintained, then there will be a near constant release rate until M_t becomes a significant fraction of M_∞. This secondary condition can be met by making the drug content of the matrix phase large compared with the desired total dose (and removing the device when its function has been served) or by repeated injection of drug into the device matrix. The latter arrangement is termed a reservoir or sustained release device.

However, actual or practical devices involve more complexity than this simple example. Figure 3.5 also schematically depicts (right side) a practical design for an external skin (transdermal) release device, such as the familiar nicotine patches for assistance in quitting smoking. (Note that the dimension perpendicular to the skin is greatly expanded for clarity.) Fundamentally, the same two elements are present: a barrier membrane (B1) and a matrix with the drug (M). However, two other elements are necessary:

- B2: a protective barrier to prevent the loss of the drug or filler from the backside or the diffusion of air or water into the device. For cosmetic reasons, this barrier may also be colored and include printing, such as a trademark or instructions for use.
- A: an adhesive layer to secure the device on the patient's skin. Because this layer is between the reservoir and the tissue, its diffusional properties must be taken into account in the selection and dimensioning of B1.

This is a schematic example of a device that utilizes diffusional leaching to produce controlled drug release. Simpler designs are possible, such as application of a drug-impregnated single- or multilayer coating to a structural implant. In addition, for complex devices such as the example given, adjustment of geometries and the use of different forms of drugs can produce a wide range of release rate (and resultant tissue concentration) profiles with time. Combining the effects of absorption (which may alter diffusion rates by changing reservoir osmotic pressure) with changes in the composition of the solvent or the filler phase produces still more options for the drug release device designer. Finally, the designer might consider introducing active design elements, such as invoking sonopheresis by utilizing ultrasonic cavitation to alter the diffusional properties of the adjacent tissue (Mitragotri et al. 1995) or iontopheresis by taking account of ionic charge of certain drugs at or near neutral pHs' and imposing an electrical gradient across the device–tissue interface (Singh et al. 1994).

3.8   Effects of Swelling and Leaching

There are adverse aspects to large deformations that may be caused by swelling and leaching. It is possible to exceed the creep stress in the material. This will produce continual deformation and absorption, rather than the attainment of an equilibrium solute concentration. Even if this does not happen, swelling reduces the elastic limit of a material (that is, the available strain to the elastic limit) and may lead to a mode of failure termed static fatigue or "crazing," especially in brittle materials. Crazing is the development of microcracks that merge and can eventually result in fracture.

Leaching, the reverse of swelling, usually has a less pronounced effect on properties. The primary undesirable aspects of unplanned leaching are the local and systemic biological reactions to the released products. Excessive leaching (for instance, intergranular leaching in metals) can result in a reduction in fracture strength. The defects produced by leaching can coalesce into macroscopic voids. If these begin to constitute a significant percentage of the volume of rigid materials, the elastic modulus will decline. The decrease is proportional to the second power of the volume percent of voids (see Section 6.3.2).

References

Carmen, R. and Kahn, P., *In vitro* testing of silicone rubber heart-valve poppets for lipid absorption, *J. Biomed. Mater. Res.*, 2, 457, 1968.

Chien, Y.W., Rate-control drug delivery systems: controlled release vs. sustained release, *Med. Prog. Technol.*, 15, 21, 1989.

McHenry, M.M. et al., Critical obstruction of prosthetic heart valves due to lipid absorption by Silastic, *J. Thorac. Cardiovasc. Surg.*, 59, 413, 1970.

Mitragotri, S. et al., A mechanistic study of ultrasonically enhanced transdermal drug delivery, *J. Pharmaceutical Sci.*, 84(6), 697, 1995.

Pfleiderer, B. et al., Study of aging of silicone rubber biomaterials with NMR, *J. Biomed. Mater. Res.*, 29, 1129, 1995.

Refojo, M.F., Vapor pressure and swelling pressure of hydrogels, in *Hydrogels for Medical and Related Applications*, Andrade, J.D. (Ed.), American Chemical Society, Washington, D.C., 1976, 37.

Singh, P. and Maibach, H.I., Transdermal iontophoresis. Pharmacological considerations, *Clin. Pharmacol.*, 26(5), 327, 1994.

Swanson, A.B. et al., Durability of silicone implants — an *in vivo* study, *Orthop. Clin. N. Am.*, 4(4), 1097, 1973.

Bibliography

Berti, J.J. and Lipsky, J.J., Transcutaneous drug delivery: a practical review, *Mayo Clin. Proc.*, 70, 581, 1995.

Brophy, J.H., Rose, R.M. and Wulff, J., *Thermodynamics of Structure,* Vol. II of *The Structure and Properties of Materials*, Wulff, J. (Ed.), John Wiley & Sons, New York, 1964.

Crank, J., *The Mathematics of Diffusion*, 2nd ed., Oxford University Press, London, 1975.

Daugherty, A.L. and Mrsny, R.J., Emerging technologies that overcome biological barriers for therapeutic protein delivery, *Expert Opin. Biol. Ther.*, 3(7), 1071, 2003.

Edwards, D.A. and Langer, R., A linear theory of transdermal transport phenomena, *J. Pharmaceutical Sci.* 83(9), 1315, 1994.

Kost, J., Biomaterials in drug delivery systems, in *Encyclopedic Handbook of Biomaterials and Bioengineering, Part A: Materials,* Vol. 2, Wise, D.L. et al. (Eds.), Marcel Dekker, New York, 1995, Chapter 34.

Purdon, C.H. et al., Penetration enhancement of transdermal delivery — current permutations and limitations, *Crit. Rev. Ther. Drug Carr. Sys.*, 21(2), 97, 2004.

4

Corrosion and Dissolution

4.1 Chemistry of Corrosion

Everyone has an intuitive understanding of corrosion. The purpose of this chapter is to consider the principles of chemistry that underlie this understanding, to characterize and classify the types of corrosion that may occur, and to see how these considerations apply to the use of metals as implants.

The layperson tends to equate corrosion with the "rusting" of iron. However, the term has a far broader application. The word *corrosion* derives from the Latin *rodere*, to gnaw. The chemical processes that contribute to the phenomenon of corrosion can be strictly termed processes of reaction and/or dissolution in the presence of water. However, it has come to be used to describe any chemical attack on solid materials, especially metals. In the case of metals, reaction tends to dominate; for ceramic and polymeric biomaterials, dissolution dominates. The bulk of this chapter will address the corrosion of metals; Section 4.11 and Section 4.12 deal briefly with dissolution of ceramics and polymers, respectively.

In the case of metals, the following four generic reactions are the most usual (note: typical valence states and changes are given; other values are possible):

Ionization: the direct formation of cations (positively charged metallic ions) generally under acidic or reducing (oxygen-poor) conditions:

$$M \rightarrow M^+ + e^-$$
$$0 \quad +1 \text{ (= valence of metallic atom)} \tag{4.1}$$

Oxidation: the direct reaction of metal with gaseous or dissolved oxygen, without the participation of water. In the extreme examples, oxidation is recognized as burning:

$$M + O_2 \rightarrow MO_2$$
$$0 \qquad\quad +4 \tag{4.2}$$

Hydroxylation: the reaction of metal with water under alkaline (basic) or oxidizing conditions to yield a hydrated oxide or hydroxide. Because most hydroxides are only sparingly soluble in alkaline conditions, this process often leads to the formation of a passivating film, of which more will be said later:

$$2M + O_2(diss.) + 2H_2O \rightarrow 2M(OH)_2$$
$$0 \qquad\qquad\qquad\qquad\qquad\qquad +2 \qquad\qquad (4.3)$$

Reaction: the combination of metal or metallic ions with other cations and anions (negatively charged ions); this is often termed complex formation:

$$MO_2^{2-} + HCl \rightarrow MOCl^- + OH^-$$
$$+2 \qquad\qquad +2 \qquad\qquad\qquad\qquad (4.4)$$

In biomaterials' applications, the presence of specific and nonspecific organic binding molecules results in the formation of organometallic complexes as a general rule.

Each of these processes has the effect of decreasing the amount of pure metal present and of producing metal-bearing ions and compounds. Consideration of the effects of corrosion must take note of the attack on the parent metallic component as well as the formation of reaction products.

4.2   Classification of Reactions

It is necessary to make some order out of these various chemical processes that contribute to corrosion so that one can approach the prediction of corrosive attack in a systematic manner. All of these and other processes involved in corrosion can be classified by answering two questions:

- Does the reaction depend upon pH?
- Does the reaction depend upon local electrical potential?

For the purpose of discussion, the answers to these questions will be designated with "+" or "–." Thus, a reaction such as dissolution of gas, which is independent of pH and potential, would be an example of a "– –" reaction. There may be as many as several dozen possible reactions for the interaction of an elemental metal with pure water in the presence of oxygen.

A further observation simplifies these efforts of organization. For any particular combination of pH and potential, there will be a single dominant reaction for a specific metal in a specific solution; that is, of all of the possible

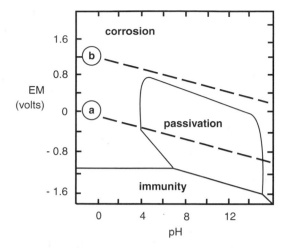

FIGURE 4.1
Pourbaix diagram for chromium in pure water.

reactions, one will be the maximum or principal contributor to the degradation of a metallic part and to the concentration of metal in solution.

4.3   The Pourbaix Diagram

4.3.1   Reactions of Chromium in Pure Water

Classification of all possible reactions between a metallic element and water (and its constituents) by their pH and potential dependence, combined with the determination from various types of experiments of those combinations that favor particular reactions provides the information needed for a graphic representation of the overall reaction system (see Figure 4.1). This is called a pH-potential or, more usually, a Pourbaix (poor BAY) diagram, after Marcel Pourbaix (Pourbaix 1966) who popularized its use. This diagram is for pure chromium in pure water and summarizes the reactions among five primary species (Cr, O_2, H_2, H^+, and OH^-).

A Pourbaix diagram has three major regions. Each of these represents combinations of ranges of pH and potential for which a reaction or a related group of reactions is dominant; each region corresponds to one of the three fundamental conditions that describe the response of metals to aqueous solutions:

- Immunity. In this region, the dominant reaction is ionization. However, throughout the region the resulting equilibrium concentration of chromium in solution, in all ionic forms, is less than 10^{-6} *M*. This concentration is generally taken as the threshold between corrosion and immunity. If reaction processes yield a total equilibrium concentration (of all metal-bearing ions) of less than this value, it is engineering practice to speak of the metal as immune from corrosion, or more simply immune, under that particular set of conditions. Because the level of 10^{-6} M (typically 50 ppb) greatly exceeds normal physiological concentrations for most of the less common ions (especially those containing trace metals), it is good practice to assume in implant applications that some metal is released for all combinations of pH and potential.

- Passivation. In this region, the dominant reactions lead to the formation of oxides and hydroxides. Because these products for chromium are largely insoluble at a pH above 4, they cling to the interface between the metal and the solution, reducing and eventually preventing further reaction. This renders the chromium passive. Throughout this region, the solubility of the oxides and hydroxides is low enough that the total concentration of chromium in solution is, as it was in the immune region, less than 10^{-6} M.

- Corrosion. In this region, a variety of processes can attack metallic chromium (at low or high values of pH) or its passive coating (if present, at intermediate values of pH). The result throughout the region is a total equilibrium concentration of chromium in solution that equals or exceeds 10^{-6} M; thus, in engineering terms, the chromium is said to corrode.

Two additional features are of interest. The diagonal dotted lines in Figure 4.1 define the reactions of gaseous oxygen and hydrogen with water. The upper line, b, is that for oxygen; the lower line, a, is that for hydrogen. Both of these reactions are of the "++" type, so the lines slope. The region between the lines is that in which water is stable. Above the oxygen line, b, oxygen is released, and below the hydrogen line, a, hydrogen is released. Dominant reactions of the "+ –" type produce vertical region boundary segments; those of the "– +" type produce horizontal segments. Reactions of the "– –" type do not produce regions of dominance on this type of diagram.

In biological systems that are pH controlled by buffering, the local oxygen or hydrogen partial pressure defines an effective local potential. Thus, tissues perfused with arterial blood and maintained at pH 7.37 have an equivalent potential of + 0.782 V. This last fact makes it possible to apply the Pourbaix approach to the prediction of metallic corrosion *in vivo*.

4.3.2   Reactions of Chromium in the Presence of Aqueous Chloride Ion

Figure 4.2 is again the Pourbaix diagram for chromium, but with two important changes:

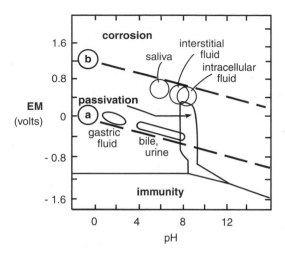

FIGURE 4.2
Pourbaix diagram for chromium in water (1 N Cl⁻).

- The solution is now water with 1.0 N chloride ion (Cl⁻) to simulate the situation *in vivo* more closely. The principal effect of this addition is to shrink the passive region radically. This results from reaction of the chloride anion with free metal ions and the passive layer to form soluble complexes, thus raising the effective solubility of chromium.

- The areas of pH and potential (as defined by pO_2) for various body fluids have been superimposed. Note that the areas for interstitial and intracellular fluids actually lie closer to pH 7.0; they are plotted as more alkaline for clarity. From this, it can be seen that pure chromium would perform satisfactorily in neutral conditions in the bile duct or urinary tract, but would be unsatisfactory in the stomach, where pH may approach 1. General tissue applications for pure chromium might be considered to be marginal because they lie on the boundary between the passivation and corrosion regions.

It should be clear that a Pourbaix diagram is useful in predicting corrosion in only a general way. The following limitations should be realized:

- As determined by local ionic conductivity and by limitations in the diffusion of oxygen, hydroxide, and hydrogen ions, the local microconditions dictate the exact equivalent potential that may be expected. Thus, the regions shown on this diagram for different physiological situations may be considered as reflecting average conditions. In particular, pericellular conditions may be radically different.

- The areas of dominance and other details of the diagrams are those that prevail after all reactions have come to equilibrium. Reactions may be very slow, as is the case for many involving chromium compounds, leading to prolonged nonequilibrium conditions.

- Reactions and their kinetics depend upon the history of the metal to some degree. Thus, a bare piece of chromium placed under conditions that lie within the passive region of the Pourbaix diagram will undergo reactions leading to formation of hydroxides; however, if its surface is pretreated* to produce an oxidized (passive) layer, the dominant reactions under the same set of conditions will be hydration and partial dissolution of this surface layer. Such reactions may be very slow; in the case of prepassivated chromium-containing alloys, they are so slow that such passive films are termed metastable and the materials may be used for some applications with conditions within the corrosion region of the diagram.

- Pourbaix diagrams are available for most elemental metals in pure water, but they do not exist for the vast majority of alloys or for other aqueous solutions. However, because the corrosion resistance of chromium-containing stainless steels and cobalt-base "super alloys" depends to a great degree on the presence of chromium hydroxide passivation films, the diagram for chromium in the presence of chloride ion (Figure 4.2) is quite useful in understanding the chemical aspects of their material response *in vivo*.

- Finally, as will be discussed in Section 4.10, the presence of active cell products *in vivo* may modify the rate of reactions and the nature of their products.

4.4   The Electrochemical Series

4.4.1   Ideal Series

It is possible to plot a complete Pourbaix diagram for any real metal or alloy in a defined solution. However, a further simplification may be made if one is only interested in the relative corrosion resistance of metals. One can begin by noting that the boundary between the immunity region and the corrosion region for acid and neutral pH is horizontal. The left-hand intercept (or more correctly, the potential for pH = 0) is a single potential value. This potential will be different for each metal alloy.

---

* Passivation by acid treatment or by anodic polarization (see Section 4.7.2) is common practice for engineering application within this pH-potential region. Many proprietary surface treatments also take advantage of control of structural and compositional features of the passive layer to gain maximum kinetic protection from dissolution.

TABLE 4.1

Ideal and Practical Electrochemical Series

Potential	Ideal	Practical
Noble or cathodic		
	Gold	Platinum
	Platinum	Gold
	Silver	Stainless steel (passive)
	Copper	Titanium
$E = 0$	Hydrogen	Silver
	Lead	Nickel
	Tin	Stainless steel (unpassivated)
	Nickel	Copper
	Cobalt	Tin
	Iron	Lead
	Chromium	Cast iron
	Aluminum	Wrought iron
	Titanium	Aluminum
	Magnesium	Magnesium
Base or cathodic		

On the left side of Table 4.1, a number of metals are ranked by this potential in an ideal (sometimes termed absolute) electrochemical series. This electrochemical series is arranged with the most noble or cathodic potentials (with respect to the II/II^+ half cell reaction) at the top and increasingly base or anodic potentials as one proceeds down the list. Note that the apparent sign of an electrode depends upon whether it is self-polarized (as in corrosion) or externally polarized (as in electroplating). A self-polarized anode is negative and an externally polarized one is positive and vice versa for the cathode. The oxidation-reduction nature of the reactions is identical in both situations: reduction takes place at the cathode and oxidation at the anode.

Despite the use of potentials obtained under acidic, oxygenated conditions, the ideal series is a reasonable measure of the relative corrosion resistance of metals under a variety of conditions in pure water. The higher the place in the list (the more cathodic the potential), the more noble or corrosion resistant the metal is. Section 4.7.2 will show that the relative position in an electrochemical series determines which of a coupled pair of dissimilar metals may undergo corrosion.

4.4.2 Practical Series

In the right-most column of Table 4.1, many of the same metals, and some alloys, are listed in a practical electrochemical series. The use of a practical series, in this case for the exposure of these metals to seawater, begins to take into account the situation peculiar to a specific application. Seawater exposure, particularly in tropical climates, is the engineering condition that most closely simulates environments encountered by implants, except for the general lack of soluble organic species. Comparison of the practical to the ideal series demonstrates some interesting differences related to the differences in environment:

- The two noblest metals in both series, platinum and gold, change their relative positions. This reflects the fact that, although neither is strongly attacked by seawater, gold forms chlorides more readily than does platinum.

- Titanium moves well up the list, reflecting the highly insoluble nature of most of its compounds, particularly its TiO_2 passivation layer that forms spontaneously in air.

- Unpassivated stainless steel, a class of alloys of iron, nickel, and chromium (as well as other minor elements), is not particularly high on this list. The choice of stainless steels as implant materials (primarily in temporary applications, such as in internal fixation devices for fractures) depends primarily upon their mechanical properties and machinability in the presence of an acceptable level of corrosion resistance (when passivated before use) and moderate local host response to its corrosion products.

A practical series begins to take factors of corrosion other than equilibrium thermodynamics into account. That is, it reflects not only the possibility of corrosion, but also details of actual attack in specific environments. Pourbaix diagrams and electrochemical series tell something about the likelihood of corrosion. They define equilibrium conditions and imply rates of corrosion as proportional to deviations from equilibrium. It is important to know something about the rates of corrosion. These rates will help to determine, for instance, the rate of release of metallic ions from an implant.

4.5   Corrosion Rate

In engineering applications, corrosion rates are expressed as rates of surface dissolution or recession per year. The common unit is the mpy (mil [0.001 in.] per year). This unit is far too big to be used to examine corrosion rates in the biological environment for the same reasons that an equilibrium concentration of 10^{-6} M is too high to be considered indicative of immunity.

A more direct measure may be obtained by examining Equation 4.1 through Equation 4.3. These are characteristic of metallic corrosion. Note that in each case the valence of the metal is reduced, with a required transfer of charge or electrons to another species. Because the sites of reduction (cathode) and oxidation (anode) are separated in space, an equivalent current must flow.

Corrosion (at the anode) of one molecular weight of metal, with an accompanying valence change of +1 (for instance, from 0 to +1), will result in the transfer of 1 faraday (F) of charge. Thus, for a corroding anode, one may determine the corrosion rate by measuring the net current flow and dividing by the area. The unit of corrosion, defined in this way, is then amp/cm².

4.6   Potential-Current Relationships in Corrosion

Briefly consider an ideal case of corrosion, taking the reaction at the anode to be Equation 4.1.

$$M \rightarrow M^+ + e^-$$

At the cathode, assume that the reaction is the reduction of dissolved oxygen:

$$O_2(d) + 2\ H_2O + 4\ e^- \rightarrow 4\ OH^- \tag{4.5}$$

An alternative reaction — the reduction of hydrogen ion with the release of gaseous hydrogen — is also possible:

$$2\ H^+ + 2\ e^- \rightarrow H_2(g) \tag{4.6}$$

The latter reaction will occur preferentially if the oxygen potential is very low or the metal is extremely active (base or non-noble). In this case, consider Equation 4.5 to be the cathodic reaction.

Now look at Figure 4.3. The initial potentials at the anode and cathode are E_{Ao} and E_{Co}. Due to the differences in potential, current begins to flow (corrosion takes place). This may be represented by moving to the right of the diagram. Due to the familiar Ohm's law relationship among current, potential difference, and resistance, the effective potential of the cathode drops and that of the anode rises. If nothing happens to intervene, the potentials become equal. This mixed potential, E_M, is then maintained, and the current, i_3, is defined by

$$\frac{E_M}{\text{Total resistance}} = i_3 \tag{4.7}$$

The current (i_3) divided by the area of the anode yields the corrosion rate.

If an external resistance, R_{ex}, that is large compared to the previous resistance is inserted between anode and cathode, the resulting current is i_2 and is defined by

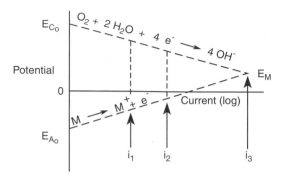

FIGURE 4.3
Potential–current (log) relationships in corrosion.

$$\frac{E_{C_o} - E_{A_o} - i_2 R_{ex}}{\text{Total resistance}} = i_2 \tag{4.8}$$

The current i_2 is less than i_3; thus, less corrosion takes place in a given period of time. This is the situation when a passivation or insulating layer can be maintained on a metal in a pH-potential region that would normally promote corrosion. If the supply of oxygen is limited by diffusion, for instance, the potentials of anode and cathode may remain more widely separated, and a still smaller current i_1, resulting in less corrosion, may flow. In either case ($i = i_1$ or i_2), the effective potential will be somewhere between E_{Co} and E_{Ao}, depending upon the relative areas of the cathode and anode.

Thus, it should be clear that the actual rate of corrosion may vary widely for a given set of equilibrium conditions. Local oxygen supply, conductivity of the bathing electrolyte, and the extent of the electrode surfaces, as well as the presence of various inhibitors and enhancers of corrosion, may affect the result.

Corrosion in real environments is not usually detected by measurement of potentials and currents or of concentrations of ions in solutions. Rather, it is recognized by the evidence of attack on the bulk material, the chemical gnawing away of the fabricated part.

4.7   Forms of Corrosion

I am indebted to Mars Fontana and Norbert Greene (Fontana 1985), who have collected many diverse descriptions of the physical appearance of corrosion and grouped them into eight categories or forms, depending upon mechanism and common features of the result of attack. The eight forms of corrosion will be briefly examined and some comments made on their mechanisms.

4.7.1 Uniform Attack

Uniform attack, or general overall corrosion, is a self-explanatory term. This is the process that is taking place in the corrosion region and, by oxide/hydroxide dissolution, in the passivation region of the Pourbaix diagram. It is the most common form of corrosion. In the absence of equilibrium concentrations of their constituent ions in the bathing solution, it will occur for all metals. Even in the immunity region, uniform attack will result in a slow removal of metal from implants. Thus, it is fair to state that, due to uniform attack, all metals have a finite corrosion rate *in vivo*. However, uniform attack may not be noticed until, or unless, significant amounts of metal are lost. Because all metals currently used in implants are relatively highly resistant to uniform attack, little evidence of such attack is ever seen in implant applications.

Uniform attack is usually measured in terms of surface recession. An approximation to this rate may be obtained from Equation 4.9 if the surface area of an implant (A, in.^{2}), the density of the alloy used (D, g/cm^3), the exposure time (T, hours), and the total weight loss (w, mg) are known:

$$mpy = \frac{534\,w}{DAT} \tag{4.9}$$

For a typical implant alloy with a density near 8 g/cm^3, 1 mpy ≈ 0.7 mg/cm^2/day. *In vivo* uniform corrosion rates for well-passivated alloys are thought to be about 1/100 of this value (Steinemann 1980), reinforcing the prior statement of the low utility of this measure in biomedical applications.

4.7.2 Galvanic Corrosion

Galvanic (or two-metal) corrosion takes place when two different metals are in physical (electronic) contact and are immersed in an ionic conducting fluid medium such as serum or interstitial fluid. This is also referred to as couple corrosion. An example of a situation that may lead to this is shown in Figure 4.4. The "difference" between the screw and plate, responsible for the galvanic process, may be due to different compositions (major and/or minor constituents) and/or processing.

For a particular combination of pH and potential (defined by pO$_2$), the two metals will have different electrochemical potentials. The one that is less noble than the other — that is, below it on a suitable practical electrochemical series — becomes anodic. The surface of the less noble metal that is in contact with the solution will experience attack, of a uniform nature, with a release

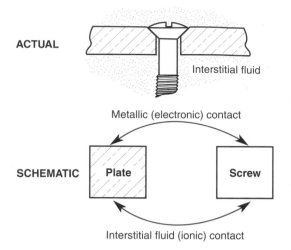

FIGURE 4.4
Conditions for galvanic corrosion.

of metallic ions. The other metal becomes cathodic. Electrons move to it through the physical connection, driven by the intermetallic potential difference. The electrons may then reduce dissolved oxygen or hydrogen ions, depending upon local conditions. Although the less noble metal of the pair may not corrode because it is in a passive region in its respective Pourbaix diagram, the more noble metal cannot corrode under any conditions. Thus, because it is cathodic, it is said to have cathodic protection.

The actual details of galvanic corrosion depend upon a large number of complicating factors, including the relative size of the areas of electronic and ionic contact, as well as on the actual metal pair involved. However, although some exceptions occur in actual practice, it is safe to assume that galvanic corrosion can occur in any metal pair in acid pH. Note that all three conditions must be met for galvanic corrosion to take place; thus, the presence of two or more different compositions of metallic implants within an animal or patient will not produce galvanic effects unless the implants are in direct physical contact so that an electron current may flow between them.

4.7.3   Crevice Corrosion

Crevice corrosion is one of a number of forms of corrosion related to structural details. The basic requirement for the occurrence of this process is the presence of a crevice (a narrow, deep crack): an interface between parts of a device, such as between plate and screw head, or a defect such as an incomplete fatigue crack. The details of the initiation of crevice corrosion are not yet clear. Once begun, however, it is characterized by oxygen depletion in the crevice, anodic metallic corrosion along the crevice faces, and cathodic protective conditions on the metal surface around its mouth.

Static nonflowing conditions in the solution seem to favor crevice corrosion, perhaps because of the formation of a metallic ion concentration gradient away from the open end of the crevice. Because the areas of attack are concentrated, evidence of crevice corrosion can easily be seen in the mating areas in multipart devices, such as between screw and plate in retrieved fracture fixation devices (Colangelo and Greene 1969). This is a frequently observed effect; the majority of multipart fracture-fixation devices retrieved from patients show crevice corrosion and/or pitting corrosion (see Section 4.7.4) (Cook et al. 1985). High local concentrations of corrosion products may also result in precipitation of oxides, hydroxides, or phosphates in adjacent tissues (Jacobs et al. 1995). In conjunction with stress corrosion, crevice corrosion may change the mechanical behavior of metals subjected to cyclic loading (see Section 6.5.2).

4.7.4 Pitting Corrosion

Pitting corrosion is a special case of crevice corrosion. It is a more isolated, symmetric form of attack; inclusions, scratches, or handling damage may initiate it. Pitting corrosion proceeds through processes similar to those for crevice corrosion, although static conditions and reduced oxygen potential seem less important and autocatalysis may play an important role (Punckt et al. 2004). Thus, pits often occur in large numbers, like freckles, and grow down in the direction of gravity in unstirred solutions.

It would be desirable to avoid pits in highly stressed implants because they constitute points of stress concentration and may serve as the starting points for mechanical cracks to develop. Like the effects of crevice corrosion, pits are easy to see. When they are very small, they change the surface finish, often producing a "frosted" or matte appearance. Larger, more developed pits often have accumulations of colored corrosion products in them and may show up as green, brown, or black spots against the otherwise polished surface of the implant. For this reason, it is inadvisable to clean implants vigorously after removal before they have been examined for evidence of corrosion. In practice, it may be difficult to distinguish between pitting and crevice corrosion at early stages of attack. Multiple part implants have, in the past, often shown evidence of crevice, pitting, and fatigue corrosion (Cohen and Lindenbaum 1968); however, as alloy cleanliness has improved with time, the prevalence of these effects has declined.

4.7.5 Intergranular Corrosion

Intergranular corrosion is somewhat related to crevice corrosion but has different origins and produces different effects. It is more common in devices that are made by casting. Cast metals have multiple crystals or grains, with impurities preferentially deposited between the grains during solidification. As a result, the chemistry of a grain boundary will be different from that of the grains on either side and will probably have a different, and generally less noble, electrochemical potential. The consequence in a corrosive environment is an intergranular attack resembling crevice corrosion. A part may appear essentially normal and then suddenly crumble into grains under a mechanical stress. A less radical effect is sometimes seen in brass doorknobs in old houses. Because of the perspiration left on the knob by generations of hands, the intergranular corrosion of zinc precipitates "etches" the surface and makes the individual grains visible.

Intergranular corrosion is obviously more common in alloys than in pure metals and is favored by high levels of impurities and inclusions. If not properly heat treated, stainless steel may corrode by this mechanism due to a relative depletion of chromium from the grain boundaries. Welding of alloys that results in local melting and resolidification can also lead to a variant of this called knife-edge attack. The name derives from the appearance of the failure: a straight crack through the metal parallel to and near the weld. Again, proper heat treatment after welding will restore the right compositional distribution and reduce or prevent this type of attack.

4.7.6 Leaching

Leaching is similar to intergranular corrosion. However, in this case the components of a particular alloy are sufficiently weakly bound to each other and differ enough in chemical reactivity so that there is a large difference in the rate of loss of the alloy components by uniform attack. Thus, leaching as a form of corrosion is a special case of leaching (discussed in Chapter 3), with an accompanying chemical reaction. Attack of this kind will remove metal with a regular periodic variation of effect at a microscopic level. It is peculiar to certain alloy systems but can be induced by two conditions:

- The introduction into the solution around the metal of an agent that attacks one component of the alloy in preference to another. For instance, fluoride ion (F^-) will selectively remove aluminum from copper–aluminum alloys.

- The presence of more than one phase in the alloy. Usually, all of the grains in an alloy have the same composition. The alloy is then said to have a single phase. However, it is possible for individual grains to be of two or more different, discrete compositions. Such an alloy is said to possess multiple phases. Because electrochemical potential varies as chemical composition, these phases may have a different susceptibility to various forms of corrosive attack. Note that heat treatment to reduce the size of the grains will not change this situation. For this reason, multiphase alloys are not usually used in corrosive applications. Thus, considerable academic concern arose when ASTM F-562 — a multiphase alloy of cobalt, nickel, chromium, and molybdenum containing 35% nickel — was introduced for use in implants. However, experience suggests that, despite the differences in the phase compositions, all of the phases are sufficiently passive under the conditions experienced in soft and hard tissue implant sites so that leaching does not occur in this alloy.

Leaching produces surface appearances similar to those produced by pitting or intergranular attack.

4.7.7 Erosion Corrosion

Erosion corrosion is a rare form of corrosion. This is an acceleration of attack on a metal because of relative movement between the surrounding fluid and the metallic surface. It is not a unique process, but it serves to increase the rate of attack by several other mechanisms. This happens because many corrosion processes tend to be self-limiting. That is, the accumulation of the products of corrosion at the interface between metal and solution tends to reduce the rate of reaction. Flowing solution will sweep away these corrosion end products as well as provide new amounts of dissolved reactants, such as chloride ion and oxygen. In extreme cases, the solution may physically erode the passive layer in regions of passivity. The reformation of this layer and its removal by continued flow produces progressive attack on the metal and renders that region of the pH-potential diagram corrosive rather than passive as predicted.

The physical damage resembles pitting, except that these pits are elongated in the direction of flow and are generally larger and less symmetric than those seen in pitting corrosion under static conditions. The peculiarities of flow, especially if it is a stable pattern, will often result in etching a clear picture of the course of the flow on the surface of the metal.

4.7.8 Stress and Fatigue Corrosion

Stress corrosion is the last of the eight forms of corrosion. Simply stated, tensile stress increases the chemical activity of metals. A flexed metal component will sustain a tensile stress on one side and a compressive stress on the other side. This produces a difference in electrochemical potential that renders the convex surface anodic with respect to the concave one. As an acceleration of uniform attack or, perhaps, secondary to tensile rupture of the passive film, corrosion may then attack the convex surface. Local corrosion rates (as measured by corrosion current) may be two- to threefold elevated over the uniform corrosion rate (Bundy et al. 1991)

Because the formation of even a small crack in a loaded structure, such as a flexed plate, will concentrate stress, this attack tends to initiate cracks that grow rapidly, leading to possible structural failure. The cracks extend between grains; however, this process can be differentiated from intergranular cracking due to the small number, relative isolation, and branched structure of stress corrosion cracks.

Many metals display an endurance limit to cyclic loading. In the presence of crevice corrosion in physical cracks or in crack-like defects in a passive surface layer produced by single or repeated cyclic loading, this limit may be abolished. That is, the maximum stress that can be reached without failure continuously decreases as the number of load cycles increases instead of reaching a lower limit. This phenomenon, which is a dynamic form of stress corrosion, is termed fatigue corrosion and may be an important limit on the life of metallic implants undergoing cyclic mechanical deformation.

4.8   Corrosion in Implant Applications

Which of these eight forms of corrosive attack are important in implant applications? As a general rule, corrosive attack is more common on multipart implants than single part devices. Some studies indicate that a majority of multipart orthopaedic fracture fixation devices show evidence of corrosion after recovery at the end of treatment (Cook et al. 1985). Uniform attack occurs on these as on all other implants. The primary physical evidence suggests that crevice and pitting corrosion are the next most important forms (Cohen and Lindenbaum 1968). Crevice corrosion occurs in the gap between the screw and the plate in screw–plate assemblies. The attack is most often seen on the plate — within the hole, but near the longitudinal surfaces. Occasionally, crevice attack will be noted on the portions of the screw opposite these areas. Due to the reduction in the cross section of the plate at the hole, these areas have a high stress concentration. Frank mechanical fracture of the plate through a screw hole can often be associated with microscopic evidence of crevice corrosion. The introduction of modularity into joint replacement devices has produced a range of apparent crevice and related corrosion effects, with occasional but rare component failure, which have not previously been seen (Gilbert et al. 1993).

Pitting most often occurs on the underside of screw heads. Despite the characteristic freckle appearance of the pits, they may be hard to distinguish from mechanical scoring of the screw head and shaft during insertion and/ or removal. Such scoring may result from rubbing against a burr in the hole in the plate or against a fragment of bone caught between plate and screw during removal.

Galvanic corrosion may also occur between plates and screws. There is a slight tendency for this naturally because the plates and screws are fabricated by different processes; thus, if they are not properly heat treated, they may have slightly different electrochemical potentials. Mixing screws and plates from different manufacturers may also produce galvanic effects because each manufacturer uses a slightly different heat treatment schedule. Screws of a different composition from the plate, as well as metallic foreign bodies such as drill bit fragments inadvertently introduced into an implant site, may also cause galvanic corrosion (Fothi et al. 1992).

Attack of this sort is often discovered through reports of persistent, very localized operative site pain. It may occur, however, as judged by frequent observations of tissue discoloration during routine device removal procedures, without any apparent sensation. Galvanic corrosion may leave a discoloration with a "burned" or sooty appearance on the screw or the plate in the area of contact.

Stress corrosion is also possible but extremely rare. Intergranular corrosion, leaching, and erosion do not occur to any real extent in modern multipart devices in orthopaedic applications. A solid-state version of erosion corrosion may occur if an interface is loose or fixation is poor. Relative motion between plate and screws may result in physical removal of material, or fretting. This may disrupt the passive film and produce accelerated corrosion in much the same way that erosion corrosion takes place. This phenomenon is difficult to distinguish from simple wear and is called fretting corrosion (Brown and Merritt 1981).

In single part devices such as cranial plates, intramedullary rods, endoprostheses, pins, and cerclage wire, the effects are rather more limited. Uniform attack does occur, as previously noted. Stress corrosion or, more generally, stress enhancement of fatigue failure (fatigue corrosion) is probably the most common destructive form. Although rare in prostheses, its incidence is very high in the highly stressed cerclage wire used for uniting bone fragments. Intergranular corrosion does occur occasionally and is probably most often associated with surface inclusions or casting defects in cast prosthetic sections. It is rarely active enough to lead to mechanical failure in the absence of cyclic loading.

Corrosion in blood contact areas is much more complex. The abundant supply of oxygen and the continued flow of electrolytes render most processes highly active. In addition, the presence of many small organic molecules influences rates. Sulfur-bearing molecules such as cystine appear to accelerate corrosion; neutral molecules such as alanine may inhibit corrosion (Svare et al. 1970) in much the same way as rust inhibitors in engineering applications. Furthermore, corrosion may profoundly affect surface properties and thus influence thrombogenic behavior; this will be discussed in Section 9.3.2.

Corrosion is generally considered to be undesirable. However, in some biomaterial applications the response to local concentrations of corrosion products is necessary to the successful function of an implant. For instance, the copper IUD (intrauterine device) depends for its contraceptive properties on the release of copper ions by a corrosion process.

It may also be desirable to accept a higher corrosion rate because of other more critical properties of an alloy. In a surgical setting, the stainless steel spring clips used for the repair of large cranial aneurismal defects have been deliberately fabricated from type 301, 416, and 420 steel alloys (McFadden

1969). These alloys corrode at a more rapid rate than the more usual grade of stainless steel used in implants, 316L (ASTM F 138). However, these alloys are superior to 316L for spring fabrication. One feature of local response to these products is undoubtedly an increased fibroplasia — perhaps producing a more rapid and mechanically sound scarring process — but otherwise they appear to be adequately tolerated.

4.9 Engineering Variables Affecting Corrosion Rates

Despite the prevalence of corrosive attack on implanted devices, the rate of failure of structure or of function is quite small. Why is it that a particular device can perform well in 99 patients and then cause problems in the 100th? Conversely, why do materials known to be prone to corrosion occasionally survive for very long periods *in vivo* (Blackwood and Periera 2004)? The answers are not simple. To all of the normal biological variables of human health and disease, at least four "engineering" variables must be added:

- Composition of the implants — in particular, variations within the implant and extremes of implant-to-implant variation — can affect corrosion rates in many ways, as has been discussed.

- Manufacturing variables, including casting conditions, metal purity, amount of cold work, and the degree and type of heat treatment, have a profound effect on corrosion rates (Sutow et al. 1976). Corrosion rates, at least initially, are markedly affected by the details of the passivation process used (Browne and Gregson 1994; Callen et al. 1995).

- Handling in manufacture, delivery, and insertion can affect results. Occasionally, corrosion initiation can be traced to unintended physical damage (Gray 1974).

- Positioning of the implant will affect the stresses upon it as well as the local environment that it experiences. Anatomical location and small differences in it may have an important effect (Oron and Alter 1984), primarily due to local differences in pH and pO_2 (Morita et al. 1992).

4.10 Corrosion Factors Peculiar to Biological Environments

In addition to the factors just discussed, it is apparent that organic molecules present in implant sites may affect corrosion rates. These are thought to act in four ways:

- Formation of organometallic complexes. If conditions at any point in the pH-potential region of interest favor the formation of organo-metallic complexes, the metallic content of these represents an addition to the corrosion rate.

- Alteration of charge of corrosion products. Many organic molecules are potent oxidizing agents, producing the possibility of different ionic valences than predicted by pH-potential considerations. For example, in the presence of serum proteins, it is probable that significant amounts of chromium may be released from alloys as Cr^{+6} rather than Cr^{+3} (Rogers 1984). Despite the high degree of oxidation, Cr^{+6} may persist for several minutes (Liu and Shi 2001) before even partial reduction occurs.

- Modification of the passive layer. Combination of organic species with the passive layer, in the passive region or in adjacent regions of metastability (low passive film-dissolution rate), may alter the nature of the passive film. These may act to stabilize or destabilize the film or to change its electrical conductivity, thus altering corrosion rates (Svare et al. 1970).

- Changes in wear conditions. Although the presence of serum proteins generally elevates corrosion rates, in *in vitro* experiments, it markedly reduces fretting corrosion rates of stainless steel (Brown and Merritt 1981; Merritt and Brown 1988).

Previously, I have emphasized the need to distinguish among physiological, biophysiological, and pericellular environments (Section 2.3). The addition of cells and bacteria to a biological environment produces the possibility of true "bio" corrosion phenomena. Degradative cells such as macrophages (Yang et al. 1992), as well as a wide range of bacteria (Wilson et al. 1997), can directly corrode metals without phagocytosis (see Section 8.2.3), primarily by modification of the pericellular environment. This latter phenomenon mirrors that encountered in marine environments (Thomas et al. 1988).

4.11 Ceramic Dissolution

As a class of materials, ceramics are most generally defined as inorganic, nonmetallic solids. This category contains a wide range of compounds and mixtures, primarily compounds of metals, such as oxides, carbonates, sulfates, etc. They may be crystalline or amorphous; if they contain chain formers, such as elemental carbon or silica (SiO_2), amorphous materials may be glassy. Multiphase physical mixtures and, in the presence of glassy phases, compound alloys, are also possible.

Metals under immune conditions, whether deliberately passivated or not, have surface films composed of oxides or hydroxides. In the most common biomaterial alloy systems, the surfaces of stainless steels and cobalt-base super alloys are primarily chromium oxide and hydroxide, while the surfaces of titanium-base alloys are primarily titania (titanium dioxide, TiO_2). Thus, the behavior of metals (with or without prior passivation), under chemical conditions producing immunity for the underlying alloy, is essentially that of dissolution of a ceramic. In fact, very small metallic wear debris may be completely ceramic in nature and their reactions with biological environments may be better considered in this light.

Two main classes of ceramics are used as biomaterials: structural (or technical) and resorbable (or soluble); the latter includes so-called "bioceramics." Structural ceramics such as alumina (Al_2O_3) and zirconia (ZrO_2) are selected for, among other properties, their low chemical reactivity and essential insolubility in water. Along with some forms of carbon — especially vitreous carbon — these materials may be regarded as insoluble in biomaterial applications. In general, reports of dissolution products from solid structural ceramic biomaterials should be regarded as artifactual; however, very large surface area/volume ratio ceramic materials, such as aggregations of small (submicron) wear debris, may be able to release measurable amounts of dissolution products. No evidence indicates that biophysiological, biological, or pericellular conditions affect this conclusion.

Soluble ceramics are an example of type 2 or interactive biomaterials (see Section 1.4). The most common types are those that resemble calcium-based minerals that naturally occur in mammalian bodies, such as calcium hydroxyapatite ($Ca_{10}(PO_4)_6(OH)_2$), tricalcium phosphate ($Ca_3(PO_4)_2$), octacalcium phosphate ($Ca_8H(PO_4)_6 \cdot 5H_2O$), etc. However, other resorbable materials, such as hydrated calcium sulfate ($CaSO_4 \cdot 2H_2O$), Bioglass™ (see Section 10.3.4.3), etc., are in use as biomaterials.

The dissolution behavior of these more soluble ceramic materials depends upon their composition, processing, and final form, as well as on local pH and pO_2 (but not on local applied potential because, as a class [with the exception of carbons and graphites], these materials are electrical insulators). In addition, phagocytic cells (see Section 8.2.3) are able to attack many of these materials, thus raising their solubility in pericellular environments.

Although general rules are hard to draw, the following principles may be useful:

- Crystalline (polycrystalline) forms tend to be less soluble than glassy or amorphous ones of the same composition.
- Polycrystalline forms tend to be more soluble than single crystal forms of the same composition.
- Hydrated forms tend to be more soluble than nonhydrated forms of the same composition.
- Mass loss per unit time depends significantly on specific surface area; thus, porous or fine particulate materials tend to dissolve more rapidly than equal weights of the same material in a solid, nonporous form.
- Cellular attack, when successful, is more rapid on small particles (<25 μm) than on solid bodies of the same composition.

4.12 Polymer Dissolution

Polymers possess such a wide range of compositions, structures, and molecular weight that it is difficult to make any generalizations concerning their dissolution behavior. One worthwhile distinction is whether a polymeric material is hydrophilic or hydrophobic. Dissolution of hydrophilic polymers, especially low molecular weight, resembles uniform corrosion of metals, in that the result is a surface recession (Figure 4.5, right). By contrast, hydrophobic polymers, which will nevertheless absorb polar fluids such as water, may undergo a form of internal attack in which amorphous regions dissolve preferentially to crystalline ones (Figure 4.5, left). The effect is to produce increased surface area, increasing the effective dissolution rate and leading, perhaps, to structural effects similar to those of intergranular corrosion, with sudden loss of integrity and release of small particles.

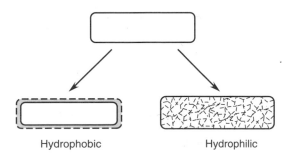

Hydrophobic   Hydrophilic

FIGURE 4.5
Comparison of dissolution of hydrophobic and hydrophilic polymers.

4.13   Final Remarks

The one certain thing that can be said about corrosion is that it results in the release of cations from all metallic implants. Cations also form a wide variety of organometallic complexes. Some of these soluble products, such as the ferric and ferrous ions, are familiar parts of the internal environment. Some are trace elements with known biological roles, such as trivalent chromium ions. Others are rare enough in nature that they do not have known metabolic roles and are released in the body — even in the absence of abnormal corrosion processes — at concentrations orders of magnitude above their normal *in vivo* occurrence. Under certain conditions, small particles also may be released or formed by precipitation, locally or at remote sites, of soluble products. Dissolution of nonmetallic materials is still more complex and difficult to summarize, but it too results in release of soluble and particulate materials of a wide range of compositions. The consequences of such release will be considered at length in later chapters.

References

Blackwood, D.J. and Pereira, B.P., No corrosion of 304 stainless steel implant after 40 years of service, *J. Mater. Sci.: Mater. Med.*, 15, 755, 2004.

Brown, S.A. and Merritt, K., Fretting corrosion in saline and serum, *J. Biomed. Mater. Res.*, 15, 479, 1981.

Browne, M. and Gregson, P.J., Surface modification of titanium alloy implants, *Biomaterials*, 15, 894, 1994.

Bundy, K.J., Williams, C.J. and Luedemann, R.E., Stress-enhanced ion release — the effect of static loading, *Biomaterials*, 12, 627, 1991.

Callen, B.W. et al., Nitric acid passivation of Ti6Al4V reduces thickness of surface oxide layer and increases trace element release, *J. Biomed. Mater. Res.*, 29, 279, 1995.

Cohen, J. and Lindenbaum, B., Fretting corrosion in orthopedic implants, *Clin. Orthop. Rel. Res.*, 61, 167, 1968.

Colangelo, V.J. and Greene, N.D., Corrosion and fracture of type 316 SMO orthopedic implants, *J. Biomed. Mater. Res.*, 3, 247, 1969.

Cook, S.D. et al., Clinical and metallurgical analysis of retrieved internal fixation devices, *Clin. Orthop. Rel. Res.*, 194, 236, 1985.

Fontana, M.G., *Corrosion Engineering*, 3rd ed., McGraw–Hill, New York, 1985, Chapter 4, 137.

Fothi, U., Perren, S.M. and Auer, J.A., Drill bit failure with implant involvement — an intraoperative complication in orthopedic surgery, *Injury 23* (Suppl 2), S17, 1992.

Gilbert, J.L., Buckley, C.A. and Jacobs, J.J., *In vivo* corrosion of modular hip prosthesis components in mixed and similar metal combinations. The effect of crevice, stress, motion, and alloy coupling, *J. Biomed. Mater. Res.*, 27, 1533, 1993.

Gray, R.J., Metallographic examinations of retrieved intramedullary bone pins and bone screws from the human body, *J. Biomed. Mater. Res. Symp.*, 5(1), 27, 1974.

Jacobs, J.J. et al., Local and distant products from modularity, *Clin. Orthop. Rel. Res.*, 319, 94, 1995.

Liu, K.J. and Shi, X., *In vivo* reduction of chromium (VI) and its related free radical generation, *Mol. Cell. Biochem.*, 222, 41, 2001.

McFadden, J.T., Metallurgical principles in neurosurgery, *J. Neurosurg.*, 31(4), 373, 1969.

Merritt, K. and Brown, S.A., Effect of proteins and pH on fretting corrosion and metal ion release, *J. Biomed. Mater. Res.*, 22, 111, 1988.

Morita, M. et al., Influence of low dissolved oxygen concentration in body fluid on corrosion fatigue behaviors of implant metals, *Ann. Biomed. Eng.*, 20, 505, 1992.

Oron, U. and Alter, A., Corrosion in metal implants embedded in various locations of the body of rats, *Clin. Orthop. Rel. Res.*, 185, 295, 1984.

Pourbaix, M., *Atlas of Electrochemical Equilibria*, Pergamon Press, Oxford, 1966.

Punckt, C. et al., Sudden onset of pitting corrosion on stainless steel as a critical phenomenon, *Science*, 305, 1133, 2004.

Rogers, G.T., *In vivo* production of hexavalent chromium, *Biomaterials*, 5, 244, 1984.

Steinemann, S.G., Corrosion of surgical implants — *in vivo* and *in vitro* tests, in *Evaluation of Biomaterials*, Winter, G.D., Leray, J.L. and deGroot, K. (Eds.), John Wiley & Sons, Chichester, U.K., 1980, 1.

Sutow, E.J., Pollack, S.R. and Korostoff, E., An *in vitro* investigation of the anodic polarization and capacitance behavior of 316-L stainless steel, *J. Biomed. Mater. Res.*, 10, 671, 1976.

Svare, C.W., Belton, G. and Korostoff, E., The role of organics in metallic passivation, *J. Biomed. Mater. Res.*, 4, 457, 1970.

Thomas, C.J., Edyvean, R.G.J. and Brook, R., Biologically enhanced corrosion fatigue, *Biofouling*, 1, 65, 1988.

Wilson, M. et al., Corrosion of intraoral magnets by multi-species biofilms in the presence and absence of sucrose, *Biomaterials*, 18, 53, 1997.

Yang, J. et al., Human neutrophil response to short-term exposure to F-75 cobalt-base alloy, *J. Biomed. Mater. Res.*, 26, 1217, 1992.

Bibliography

Bundy, K.J., Corrosion and other electrochemical aspects of biomaterials, *Crit. Rev. Biomed. Eng.*, 22, 139, 1994.

Deltombe, E., De Zoubov, N. and Pourbaix, M., Chromium, in Pourbaix, M., *Atlas of Electrochemical Equilibria*, Pergamon Press, Oxford, 1966, 256.

Fraker, A.C. and Griffin, C.D. (Eds.), *Corrosion and Degradation of Implant Materials: Second Symposium, STP 859*, American Society for Testing and Materials, Philadelphia, 1985.

Fusayama, T., Katayori, T. and Nomoto, S., Corrosion of gold and amalgam placed in contact with each other, *J. Dent. Res.*, 42, 1183, 1963.

Hofmann, G.O., Biodegradable implants in traumatology: a review on the state-of-the-art, *Arch. Orthop. Trauma Surg.*, 114, 123, 1995.

Jacobs, J.J., Gilbert, J.L. and Urban, R.M., Current concepts review: corrosion of metal orthopedic implants. *J. Bone Joint Surg.*, 80A, 268, 1998.

Luckey, H.A. and Kubli, F., Jr. (Eds.), *Titanium Alloys in Surgical Implants*. STP 796. American Society for Testing and Materials, Philadelphia, 1983.

Marcus, P. and Oudar, J. (Eds.), *Corrosion Mechanisms in Theory and Practice*, Marcel Dekker, New York, 1995.

Pohler, O.E.M., Degradation of metallic orthopedic implants, in *Biomaterials in Reconstructive Surgery*, Rubin, L.R. (Ed.), C.V. Mosby, St. Louis, 1983,158.

Pourbaix, M., Electrochemical corrosion of metallic biomaterials, *Biomaterials*, 5, 122, 1984.

Ravaglioli, A. and Krajewski, A. (Eds.), *Bioceramics*, Chapman & Hall, London, 1992.

Scully, J.C., *The Fundamentals of Corrosion*, 3rd ed., Pergamon Press, Oxford, 1990.

Shahgaldi, B.F. et al., *In vivo* corrosion of cobalt-chromium and titanium wear particles, *J. Bone Joint Surg.*, 77B, 962, 1995.

Schweitzer, P.A. (Ed.), *Corrosion Engineering Handbook*, Marcel Dekker, New York, 1996.

Syrett, B.C. and Acharya, A. (Eds.), *Corrosion and Degradation of Implant Materials*, STP 684, American Society for Testing and Materials, Philadelphia, 1979.

Tengvall, P. and Lundström, I., Physicochemical considerations of titanium as a biomaterial, *Clin. Mater.*, 9, 115, 1992.

Vermilyea, D.A., Physics of corrosion, *Physics Today*, Sept. 1976, 23.

Williams, D.F., Corrosion of implant materials, *Ann. Rev. Mater. Sci.*, 6, 237, 1976.

Zitter, H. and Plenk, H., Jr., The electrochemical behavior of metallic implant materials as an indicator of their biocompatibility, *J. Biomed. Mater. Res.*, 21, 881, 1987.

5

Reactions of Biological Molecules with Biomaterial Surfaces

5.1 Introduction

Strictly speaking, in a biomaterials–tissue system, there are no surfaces; as Andrade (1973) has pointed out, there are only interfaces. In this chapter, the solid–liquid interface produced by the contact of a solid biomaterial with body fluids will be considered briefly. The solid–liquid interface can affect dissolved species in the surrounding fluid at two levels of characteristic dimension:

- The molecular level (3 to 15 Å): these effects are essentially chemical.
- The macromolecular level (15 to 500 Å): these effects are more of a mechanical nature.

Chemical effects depend upon the detailed chemistry and ionic charge distribution of the surface. The effects that local chemistry can have on some of the events of coagulation (Section 9.3.2) and on adaptation (Chapter 10), immune response (Section 12.2.1), and carcinogenesis (Section 13.2) will be considered. These effects can be undesirable side aspects of the biomaterial selected for other properties (as in the general blood conduit problem) or deliberately induced effects required to mediate a cellular response. Examples of induced effects are common in the results of various surface treatments used to reduce or eliminate thrombus formation on the surface of blood contact materials. A less common induced effect is the production of surface activity (in the chemical sense) to stimulate directly adaptive cellular response.

In addition to the direct chemical (inorganic) effect of surface modification on cellular activity, local changes in composition, pH, and molarity will produce a variety of physiochemical changes in proteins, including dissociation and denaturation. The observed cellular response may be secondary to these physiochemical changes in proteins.

Dissociation is understood in the general chemical sense as the separation of ions from molecular species. In addition, it refers to the disaggregation of multimolecular organic complexes, such as enzyme-cofactor complexes.

These associations, like all chemical bonding processes, depend upon free energy considerations and may be affected by local pH and ionic concentration. On the other hand, denaturation can be viewed as a purely topological and mechanical process and will be discussed in the next section.

5.2 Denaturation

Denaturation is a problem peculiar to large organic molecules such as proteins. Four levels (or orders) of structure are recognized in these molecules:

1° The chemical composition as defined by atomic content and primary bonds between atoms

2° The spatial arrangement of portions of a molecule as defined by the requirements of bond angulation at each atomic center and by the intramolecular bonds other than main chain bonds

3° The spatial arrangements determined by strong intramolecular bonds and secondary folding to produce stable domains

4° The aggregation of three structures by weak associative bonding (hydrogen or Van der Waals bonds)

The primary and, to some degree, secondary levels of structure are determined during synthesis. The tertiary may be produced by a self-assembly process or occur secondarily to a usually extracellular, one-time cleavage of a portion of the synthesized molecule. Thus, if these structures are disturbed by heat or local chemical activity, the molecule may not be able to revert to its original or native structure. Such a molecule is said to be denatured and may arouse a variety of biological responses despite a normal or near normal chemical composition (primary structure). Finally, because it depends upon weak bonds, the quaternary of structure is quite sensitive to pH and concentration changes. The results of these changes may be as simple as slight alterations in configuration or as profound as the dissociation of multimolecular structures, such as those formed by enzymes and cofactors.

5.3 Organometallic Compounds

5.3.1 Definitions

Beyond the effects on structure, surfaces may obviously be chemically reactive. As a class, metals are the most reactive implant materials. They may provoke a host response due to the formation of corrosion products (discussed in Section 8.2.5). However, many of these corrosion products are organometallic complexes or compounds and, as such, have a special behavior of biological importance.

As the name implies, organometallic compounds have two components: one is an organic moiety and the other is the metallic moiety. The association between the two can be a weak interaction or, at the other end of the spectrum, a very strong interaction, as in the case of the Fe-containing porphyrin heme in the hemoglobin complex. There also can be a degree of specificity of structure, again as seen in the heme molecule. If another metallic ion were to replace the iron, the function of oxygen transport would be impaired. This is apparently the case when elevated chromium levels are present in heme synthesis sites (Smith 1982).

Three terms are useful in discussions of organometallic compounds:

- Chelation: a type of interaction between an organic compound (having two or more points at which it may coordinate with a metal) and the metal to form a ring-type structure
- Coordination: the joining of an ion or molecule to a metal ion by a nonionic valence bond to form a complex ion or molecule
- Ligand: any ion or molecule that, by donating one or more pairs of electrons to a central metal ion, is coordinated with it to form a complex ion or molecule, as in the cobalt complex $[CoCl(NH_3)_5]Cl_2$, in which Cl and NH_3 in the bracketed portion are ligands coordinated with Co

5.3.2 Stability

In a free metal cation, all of the five d orbitals have the same energy level. However, in a chelate or complex, some of the filled orbitals are oriented toward the chelating atoms. Repulsion between nonbonding electrons in a d orbital and those of the chelating atom causes electrons in these orbitals to be less stable with respect to the other orbitals. In addition, bonding can preferentially stabilize one orbital with respect to the others. The theory dealing with repulsion from the field produced by the chelating atoms is called crystal field theory; the total effects are dealt with in ligand field theory.

By preferentially filling low-energy orbitals in organic ions, the metallic d orbitals can stabilize the molecular system. For example, if three orbitals have a low energy and two have a higher energy, as in an octahedral complex, the configuration would be much more stable with six electrons occupying the low-energy levels than with the electrons spread throughout all five orbitals. The gain in bonding energy achieved in this manner is referred to as the crystal field stabilization energy (CFSE).

Complexes with more of the electrons in the lower energy levels are more stable than those with all the d orbitals equally filled. Trivalent chromium and cobalt, for example, with three and six electrons, respectively, will form very stable complexes or ions. Consequently, the tendency of these ions to form complexes is very great. A complex of univalent copper, on the other hand, has zero CFSE because the five orbitals are completely filled. As a result, cuprous complexes will be less stable than those of trivalent cobalt or trivalent chromium.

Crystal field effects are important in predicting the rates and mechanisms of reactions of coordination compounds. The essential feature here is that ions that are strongly crystal-field stabilized will be slow to react, and nonstabilized ions will be more liable (reactive). This explains why Co^{+3}, which has considerable CFSE, is so nonreactive. In order for Co^{+3} to react, the octahedral configuration, which creates the large CSFE, must first be disrupted.

5.3.3 Production

The production of the organometallic compounds by implants is controlled by a dynamic equilibrium that occurs after implantation of a metallic specimen or device. This equilibrium is established between the alloy and the intermediate organometallic compound, as well as between the alloy and the more traditional inorganic ions. The rate of corrosion will then depend on the removal of the intermediate compound. If more is removed by deposition in tissues, then corrosion could proceed at an increased rate. Because the removal of the intermediate is the rate-limiting step, differences seen between biological response to powder and bulk implants probably reflect different surface (interface) reaction conditions.

The equilibrium will also depend upon three other factors:

- The organometallic complex may be formed on the surface or in solution. If it is formed on the surface, the ratio of the implant surface area to the fluid volume available for equilibrium (SA/FLV) will govern the formation rate and the equilibrium concentration. This is apparently the case for complexes formed between chromium or nickel and serum proteins (Woodman et al. 1984). If the complex forms preferentially in solution, then SA/FLV affects only the rate of formation, as is apparently the case for cobalt.

- The chemical composition of the surface may affect the strength of the initial association and the rate of loss (desorption) of complexes that form at the interface. Table 5.1 presents data for absorption and desorption of albumin, the most common serum protein, by a variety of materials. A single monolayer corresponds to 0.2 to 0.7 µg cm^{-2}, depending upon packing of molecules. "Desorption" in this context is actually exchange because release in the absence of proteins in solution (a highly unphysiological condition) may be different. In particular, under these conditions, polyethylene releases no measurable albumin into an albumin-free solution (Brash et al. 1974). Fluid

TABLE 5.1

Albumin Absorption and Desorption from Surfaces

Material	Absorption (μg.cm^{-2}/24 h): (Conc.: 2 mg/ml)	Desorption (%/24 h): (Conc.: 1 mg/ml)
Metals		
Silver	2.01 ± 0.22	23
Vanadium	0.13 ± 0.06	73
Titanium	0.05 ± 0.02	86
Oxides		
TiO$_2$	0.15 ± 0.02	70
Al$_2$O$_3$	0.06 ± 0.01	83
Polymers	(Conc.: 3.7 mg/ml)	(Conc.: 0.1 mg/ml)
Polyethylene	0.28	42
	(Conc.: 1 mg/ml)	(Conc.: 0.2 mg/ml)
Cuprophane™	0.28 ± 0.05	90+
Polyurethane	1.0–2.8	Undetermined

Note: Metals and oxides: absorption/desorption in 0.01 M citrate/phosphate buffered saline (pH = 7.4) at 37°C using ^{125}I-labeled human albumin.

Polymers: absorption/desorption in Tyrodes solution (pH = 7.4) at 25°C using ^{125}I-labeled human albumin.

Source: Williams, R.L. and Williams, D.F., *Biomaterials*, 9, 206, 1988.
Brash, J.L. et al., *Trans. Am. Soc. Artif. Int. Organs*, XX, 69, 1974.

flow near the interface also has an effect, with release/exchange rates increasing with increasing flow rate. The situation at the implant–tissue interface is more complex than this, due to competition between proteins (see Section 5.5).

• The surface energy, which expresses not only chemical composition, but also local spatial arrangement of atoms and bonds as well, also may affect the adsorption/desorption rate (Baszkin and Lyman 1980).

5.4 Mechanical Aspects of Interfaces

Far more important than these chemical effects that take place at atomic dimensions are the mechanical effects that occur on a larger scale. These are primarily associated with the fact that the solid–liquid interface is a phase boundary. As such, it has an interfacial energy proportional to its area associated with it.

Consider the following situation (Figure 5.1). Five molecules of identical composition are shown; however, kinetic and other local affects may produce transient changes in shape, despite the fact that a sphere presents the lowest area, and thus the lowest energy state, of the phase interface. For simplicity, a molecule, *P*, will be considered to be spherical as it approaches a solid

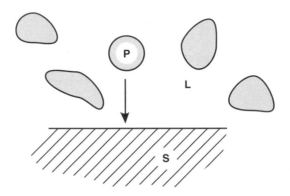

FIGURE 5.1
Molecules near a liquid (L)–solid (S) interface.

surface, S, in liquid, L. Suppose that it will stick or adhere to the surface; the work of adhesion is then (for adhesion of phase A to B):

$$W_{AB} = \gamma_A + \gamma_B - \gamma_{AB} \tag{5.1}$$

where

γ_A, γ_B = "free" surface tensions
γ_{AB} = interfacial surface tension

For this situation, one can write:

$$W_{SP} = \gamma_{SL} + \gamma_{PL} - \gamma_{PS} \tag{5.2}$$

Remember that the surface tensions are negative and that W_{SP} must be negative for adhesion to take place. For example, suppose:

$$\gamma_{SL} = 70 \text{ dyn/cm}$$

$$\gamma_{PL} = 40 \text{ dyn/cm}$$

$$\gamma_{PS} = 50 \text{ dyn/cm}$$

then,

$$W_{SP} = -70 - 40 + 50 = -60 \text{ (a change from } -110 \rightarrow -50) \tag{5.3}$$

Thus, adhesion would result.

However, now look more closely at the interface between the molecule and the solid (Figure 5.2). The normal interfacial equilibrium condition (the Young–Dupree equation) must be satisfied:

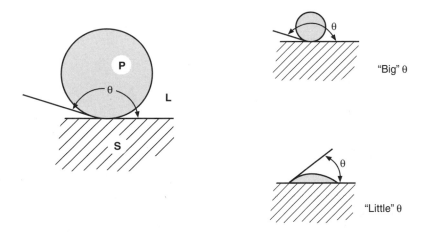

FIGURE 5.2
Conditions for molecular adhesion at an interface.

$$\gamma_{SL} = \gamma_{PS} + \gamma_{PL}\cos\theta \tag{5.4}$$

Note that, for any degree of adhesion ($W_{SP} \leq 0$), θ will be less than 180°. Because the molecule was initially considered to be a sphere, this condition can only be achieved by deformation of the natural (free) shape. A careful analysis combining the Young–Dupree equation with the restoration forces resulting from this molecular deformation would permit a more exact calculation of θ. However, the simple form can be taken as an estimator of the deformation. Thus, the larger the value of θ is, the smaller the deforming force and the likelihood of permanent mechanical damage to the molecule are.

An interesting point concerns the opposite extreme, i.e., when θ goes to zero ($\cos\theta = 1$). This is called full wetting and requires that:

$$\gamma_{PS} = \gamma_{PL}; \ \gamma_{SL} = 2\gamma_{PL} \tag{5.5}$$

This value of surface tension is called the critical surface tension (γ_c). It can be determined by measuring θ for a variety of structurally related liquids and extrapolating the data to determine the limiting value of surface tension (γ_c) as θ approaches zero. A plot of $\cos\theta$ vs. γ_{LV} is called a Zisman plot. The critical surface tension, γ_c, is determined by the intercept at $\cos\theta = 1$. A schematic result is shown in Figure 5.3 for a material surface with $\gamma_c = 28$ dyn/cm.*

---

* See Section 9.3.3 for a discussion of the supposed role of γ_c in cell–surface interactions; de Palma et al. (1972) present interesting examples of Zisman plots obtained on metallic implants before and after blood contact.

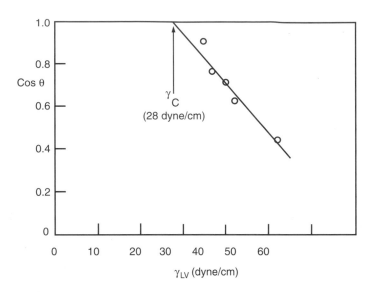

FIGURE 5.3
Model Zisman plot (five fluids). (Note: 1 dyn/cm = 1 erg/cm²)

5.5   Results of Interfacial Adhesion of Molecules

A few of the effects that can result from molecular adhesion to biomaterials or tissues are:

- Enzyme activity and rate constants depend closely upon details of the 3° and 4° molecular structure of enzymes. Accidental or deliberate enzyme adhesion at interfaces can be expected to modify their functional behavior significantly.

- Organic substrate response to enzymatic action is also structure specific. Many substrate molecules have a degree of orientational freedom, possessing features such as saturated bonds about which free rotation is possible. Association of this type of substrate with a surface could hinder or prevent such rotation. Depending upon the configuration in which the molecule is "frozen," enzymatic attack might be accelerated or inhibited.

- Many complex organic molecules, as synthesized, have a "tail" portion that serves to inactivate them. In the normal course of events, enzymatic processes act to strip this small segment and release the molecule into an active substrate pool. Contact with surfaces and the forces resulting from adhesion may cause premature activation.

Some molecules are apparently designed specifically to become activated in this manner by contact with foreign surfaces. An example is fibrinogen, which is reduced slightly in molecular weight and converted to the active protein, fibrin, by surface contact-induced cleavage.

- Immunological response to proteins also depends strongly upon 2°, 3°, and 4° structure. Contact with surface by native proteins produces unnatural configurations of the following types:

  - Conversion or activation of molecules (as mentioned above)

  - Transient deformations during surface contact that are restored upon subsequent desorption

  - Partial or total denaturation due to surface adhesion forces

  Considerable evidence indicates that molecular deformations of each of these three types can excite antibody production and trigger a variety of immune responses, directly or on a subsequent challenge.

In an effort to study the possible immunological results of the surface denaturation of proteins, Stern et al. (1972) exposed a series of polymers, including epoxies, silicones, and poly(acryl)amide), to fresh rabbit serum. The serum was then injected into the host animals, and the production of antibodies was investigated. Unless the *in vitro* exposure included exposure to macrophages as well as serum, no antibody titers were developed. However, in the presence of peritoneal macrophages, a number of these materials produced positive titers. This is evidence of a cell-mediated response to denatured serum proteins, recognized as foreign bodies (see Section 12.4.1). The absence of effect (antibody production) when the serum was directly injected suggests that the denaturation was reversible and present only when the serum proteins were adsorbed to the test surfaces.

This experiment reminds one of a further complication. The data in Table 5.1 were obtained from pure albumin (one protein) solutions. The actual exposure in the biological environment involves many proteins, as in Stern's use of serum *in vitro*. In such a situation, proteins encounter the surface depending upon the product of their concentration and their self-diffusion velocity, which is approximately inversely related to the square root of their molecular weight. (Additional factors, such as molecular shape, also affect self-diffusion rates.)

Thus, protein–surface interactions *in vivo* (or *in vitro* from mixed solutions) should be thought of as a succession of events; early arrivers (low molecular weight/high concentration) may be potentially displaced by late arrivers (high molecular weight/low concentration). This process, first recognized by Leo Vroman in the blood coagulation process (see Section 9.2) and termed by others the Vroman effect, is shown schematically in Figure 5.4:

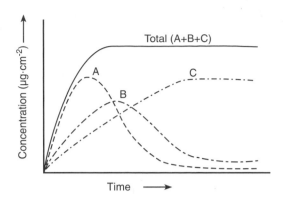

FIGURE 5.4
Vroman effect (schematic).
See Section 9.3.3 for a discussion of the supposed role of γ_c in cell–surface interactions; de Palma et al. (1972) present interesting examples of Zisman plots obtained on metallic implants before and after blood contact.

Here, even after the total surface concentration of protein (solid line) reaches a steady state value, the composition of the film continues to change, as molecules of B displace those of A and, in turn, are displaced by molecules of C. Remember also that these are equilibrium surface concentrations; the data of Table 5.1 suggest that continuing exchange of each species may take place.

5.6   Effects of Charged Interfaces and Ions

The discussion so far has focused upon interfaces considered to be electrically neutral. That is, the deforming force on molecules results simply from interfacial free energy and the equilibrium requirements for adhesion. If there is a net surface charge, then a potential gradient will exist in the vicinity of the surface. This has four major consequences:

- Uncharged molecules will suffer deformation in structure due to the interaction of their internal dipoles (primarily associated with covalent bonds) with the electrical field.

- Charged molecules and zwitterions (molecules with no net charge but with equal amounts of negative and positive charge) will undergo an additional set of constraints due to attraction or repulsion of their charge centers. These additional forces will produce additional structural deformation.

- Charged molecules and ions will also move along the electrical field gradient, attracted to surfaces of opposite charge. This motion, called electrophoresis, is utilized in analytical processes to separate ions with different ratios of charge to ionic mobility. Electrophoresis can act *in vivo* to change the concentration of ions as well as pH, thus potentially altering 3° and 4° structure.

- Finally, charged molecules and ions may interact with magnetic fields. Moving charges experience a transverse force from constant magnetic fields; time-varying magnetic fields can produce oscillatory rotation of zwitterions and local current flow through motion of ions and molecules with net charge.

One should also remember that net (nonzero) surface potentials may arise (1) by electrochemical equilibria; (2) from differences in dielectric constant across the interface; (3) from external sources such as direct potential imposition (as suggested by the experiments of Sawyer et al., 1965, in the reduction of thrombogenic behavior by changing surface potential; see Section 9.3.2); or (4) from the other member of a galvanic (corrosion) couple (see Section 4.7.2).

5.7 Final Comments

The reader will note that much of the material cited in this chapter does not have recent publication dates. This is due to the fundamental nature of the considerations and to the lack of broad interest in the topic of nonchemical physiochemical events at interfaces, other than in the issues of blood coagulation and hemolysis. However, recent developments in several areas, including design, evaluation, and, in some cases, clinical application of so-called "bioactive" materials — as well as the rising interest in cellular and tissue engineering (see Chapter 11) — suggest that this will become a much more vigorous research area. This is especially true because the combination of ultrahigh speed chemical analysis and large capacity very fast computers now permits gathering molecular configuration data and fitting it to models of molecule–surface interaction (West et al. 1997). These developments are certain to have a profound effect on knowledge of the fundamental mechanics of biological performance of materials; once again, they emphasize the need for biomaterials investigators to maintain a high level of alertness for scientific and technical advances in fields seemingly far removed from their day-to-day concerns.

References

Andrade, J.D., Interfacial phenomena and biomaterials, *Medical Instrumen.* 7, 110, 1973.

Baszkin, A. and Lyman, D.J., The interaction of plasma proteins with polymers. I. Relationship between polymer surface energy and protein adsorption/desorption, *J. Biomed. Mater. Res.*, 14, 393, 1980.

Brash, J.L., Uniyal, S. and Samak, Q., Exchange of albumin adsorbed on polymer surfaces (1974), *Trans. Am. Soc. Artif. Int. Organs*, XX, 69, 1974.

dePalma, V.A. et al., Investigation of three-surface properties of several metals and their relation to blood compatibility, *J. Biomed. Mater. Res. (Symp.)*, 3, 37, 1972.

Sawyer, P.N. et al., Electrochemical precipitation of blood cells on metal electrodes: an aid in the selection of vascular prostheses, *Proc. Natl. Acad. Sci.*, 53, 294, 1965.

Smith, G.K., Systemic transport and distribution of iron and chromium from 316l stainless steel implants, Ph.D. thesis, University of Pennsylvania, Philadelphia, 1982.

Stern, I.J. et al., Immunogenic effects of foreign materials on plasma proteins, *Nature*, 238, 151, 1972.

West, J.K., Latour, R., Jr. and Hench, L.L., Molecular modeling study of the adsorption of poly-L-lysine onto silica glass, *J. Biomed. Mater Res.*, 37, 585, 1997.

Williams, R.L. and Williams, D.F., Albumin adsorption on metal surfaces, *Biomaterials*, 9, 206, 1988.

Woodman, J.L., Black, J. and Jiminez, S.A., Isolation of serum protein organometallic corrosion products from 316LSS and HS-21 *in vitro* and *in vivo*, *J. Biomed. Mater. Res.*, 18, 99, 1984.

Bibliography

Adamson, A.W. and Gast, A.P., *Physical Chemistry of Surfaces*, 6th ed., John Wiley & Sons, New York, 1997.

Andrade, J.D. et al., Proteins at interfaces: principles relevant to protein-based devices, in *Proc. 2nd Intern. Symp. Bioelectron. Molecular Electron. Devices*, Dec. 12–14, 1988, Fujiyoshida, Japan (unpaginated), 1988.

Bamford, C.H., Cooper, S.L. and Tsurta, T. (Eds.), *The Vroman Effect*, VSP, Utrecht, 1992.

Bernabeu, P. and Caprani, A., Influence of surface charge on adsorption of fibrinogen and/or albumin on a rotating disc electrode of platinum and carbon, *Biomaterials*, 11, 258, 1990.

Elwing, H., Protein absorption and ellipsometry in biomaterial research, *Biomaterials*, 19(4–5), 397, 1998.

Friedberg, F., Effects of metal binding on protein structure, *Q. Rev. Biophys.*, 7(1), 1, 1974.

Gabler, R., *Electrical Interactions in Molecular Biophysics*, Academic Press, New York, 1978.

Gray, J.J., The interaction of proteins with solid surfaces, *Curr. Opin. Struct. Biol.*, 14(1), 110, 2004.

Hallab, N.J. et al., Systemic metal–protein binding associated with total joint replacement, *J. Biomed. Mater. Res.*, 49, 353, 2000.

Hench, L.L. and Wilson, J., Surface-active biomaterials, *Science*, 226, 630, 1984.

Ivarsson, B. and Lundstrom, I., Physical characterization of protein adsorption on metal and metaloxide surfaces, *Crit. Rev. Biocompatibil.*, 2(1), 1, 1986.

Lomer, M.C.E., Thompson, R.P.H. and Powell, J.J., Fine and ultrafine particles of the diet: influence on the mucosal immune response and association with Crohn's disease, *Proc. Nutr. Soc.*, 61, 123, 2002.

Manly, R.S. (Ed.), *Adhesion in Biological Systems*, Academic Press, New York, 1970.

Morra, M. (Ed.), *Water in Biomaterials Surface Science*, New York, John Wiley & Sons, 2001.

Tanford, C., *Physical Chemistry of Macromolecules*, John Wiley & Sons, New York, 1961.

Vogler, E.A., Structure and reactivity of water at biomaterial surfaces, *Adv. Colloid Interface Sci.*, 74, 69, 1998.

Zangwill, A., *Physics at Surfaces*, Cambridge University Press, Cambridge, 1988.

6

Mechanics of Materials: Deformation and Failure

6.1 Introduction

Mechanical integrity is a nearly universal requirement for biomaterials. All materials must cohere or "hold together" if they are to be expected to stay in one shape and in one location, and to perform their designed function. The requirement may be only that they withstand the various stresses that exist in an implant site. A more rigorous requirement exists if part of the intended function for the implant is a mechanical one, such as a heart valve replacement or a fracture fixation device. Then, the application may require the preservation of a minimum value of a property, such as ability to withstand permanent deformation, or of a design (mean) value of another one, such as possessing a particular spring constant. These are extrinsic behaviors but they depend in part on intrinsic properties: in this case, on yield strength and elastic modulus, respectively.

Unfortunately, environmental exposure of materials alters their mechanical properties in a variety of ways. As discussed in Section 2.2, the chemical and physical environment of the human body is different from external engineering environments and is, by comparison to many, quite severe. This chapter will briefly consider the origin of intrinsic mechanical properties of materials. It will also consider how materials fail in mechanical applications and how the biological environment affects these properties and types of failure.

6.2 Mechanics of Materials

The simplest experiment that can be performed to characterize the mechanical properties of a solid material is to machine a specimen with well-defined dimensions (a "standard" specimen) and load it to failure in tension. Figure 6.1 shows the result of such a model experiment, obtained by plotting the

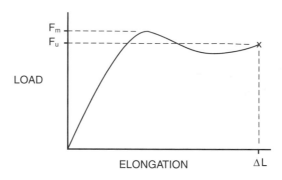

FIGURE 6.1
Load-elongation curve.

applied load directly against the resulting elongation. The following points characterize this load-elongation curve:

F_m: maximum load that can be sustained

ΔL: elongation to failure

F_u: load at failure

Unfortunately, these numbers are extrinsic (dependent upon the specific dimensions of the specimen). It is common practice to transform the load-elongation curve into a stress–strain curve. Stress, σ, is given by the force divided by the cross-sectional area perpendicular to the direction of force application:

$$\sigma = \frac{F}{A} \qquad (6.1)$$

Strain, ε, is given by the ratio of the change in length, ΔL, to the original length, L_o:

$$\varepsilon = \frac{\Delta L}{L_o} \qquad (6.2)$$

These conversions produce intrinsic values that are independent of specimen dimensions as long as certain basic rules are obeyed in the design of the specimen. In particular, it is necessary to assure that the specimen is uniform in cross section in the region in which L_o, ΔL, and A are measured. Figure 6.2 shows a stress–strain curve that might be obtained by conversion of the model load-elongation curve of Figure 6.1. This curve is characterized by several intrinsic parameters (Table 6.1).

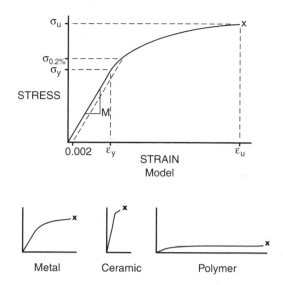

FIGURE 6.2
Stress–strain curves.

TABLE 6.1

Intrinsic Parameters from a Stress–Strain Curve

Symbol	Name	Units	Definition
σ_y	Yield stress	MPa	Stress to start permanent (plastic) deformation
ε_y	Yield strain	MPa	Strain at the moment of yielding
$\sigma_{0.2\%}$	0.2% offset stress	MPa	Stress to produce 0.002 strain
σ_u	Ultimate stress	MPa	Stress to produce fracture
ε_u	Ultimate strain	None	Total strain to fracture
M	Modulus	GPa	Ratio of stress divided by strain (slope of line in elastic (proportional) region (= σ_y/ε_y))
E	Young's modulus	GPa	Modulus determined in tension
--	Work of fracture	J/m³	Area under the stress–strain curve

Notes: MPa: megapascals; GPa: gigapascals; J/m³: joules/cubic meter.

Of course, other intrinsic parameters characterize materials, and these may be determined in forms of load application other than pure tension. However, this chapter will concentrate on tensile behavior and, in particular, the elastic modulus, E, the yield stress, σ_y, and the ultimate stress, σ_u. These three parameters tend to dominate mechanical design. The relationship of these parameters to mechanical design may be summarized as follows:

- Elastic modulus is the intrinsic "spring constant" of the material; thus, it specifies the proportional deformation as a result of stress within the limit of recoverable deformations.

- Yield stress sets the upper stress limit for the design of a body fabricated from a plastically deformable material that under load must not undergo permanent deformation from its original shape.

- Ultimate stress defines the stress that produces fracture and thus sets the maximum stress, termed the strength, that the material can withstand.

Taken together, these three parameters provide a measure of stiffness, deformability, and strength of a material.

It should be noted that the model stress–strain curve (Figure 6.2) is only a schematic. The relative values of these three parameters are governed to a large degree by the nature of the atomic bonds within a material; thus, classes of materials tend to have different general shapes of stress–strain curves. These are shown schematically for metallic, ceramic, and polymeric materials in the lower part of Figure 6.2.

6.3   Elastic Modulus

6.3.1   Fundamental Aspects

The elastic behavior of materials has its origin in the basic chemical bond structure at the atomic level. That is, for deformations below the yield point, the major effect is the elastic (recoverable) deformation of interatomic bonds. Each of the four major materials classes — metals, ceramics, polymers, and composites — possesses its characteristic bond structures.

The metals are characterized by the looseness of binding of their valence electrons. Thus, solid metals are thought of as aggregates of positively charged ions with a neutralizing negative electron cloud. The resulting cohesion is high but the individual bonds lack strong directionality. In real metals, regions of high order with almost exclusively metallic bonding (grains) are separated by zones of disorder (grain boundaries) that contain impurities and other forms of bonding.

Ceramic materials, on the other hand, are primarily ionically bonded. They are made up of geometric arrays of cations and anions with strong ordering and a resulting high directionality of bonds. Again, real (nonideal) ceramics contain grains (ordered) and grain boundaries (disordered) in combination, as do metals. In this case, ionic bonding is possible in the boundary regions, but is usually weaker than within the grains because of inclusions, mismatches between adjacent grains, and disorder effects.

Polymers exhibit the third type of bond, the covalent bond. Although it is not particularly strong, this bond, formed by orbital sharing of electrons between atoms, is highly directional. Engineering polymers consist of long-chain molecules with covalently bonded "backbones." The chains may be ordered in a regular array in regions, forming crystals, or may be uniformly amorphous; the more usual structure is, again, a combination of order and disorder. The overall structure is stabilized by occasional interchain covalent bonds or ionic bonds between charged side groups (cross links) and by diffuse attraction of hydrogen, oxygen, and nitrogen atoms to –OH groups (Van der Waals bonds).

In order of strength, these bonds may be classified as follows:

Ionic > metallic > covalent > Van der Waals

Thus, it should come as no surprise that elastic moduli can be ranked as:

Ceramic > metallic > polymeric

Composite materials do not appear in this range because they can be particle- or fiber-reinforced ceramics, metals, or polymers and thus display a wide range of elastic moduli, depending upon the arrangements and relative moduli of their components. A further complication is introduced by the nature of the bonding between the matrix and the reinforcing material. This bonding depends on the chemistry and microstructure of the interface; it affects yield and failure but has little effect upon elastic behavior. The ability to adjust the modulus (and other properties) to meet the requirements of a specific application is, of course, one of the great attractions of composites.

6.3.2 Environmental Effects

Practically speaking, the elastic moduli of metals and ceramics are unaffected by exposure to biological environments. This is due to the great strength of internal bonding in these materials, to the relative simplicity of their structure when compared with polymers and composites and to the typical temperatures encountered *in vivo*. Polymers may experience profound changes in elastic moduli in response to the internal environment. Table 6.2 summarizes the principal mechanisms and their effects.

TABLE 6.2

Environmental Effects on Mechanical Properties of Polymers

	Effects on	
Phenomenon	**Modulus (E)**	**Yield stress (σ_y)**
Absorption	Decrease ("plasticizing")	Increase
Leaching	Increase ("antiplasticizing")	Decrease
Chain scission	Decrease	Decrease
Cross linking	Increase	Increase

Absorption and leaching have been discussed in Section 3.3 and Section 3.6. The principal effect of absorption of low molecular weight species is to swell the amorphous matrix, moving the crystalline "islands" further apart and thus weakening the already weak bonds between them. This permits easier deformation in the same way that lubrication makes it easier for surfaces to move over each other. However, many polymers already contain plasticizers in the form of low-molecular-weight fragments of the basic polymer, deliberately added low-molecular-weight agents, and water. Thus, the loss of these by leaching would be expected to reverse the effect of absorption and increase the elastic modulus. In real applications, there is competition. However, because biomedical polymers tend to be simple (low additive) materials due to host response considerations and tend to have high molecular weight due to strength and stability considerations, the usual effect of exposure to physiological fluids is to lower the effective elastic modulus. Elastic moduli of highly crystalline or highly cross-linked polymers should be less sensitive than amorphous, low-molecular-weight ones.

An illustration of plasticizing and antiplasticizing effects can be seen in data on the elastic moduli of polymers in compression in Table 6.3. In this study (Jacobs 1974), standard compression test cylinders were made of a commercial poly(methyl)methacrylate (PMMA) surgical cement, a duplicate formulation compounded in the laboratory, and a commercial medical grade of ultrahigh molecular weight polyethylene (UHMWPE). These were tested as fabricated (except for UHMWPE, for which the fabrication date was

TABLE 6.3

Variation of Compressive Moduli of Polymers with Environmental Exposure

Test condition:	PMMA (raw materials) $E_1\%$ ($\times 10^5$ psi)	PMMA (commercial)[a] $E_1\%$ ($\times 10^5$ psi)	UHMWPE (commercial)[b] $E_1\%$ ($\times 10^5$ psi)
As fabricated	3.0 ± 0.2[c]	3.4 ± 0.2	NA
Postlaboratory storage (24°C/120 days)	3.9 ± 0.2	3.8 ± 0.5	0.83 ± 0.06
Post humid storage (97%RH/37°C/120 days)	2.7 ± 0.3[d]	2.6 ± 0.2[d]	0.81 ± 0.05
Post saline storage (0.9% NaCl/37°C/120 days)	2.7 ± 0.4[d]	2.8 ± 0.2[d]	0.80 ± 0.06
Post implantation (rabbit, subcutaneous/120 days)	3.2 ± 0.2[d]	3.1 ± 0.4	0.80 ± 0.05

Notes: $E_{1\%}$ = tangent modulus at 1% strain; NA = not available.

[a] Simplex-P™ (North Hills Plastics, Ltd.).
[b] Zimmer-USA.
[c] ±95% confidence interval.
[d] Different from "post laboratory storage" ($p < 0.05$).

Source: Adapted from Jacobs, M.L., M.S. thesis, University of Pennsylvania, Philadelphia, 1974.

unknown) and after 120 days' exposure to a variety of environments, including subcutaneous implantation in the rabbit. The slope of the stress–strain curve at 1% strain, $E_{1\%}$, was used for comparison because, in common with most other polymers, these polymers do not possess a single well-defined elastic modulus in the elastic region of the stress–strain curve. Exposure of both PMMA formulations to high humidity or saline solutions that duplicated the ionic concentration of serum at 37°C produced a reduction of ~30% in $E_{1\%}$ when compared with dry, room-temperature storage. This illustrates the plasticizing effect of absorbed water. Although it produced a similar reduction, implantation was much less damaging. This could be interpreted in one of two ways:

- Implantation might have prevented the loss of residual monomer by leaching. An effect similar to leaching — loss of monomer by evaporation — is probably responsible for the increase of $E_{1\%}$ due to dry storage when compared with the as-fabricated value. Residual monomer would serve as a plasticizer; however, because it is hydrophobic, it might exclude the more efficient plasticizer, water.

- A cross-linking agent or an antiplasticizer might be absorbed from serum in the animal, counteracting the plasticizing effects of water absorption.

On the other hand, UHMWPE, with its more crystalline nature and far higher average molecular weight ($\approx 2 \times 10^6$ vs. 2×10^4), is unaffected by the environmental exposures used in this experiment.*

Chain scission is the polymeric equivalent of the processes of corrosion and dissolution of metals discussed in Section 4.1 and Section 4.2. The principal mechanisms are intrinsic scission (no external chemical species involved), oxidation, hydrolysis, or chemical attack. Figure 6.3 summarizes these mechanisms and provides some generic examples.

Chain scission reduces the elastic moduli of polymers through three routes:

- The scission reaction may release a very small molecular fragment, such as a water molecule, that can act as a plasticizer.

- Although the principal resistance to small deformations in polymers is due to stretching and/or disruption of weak bonds, some contribution is due to "tangling" of long molecules. In much the same way that long strands of spaghetti tend to entrap each other, this tangling forces an elongation of a portion of the strong, covalently bonded molecules, even at modest deformations. Thus, scission of molecules by reducing average molecular weight releases these

---

* In this study, the implants were sterilized chemically. If they had been irradiated, chain scission, cross-linking, and oxidation of residual free radicals would have affected the results. See the subsequent part of this section.

INTERNAL MECHANISMS

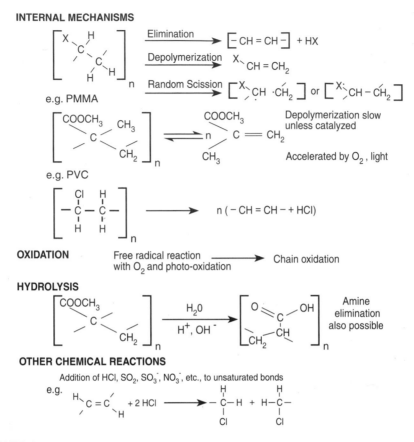

FIGURE 6.3
Mechanisms of chain scission in polymers. (Adapted from Adams, R. and McMillan, P.W., *J. Mater. Sci.*, 12, 643, 1977.)

> trapped molecules and permits greater strain before covalent bond stretching can contribute significantly to the elastic modulus.

- The disorder associated with shorter chain length may reduce crystallinity and thus reduce the average strength of bonding, leading to lower moduli.

Cross linking is the reverse of scission. The formation of new bonds between chains increases the effective molecular weight, further tangles and traps molecules, and may reduce the effective concentration of plasticizers by chemical combination. A common mechanism for cross-linking polymers in the laboratory is exposure to ionizing radiation. This produces active free radicals, as in chain scission, that link with free radicals in neighboring chains, forming covalent cross links. Although clinical doses of x-radiation do not produce measurable changes in the properties of polymeric implants in patients (Eftekhar and Thurston 1975), high-dose γ-radiation in the laboratory is a convenient process to enable studying the mechanical consequences of cross linking.

Irradiation of simple pure polymers such as polyethylene suggests a linear increase of modulus with the number of cross links (Grobbelaar et al. 1978), and a more pronounced effect may occur if a number of low-molecular-weight agents that can be incorporated are present during irradiation. Furthermore, unless they are removed by annealing or doping with reducing agents such as vitamin E, residual free radicals produced by γ or electron beam irradiation may produce progressive *in vitro* and *in vivo* property changes by continuing reaction with polymer molecules and diffusible small molecules, such as water or oxygen.

The environmental effects on the elasticity of composites are more difficult to generalize. In an ideal model, the elastic modulus of a randomly oriented composite, E_C, made of materials A (matrix) and B (reinforcing or filler phase) can be calculated from

$$E_C = E_A V_{fA} + E_B V_{fB} \qquad (6.3)$$

where V_{fi} = volume fraction of material (phase) i. Then, any effect on the modulus of either material is seen as a proportional effect on the modulus of the composite. A special case would be the formation of voids in a material, by leaching of a second phase or by aggregation of internal defects. Because the modulus of a void is zero, the modulus of a porous material, for small pore volumes, can be given by

$$E = E_o(1 - V_{fp}) \qquad (6.4)$$

where E_o = elastic modulus of fully dense material. Thus, the modulus would be expected to decrease linearly with increasing volume fraction of pores.

In real materials, the effect is somewhat greater at small void volume fractions but becomes less pronounced for more porous materials. Equation 6.5 was derived for rigid ceramics (MacKenzie 1950) and has been shown experimentally to describe effects in materials with Poisson ratios near 0.3:

$$E = E_o(1 - 1.9\, V_{fp} + 0.9\, V_{fp}^2) \qquad (6.5)$$

There is a further problem in describing the effects of environment on the elastic moduli of composites. Equation 6.3 is based upon an assumption that a perfect bond exists between the phases so that each phase experiences an equal internal strain for a given external uniform deformation of the composite material. Real composites rarely display such perfect bonding, and the bond is often the weak point for environmental attack. The consequences of this are unpredictable but the usual effect is a reduction in modulus.

6.4   Yield Strength

6.4.1   Fundamental Aspects

The yield strength is defined by the stress necessary to produce unrecoverable deformation in a material. Deformation at lower stresses may be linear in the case of a simple solid or increasingly nonlinear as strain increases, as in the case of many polymers. Recovery may be rapid at lower strains and become slower as peak strain increases. Finally, at the yield stress, conditions of deformation are such that a residual unrecoverable strain remains, even after long times at zero stress.

Within crystals, unrecoverable strain is produced by migration and aggregation of defects and by the slippage of material along defect planes. However, in complex materials and composites, slip, leading to unrecoverable deformation, may occur preferentially along grain and phase boundaries.

6.4.2   Environmental Effects

At room and body temperature, the processes leading to crystalline deformation or grain boundary slip in metals and ceramics are little affected by environmental exposure because of the relatively high bonding energies. However, the situation for polymers and polymer-based composites is different, as noted in the earlier discussion of elastic modulus. The effects are summarized in Table 6.1.

Absorption and leaching produce what appear to be paradoxical effects on yield strength. That is, a lower modulus, as results from absorption of a plasticizer, might be expected to accompany a lower yield strength. In general, however, the yield strength is raised. Motion along a particular grain boundary may become easier; however, this may lead to increased load sharing with adjacent material and, in fact, may produce modest elevations of yield stress in inhomogeneous materials. A similar but inverse effect is seen when plasticizers are leached from the material.

On the other hand, chain scission produces an overall reduction in molecular weight, making plastic deformation more dependent upon the interruption of weak bonds and thus reducing the yield stress. Cross linking increases the tangling effect of long molecules, thus substituting strong covalent bonds for weaker bonds and raising the yield stress.

The situation in composites is more complex, and no generalizations can be made. This is the case because the environment may affect the matrix and the matrix-filler bond as well. The results depend upon the details of the composite material in question and its exposure.

It is possible for materials to undergo unrecoverable deformation under constant load at stress below the yield stress. This is the familiar creep process. Creep rates are generally very slow for temperatures below one-half the melting temperature of the material. However, for temperatures above one-half the melting temperature, or in the presence of plasticizers, creep can be significant. Creep is possible in many biomedical polymers at room temperature and is generally increased at body temperature.

Creep is characterized by an initial or primary creep phase in which the creep rate diminishes rapidly. This is followed by a long secondary creep phase with a strain rate that is essentially constant in logarithmic time. In this secondary creep phase, the Dorn–Weertman equation can be used to describe the creep rate:

$$\dot{\varepsilon} = A\sigma^{n}e^{-Q/RT} \qquad (6.6)$$

where

$\dot{\varepsilon}$ = creep rate

σ = stress

n = experimentally fitted parameter ($\cong 5$)

Q = activation energy

The activation energy (Q) is usually taken to be the activation energy for self-diffusion, but may be considered more generally as an intrinsic activation energy for creep (Parsons and Black 1977). Thus, environmental effects on the creep rate can be interpreted in terms of changes in the activation requirements of the creep process.

The final or tertiary process of creep is characterized by a rapidly increasing strain rate leading to fracture. Little is known about the mechanism of this process or about environmental effects on it.

It should also be clear from this discussion that creep in biomedical applications is observed primarily in polymers and polymer-based composites. In general, secondary creep rates decrease with increasing yield stress at a given temperature, but the relationship is weak. However, they increase with increasing temperature and with the presence of plasticizers. This latter effect may dominate in polymer matrix composites, producing significant increases in creep rate (Soltész 1986).

6.5 Fracture Strength

6.5.1 Fundamental Aspects

Fracture occurs when the cohesive strength of a material is exceeded. It represents an accentuation and final stage of the processes that earlier led to yielding — if that is possible in a particular material. However, it is generally observed that ultimate strengths, such as the ultimate tensile stress,

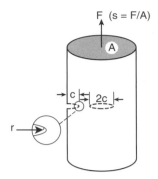

FIGURE 6.4
The ideal Griffith crack.

are small compared with those expected, based upon cohesive energy calculations.

Typical calculations of cohesive energy or theoretical maximum strength lead to values of σ_u equal to $E/10$. This would predict a tensile strength of 12.7 GPa for Ti6Al4V, a common alloy useful in implant applications. The actual value of σ_u is typically 0.9 GPa (900 MPa), that is, $\approx E/140$. This is a relatively strong material; weaker materials such as stainless steels have σ_u in the range of $E/250$ to $E/350$.

Griffith (Guy 1971) was the first to explain this observation for brittle materials (those that fail without significant unrecoverable strain) by suggesting that defects exist on the surface and within the body of real materials as seen in Figure 6.4. He calculated that the presence of an elliptical crack in brittle materials produces a stress concentration at the "point" of crack, as given by:

$$\sigma_m \cong 2\sigma \left(\frac{c}{r} \right)^{1/2} \tag{6.7}$$

where

σ = apparent or "macro" stress
σ_m = elevated stress at "point" of crack
c = 1/2 major diameter of internal elliptical crack = major width of surface crack
r = radius of curvature at "point" of crack ($r \ll c$)

Thus, Griffith suggested that, although the macrostress might be well below the true ultimate stress, the elevated local stress, σ_m, near a defect might exceed the ultimate strength, and a crack would propagate. By considering the energy required to form the crack (the difference between elastic strain energy released in the material near the newly formed crack and the increase of interfacial surface energy due to formation of the new material–environment interfacial area along the crack), he also calculated the minimum stress required to propagate the crack:

$$\sigma = \left(\frac{2\gamma E}{\pi c} \right)^{1/2} \tag{6.8}$$

where
  γ = surface tension (material–environment)
  E = elastic modulus

Fortunately, most materials undergo plastic deformation before fracture. Thus, as stresses about a defect are increased, as predicted by Equation 6.7, plastic deformation will take place before fracture, even if the macrostress is below the yield stress. Orowan (Guy 1971) dealt with this problem by replacing the term γ in Equation 6.8 with the quantity ($\gamma + p$), where p = the work of plastic deformation at the "point" of the propagating fracture. Because p is typically 1000 times γ in magnitude, Equation 6.6 then becomes approximately,

$$\sigma \cong \left(\frac{Ep}{c} \right)^{1/2} \tag{6.9}$$

Such materials will be proportionally stronger because they will require far higher stresses to propagate existing defects into fracture surfaces.

A special case of Equation 6.7 occurs for spherical pores, the situation discussed previously with respect to the reduction of elastic modulus by pores. This has been studied empirically, and the usual relationship (parallel to Equation 6.5) derived by Ryskewitsch (Kingery 1976) is

$$\sigma'_u = \sigma_e e^{\left(-n V_{fp} \right)} \tag{6.10}$$

where σ'_u is the actual fracture strength for a material with pore volume fraction V_{fp}, and n is an empirically fitted constant with a value between 4 and 7.

The difference between the stresses predicted by Equation 6.8 and Equation 6.9 results in the classification of materials as those that fail in a brittle mode and those that fail in a ductile mode. Characteristic of ceramics and of polymers at low temperatures, brittle failure occurs without significant residual deformation and is governed by relations of the form of Equation 6.8. Materials with yield stresses well below ultimate stresses tend to be ductile and fail in a manner governed by Equation 6.9. Because yielding occurs during failure, they also exhibit significant unrecoverable strain.

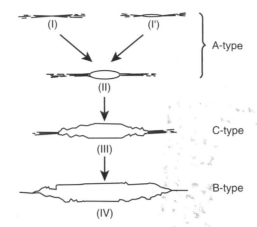

FIGURE 6.5
Plausible crack discs in section. Note: vertical dimension exaggerated. (Adapted from Taka-hashi, K., *J. Macromol. Sci. Phys.*, B8(3–4), 673, 1973.)

The existence of Griffith defects has been shown repeatedly. An elegant example is the work of Takahashi (1973) in poly(methyl)methacrylate, as shown in Figure 6.5. The A-type cracks are those seen after modest stresses, and B- and C-types after higher stresses, presumably exceeding the limit imposed by Equation 6.9.

Given that Griffith defects exist two conclusions can be drawn from this analysis:

- Equation 6.7 predicts that the magnitude of the stress concentration near a defect will vary inversely with the minimum radius of curvature, r, of the defect. Thus, a sharp crack is a more extreme stress riser than a semicircular notch. This effect is the basis of the commercial practice of drilling a hole at the advancing tip of a slowly propagating crack, as in a cracked bridge strut, to prevent further defect propagation by reducing σ_m. In implant design, this suggests that it is desirable to avoid "sharp" features, such as edges, grooves, and surface structure, to minimize stress concentration effects.

- As the defect major diameter (= 2c) increases, stress concentration increases (Equation 6.7), and the stress necessary to propagate brittle fracture (Equation 6.8) or ductile fracture (Equation 6.9) decreases. Thus, there is a critical minimum size for a Griffith defect to contribute to fracture, given that r remains constant. In practice, larger defects decrease strength to a limit beyond which the process is reversed because r begins to increase.

Calculations of minimum crack lengths in composites are much more complex. Marom (1975) has shown that the minimum or critical defect size in polymer-based composites is much greater than that in the unfilled resin and depends upon orientation of stresses with respect to the reinforcing fiber.

Attempts to improve mechanical properties of polymers by processing may lead to paradoxical results, due to the differences between brittle and ductile fracture strength. Fatigue processes require accumulation of microfractures to produce reduction in area leading to a final single cycle failure. Thus, cross linking a polymer, such as ultrahigh molecular weight polyethylene, can increase its ultimate and yield strengths; however, because this also reduces ductility, it may produce dramatic decreases in fatigue strength at high cycle numbers ($N > 10^6$) due to brittle rather than ductile crack propagation (Sauer et al. 1996).

6.5.2   Environmental Effects

The biological environment can have significant effects upon the details of crack propagation and, thus, upon the strength of materials. These effects will now be briefly discussed.

Any form of chemical attack, whether corrosion, oxidation, dissolution, or leaching, that can increase the size of pre-existing defects or produce new defects by preferential attack clearly weakens a material. Such an attack may take place preferentially near defects in stressed materials and is termed "stress-enhanced attack" or "stress corrosion" in the case of metals. Such effects are well recognized in metals and have been demonstrated in silicone rubber (Rose et al. 1973). Crazing due to swelling can also produce Griffith defects where none previously existed or can expand preexisting ones.

In brittle materials, the fact that $\gamma_{SL} < \gamma_{SA}$ for all but hydrophobic materials reduces the required propagation stress predicted by Equation 6.8. Thus, any of the degradative phenomena discussed in Chapter 3 and Chapter 4 can be expected to reduce the ultimate strength of biomaterials, and all classes of materials are susceptible.

Table 6.4 summarizes behavior for a range of typical polymeric implant materials, nonabsorbable sutures, during a 24-month experiment in rabbits (Postlethwait 1970). The data given in the table are the ultimate tensile loads normalized by dividing by the strength of materials retrieved after 1 week of implantation (in the abdominal wall) to remove the effect of differing diameters of specimens.

Absorbable materials, such as gut (natural) or polygalactic acid (synthetic) sutures, will show more pronounced and rapid loss of strength. However, the rate for an individual material and surgical situation is hard to predict. The loss of strength is affected by the material composition, fabrication, and postfabrication handling (production of surface defects), and because of possible pH dependence of degradation by hydrolysis (Chu 1982) and/or enzymatic attack (Salthouse et al. 1969; Lotan et al. 1995).

In addition to failure by fracture at stresses that exceed ultimate strength, materials may fail by fatigue. Fatigue fracture — fracture at stresses below

TABLE 6.4

Degradation of Tensile Strength of Sutures *in Vivo*

	Suture Type				
	Multifilament		Monofilament		
Period of Implantation	Silk	Cotton	Polyamide (Nylon™)	Polypropylene	Polyester (Dacron™)
2 Weeks	0.87	0.98	0.98	1.05	0.92
4 Weeks	0.58	1.07	0.97	1.14	1.03
3 Months	0.20	0.67	0.88	1.03	0.91
6 Months	0.36	0.52	0.79	0.93	0.70
12 Months	0.58	0.50	0.89	0.97	0.96
24 Months	Dis.	0.58	0.72	0.99	0.96
Comments	Slow dissolution	Separated	Swollen	No visible change	No visible change

Note: Data normalized by 1-week value of ultimate tensile stress.

Source: Adapted from Postlethwait, R.W., *Ann. Surg.*, 171, 892, 1970.

ultimate after a number of cyclic deformations — is recognized as one of the major sources of mechanical failure of implants. Fatigue failure is characterized by the construction of an S–N (stress vs. number of cycles) curve as shown in Figure 6.6. The ultimate (fracture stress) decreases with cyclic loading in air until an apparent limit, termed the "endurance limit," is reached. In this example, the endurance limit is reached between 10^6 and 10^7 cycles. However, in an aqueous or corrosive environment where stress corrosion is possible during the high-stress part of each cycle, this endurance limit is apparently abolished, and the fracture strength continues to decrease with cyclic loading. The presence of defects, such as surface markings, may lead to stress concentration and apparent reduction in fatigue strength; alteration of such defects by corrosion processes may accentuate the effect of their presence (Naidu et al. 1996).

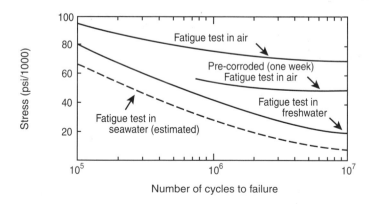

FIGURE 6.6
S–N curves for a Cr-V steel. (From Dumbleton, J.H. and Black, J., *An Introduction to Orthopedic Materials*, Charles C Thomas, Springfield, IL, 1975.)

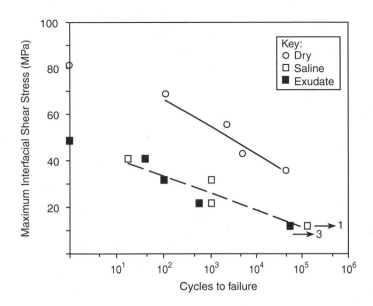

FIGURE 6.7

S–N curves for a polysulfone-carbon fiber interface (group mean values; $n = 6$ per point). --->#
= number of unbroken specimens at this stress level ($N = 2.5 \times 10^5$). (From Latour, R.A., Jr. and
Black, J., *J. Biomed. Mater. Res.*, 27, 1281, 1993.)

In polymers and polymer-based composites, similar effects are also seen,
probably secondary to plasticizing and/or "decoupling" (secondary to bond
failure) of the reinforcing phase from the matrix. This phenomenon may be
explored by using drops of polymer matrix formed on long specimens of a
fiber-reinforcing phase (Latour and Black 1993). Figure 6.7 shows the S–N
curves for such specimens, fabricated from polysulfone resin and carbon
fiber, after equilibration in various environments (37°C, 24 h). The two solutions used were physiological saline and inflammatory exudate collected
previously by implanting porous capsules of the thermoplastic matrix resin
in soft tissue in rabbits. No endurance limit was observed under dry or wet
conditions up to 2.5×10^5 cycles. The effect on shear strength of both solutions
is the same, suggesting that water is the active agent.

In polymer-based composites, a progressive reduction in modulus is also
observed as internal damage accumulates with an increasing number of load
cycles; the decrease is pronounced if the aqueous environment is such that
the fiber–matrix interface is wetted preferentially (is hydrophilic).

Ceramics display an additional fatigue problem called static fatigue, which
is a sudden failure by brittle fracture at stresses well below ultimate when
subjected to steady (noncyclic) loads. In Al_2O_3 (Krainess and Knapp 1978)
and in glasses (Adams and McMillan 1977), this effect is believed to be due
to the formation of weak bonds by absorbed water displacing stronger ionic
bonds.

Thus, it should be clearly understood that biological environments, as encountered by implants, can be expected to produce a wide range of significant changes in the mechanical properties of materials.

6.6   Final Comment

Notwithstanding the general principles discussed here, two points should be emphasized:

- Actual or real materials have more complex structures than can be dealt with here in this brief discussion. Therefore, it should be no surprise when apparently paradoxical property changes are encountered as a consequence of exposure to biological environments.

- Because it is extremely difficult to predict quantitative mechanical property changes, care should always be taken to determine the properties of materials before environmental exposure, whether simulated or by implantation. This should be performed on actual specimens, from the same batches of materials to be tested, treated identically to the specimens to be exposed (including sterilization and other postfabrication treatments), concurrently with initiation of testing, because it cannot be assumed that properties will remain unchanged over periods of months and years during laboratory storage.

References

Adams, R. and McMillan, P.W., Review: static fatigue in glass, *J. Mater. Sci.*, 12, 643, 1977.

Allara, D.L., Aging of polymers, *Environ. Health Perspec.*, 11, 29, 1975.

Chu, C.C., The effect of pH on the *in vitro* degradation of poly(glycolide lactide) copolymer absorbable sutures, *J. Biomed. Mater. Res.*, 16, 117, 1982.

Dumbleton, J.H. and Black, J., *An Introduction to Orthopedic Materials*, Charles C Thomas, Springfield, IL, 1975.

Eftekhar, N.S. and Thurston, C.W., Effect of irradiation on acrylic cement with special reference to fixation of pathological fractures, *J. Biomech.*, 8, 53, 1975.

Grobbelaar, C.J., duPlessis, T.A. and Marais, F., The radiation improvement of polyethylene prostheses, *J. Bone Joint Surg.*, 60B, 370, 1978.

Guy, A.G., *Introduction to Materials Science*. McGraw–Hill, New York, 1971.

Jacobs, M.L. Evaluation of three polymer resins for use in polymer-based composites for hard tissue prostheses. M.S. thesis, University of Pennsylvania, Philadelphia, 1974.

Kingery, W.D., *Introduction to Ceramics*. 2nd ed. John Wiley & Sons, New York, 1976.

Krainess, F.E. and Knapp, W.J., Strength of a dense alumina ceramic after aging *in vitro, J. Biomed. Mater. Res.*, 12, 241, 1978.

Latour, R.A., Jr. and Black, J., Development of FRP composite structural biomaterials. Fatigue strength of the fiber/matrix interfacial bond in simulated *in vivo* environments, *J. Biomed. Mater. Res.*, 27, 1281, 1993.

Lotan, N., Azhari, R. and Sideman, S., Enzymic degradation of polymeric biomaterials: a review, in *Encyclopedic Handbook of Biomaterials and Bioengineering*, Part A, Vol. 1, Wise, D.L. et al. (Eds.), Marcel Dekker, New York, 1995, 757.

MacKenzie, J.K., The elastic constants of a solid containing spherical holes, *Proc. Phys. Soc. (London)*, B63, 2, 1950.

Marom, G., Calculation of effective crack length in composite materials, *Int. J. Frac.*, 11, 534, 1975.

Naidu, S.H., Warner, C.P. and Laird, C., Mechanical stamping: a cause of fatigue fracture, *Clin. Orthop. Rel. Res.*, 328, 261, 1996.

Parsons, J.R and Black, J., On the thermodynamics of the viscous deformational mechanism of articular cartilage, *Trans. SFB*, 1, 78, 1977.

Postlethwait, R.W., Long-term comparative study of nonabsorbable sutures, *Ann. Surg.*, 171, 892, 1970.

Rose, R.M., et al., The role of stress-enhanced reactivity in failure of orthopaedic implants, *J. Biomed. Mater. Res. Symp.*, 4, 401, 1973.

Salthouse, T.N., Williams, J.A. and Willigan, D.A., Relationship of cellular enzyme activity to catgut and collagen suture absorption, *Surg., Gyn. Obstet.*, 129, 691, 1969.

Sauer, W.L., Weaver, K.D. and Beals, N.B., Fatigue performance of ultra-high-molecular-weight polyethylene: effect of gamma radiation sterilization, *Biomaterials*, 17, 1929, 1996.

Soltész, U., Fracture, fatigue, and aging behavior of carbon fiber reinforced plastics, in *Materials Sciences and Implant Orthopaedic Surgery*. Kossowsky, R. and Kossovsky, N. (Eds.), Martinus Nijhoff, Dordrecht, 1986, 355.

Takahashi, K., Cracking of poly(methyl methacrylate) caused by plane stress waves, *J. Macromol. Sci. Phys.*, B8(3–4), 673, 1973.

Bibliography

Anseth, K.S., Bowman, C.N. and Brannon–Peppas, L., Mechanical properties of hydrogels and their experimental determination, *Biomaterials*, 17, 1647, 1996.

Chu, C.C., Survey of clinically important wound closure biomaterials, in *Biocompatible Polymers, Metals, and Composites*, M. Szycher, M. (Ed.), Technomic, Lancaster, PA, 1983, 477.

Coury, A.J., Chemical and biochemical degradation of polymers, in *Biomaterials Science*, 1st ed., Ratner, B.D., Hoffman, A.S, Schoen, F.J. and Lemons, J.E. (Eds.), Academic Press, San Diego, 1996, 243.

Ducheyne, P. and Lemons, J.E. (Eds.), Bioceramics: material characteristics versus *in vivo* behavior, *Ann. N.Y. Acad. Sci.*, 523, 1988.

Edidin, A.A. et al., Degradation of mechanical behavior in UHMWPE after natural and accelerated aging, *Biomaterials*, 21, 1451, 2000.

Ferry, J.D., *Viscoelastic Properties of Polymers*, 3rd ed., John Wiley & Sons, New York, 1980.

Gibson, L.J. and Ashby, M.F., *Cellular Solids: Structure and Properties*, 2nd ed., Cambridge University Press, Cambridge, 1997.

Hayden, W., Moffatt, W.G. and Wulff, J., *Mechanical Behavior*, Vol. III of *The Structure and Properties of Materials*, Wulff, J. (Ed.), John Wiley & Sons, New York, 1965.

Hertzberg, R.W. and Manson, J.A., *Fatigue of Engineering Plastics*, Plenum Press, New York, 1980.

Hull, D. and Clyne, T.W., *An Introduction to Composite Materials*, 2nd ed., Cambridge University Press, Cambridge, 1996.

Jamison, R.D. and Gilbertson, L.N. (Eds.), *Composite Materials for Implant Applications in the Human Body: Characterization and Testing* STP 1178, American Society for Testing and Materials, Philadelphia, 1993.

Jones, R.M., *Mechanics of Composite Materials*, 2nd ed., Taylor & Francis, New York, 1998.

Kronenthal, R.L., Biodegradable polymers in medicine and surgery, in *Polymers in Medicine and Surgery*, Kronenthal, R.L., Oser, Z. and Martin, E. (Eds.), Plenum Press, New York, 1975, 119.

Kurtz, S.M. et al., Degradation of mechanical properties of UHMWPE acetabular liners following long-term implantation, *J. Arthroplasty*, 18(7), Suppl 1, 68, 2003.

Ward, I.M. and Sweeney, J., *An Introduction to Mechanical Properties of Solid Polymers*, 2nd ed., John Wiley & Sons, New York, 2004.

7

Friction and Wear

7.1 Introduction

The previous chapter considered the mechanical behavior of materials under stress. The areas dealt with were those concerning the properties of singular parts or components. When devices contain more than one component or are able by design or chance to move against natural tissue, another class of mechanical effects must be considered.

The general resistance to the motion of one material body over another is termed friction. When static friction is overcome and relative motion takes place, it is accompanied by a modification of the interface by a variety of processes that are collectively known as wear. Introduction of surface treatments or interposed materials to make relative motion easier is called, collectively, lubrication. The study of these three phenomena (friction, wear, and lubrication) is the science of tribology. This chapter will consider these phenomena and their presence in and alterations by biological environments.

7.2 Friction

If an attempt is made to move one body over the surface of another, a restraining force oriented to resist motion is encountered. This restraining or frictional force, F_f, is given by

$$F_f = \mu F_\perp \tag{7.1}$$

where
 $F_\perp$ = force perpendicular to interface
 μ = coefficient of friction

The force perpendicular to the surface, $F_\perp$, may be generated by compressive or gravity forces. The coefficient of friction, μ, is a ratio or unitless number, with values usually between 0 and 1, which describes the relationship of the frictional restraining force to this perpendicular force. It is characteristic of the interface, depending upon the composition and finish of the pair of materials involved, and is affected by lubrication. Furthermore, the coefficient is greater just before surfaces begin to move (initial conditions $\rightarrow$ μ_i) than when the surfaces are in continuing or steady motion (sliding conditions $\rightarrow$ μ_s). Table 7.1 gives some typical values of μ_i and μ_s.

Frictional behavior arises from the physical situation of the surfaces having a relatively small area of contact due to microscopic surface roughness. The small size of this actual contact area, perhaps as little as 1% of the geometric interface area, leads to local yielding and bonding due to high stresses at the points of actual contact. Thus, relative motion results only when these bonded areas can be disrupted in shear and moved relative to one another. This disruption produces the frictional restraining force and also clearly leads to the wear process.

Frictional restraining forces are complex, but a number of generalizations can be made:

- The coefficients of friction, μ_i and μ_s, are essentially independent of $F_\perp$ (they may be affected, however, by tangential (lateral) forces).

- For a given value of $F_\perp$, coefficients of friction are generally independent of stress — that is, of the apparent or geometric interfacial surface area.

TABLE 7.1

Initial and Sliding Coefficients of Friction

Materials Combinations	Lubricant	μ_i	μ_s
Rubber tire/concrete	None (dry)	1.0	0.7
Rubber tire/concrete	Water	0.7	0.5
Leather/wood	None (dry)	0.5	0.4
Steel/steel	None (dry)	—	0.5
Steel/polyethylene	None (dry)	—	0.1
Steel/ice	Water	0.03	0.01
Cartilage/cartilage (hip)	Synovial fluid	—	0.002
	Ringer's	—	0.01–0.005
CoCr/CoCr (hip prosthesis)[a]	None (dry)	—	0.55
	Veronate buffer	—	0.22
	Serum	—	0.13
	Synovial fluid	—	0.12
	Albumin (sol.)		0.11
CoCr/PE(UHMW)[a]	Serum	—	0.08
Al_2O_3/Al_2O_3[b]	Ringer's	—	0.1–0.05

[a] Weightman, B. et al., *J. Lubric. Tech.*, 94, 131, 1972.
[b] Dörre, E. et al., *Arch. Orthop. Unfall.-Chir.*, 83, 269, 1975.

- Coefficients of friction depend upon surface texture, the material pair, and the lubricant involved. However, in general, coefficients are lower for a pair of unlike materials of the same roughness than for identical materials and are lower for a given material pair in the presence of lubricating agents than in their absence.

- Static and dynamic coefficients of friction are not closely related to wear rates (Galante et al. 1973). In particular, low frictional coefficients do not lead necessarily to low wear rates.

7.3   Lubrication

The principle of lubrication is to provide a film or layer to separate two surfaces during relative motion in order to reduce frictional restraining forces and wear. Lubrication modes or processes are classified by the nature and the magnitude of the average surface separation characteristic for each type. It is clear from Table 7.1 that artificial material pairs do not possess coefficients of friction that closely approach those possible in natural joints, particularly at the low velocities at which joints operate. Little can be done about this situation as long as body fluids are depended upon for lubrication. However, it is important from a design point of view to know the actual coefficients of friction that may be expected.

Table 7.1 suggests the importance of using an appropriate lubricant in laboratory determinations of friction and wear. For materials in contact with blood, such as heart valve components, the appropriate lubricant is fresh serum. For device components in soft tissue locations, a 50:50 mixture of serum and normal saline approximates the intracellular exudates. For joint replacement components, the appropriate lubricant is synovial fluid. Woodman and colleagues (1977) showed that the synovial tissue remaining in the vicinity of a joint produces essentially normal synovial fluid that is available for lubrication of the artificial joint replacement.

Differences in composition between synovial fluid and serum (Table 7.2) suggest that dilute serum:saline solutions are generally superior to saline to simulate synovial fluid. However, serum, whether human or animal, is a highly variable material. *In vitro* simulator results, especially for wear rates, most closely resemble those encountered in implanted joints when total protein concentration is in the range of 20 to 30 g/L and the albumin to globulin ratio is adjusted (by albumin addition) to a range of 1 to 1.5 (Wang et al. 2004). However, such studies, performed on metal/polymer wear pairs, may not be fully generalizable to other wear pairs because synovial fluid contains one or more so-called "surfactant" species, such as phosphatidyl choline, which avidly bind to surfaces and reduce dynamic coefficients of friction under boundary lubrication regimes (see Section 7.3.4) (Hills and

TABLE 7.2

Composition of Synovial Fluid in Comparison to Serum

Component	Synovial Fluid (g/l)	Serum (g/L)	Synovial/Serum
Protein (total)	18	70	0.26
Albumin	11.3	34.3	0.33
α_1-Globulin	1.26	4.2	0.30
α_2-Globulin	1.26	8.4	0.15
β-Globulin	1.62	11.9	0.14
γ-Globulin	3.06	11.2	0.27
Lipid (total)	2.4	7.0	0.34
Phospholipids	0.8	2.0	0.40
Urate	0.016	0.018	0.88
Glucose	0.66	0.91	0.73
Hyaluronate:	2-4	4.2×10^{-5}	$\sim 7 \times 10^4$
Albumin/globulin ratio	1.57	0.96	

Sources: Proteins: Lentner, C. (Ed.), *Geigy Scientific Tables*, Vol. 1, Ciba–Geigy, Basle, 1981; other: Levick, J.R., in *Joint Loading*, Helminen, H.J., Kiviranta, I.A., Säämänen, A.-M., Tammi, M., Paukkonen, K. and Jurvelin, J. (Eds.), Wright, Bristol, 1987, 149.

Butler 1984). In addition, laboratory testing may not faithfully reproduce *in vivo* conditions in which synovial fluid is constantly replaced, even when the lubricating bath is regularly renewed.

7.3.1   Hydrodynamic

Hydrodynamic lubrication is perhaps the most usual process encountered in human prosthetic joints *in vivo*; it occurs when the motion of one body relative to the other draws a continuous film of lubricant into the contact area. The characteristic surface separation for typical lubricants and engineering finishes is between 10^{-3} and 10^{-4} cm. In this mode, all of the work of friction is dissipated by viscous shear of the lubricant.

7.3.2   Elastohydrodynamic

Elastohydrodynamic lubrication occurs at smaller surface separations, between 10^{-4} and 10^{-5} cm. In this case, the motion of one body of the pair is able to transmit force through the lubricant to generate sufficient stress for transient elastic deformation of the other body. Although this may be satisfactory in the short term, in the long term it may lead to localized fatigue failure of one or the other surface, with an accompanying increase in wear rate.

7.3.3 Squeeze Film

Squeeze film lubrication occurs in hydrodynamic or elastohydrodynamic conditions if the lubricant is sufficiently viscous to respond elastically (rather than by increased flow) to temporarily increased normal loads. Thus, a squeeze film lubricant, although highly viscous, may reduce wear in situations in which transient overloads occur. Hydrodynamic, elastrohydrodynamic, and squeeze film conditions are collectively termed *fluid film lubrication.*

7.3.4 Boundary

Boundary lubrication occurs when the lubricant coats the opposing surfaces rather than acting as a low-shear interface. This coating acts to modify the frictional character of the surfaces to reduce frictional restraining forces and wear. Characteristic mean surface separations depend sensitively on the nature of the lubricant but are usually less than 10^{-5} cm.

7.3.5 Mixed

Mixed lubrication occurs when a fluid lubricant operating in hydrodynamic or elastohydrodynamic mode is able to coat the surfaces by an adhesive process, thus providing additional protection at high loads through bonding lubrication. Natural synovial joints in the skeletal system probably demonstrate a combination of these lubrication modes (Wright 1969):

- Boundary lubrication during motion initiation
- Elastohydrodynamic lubrication during motion
- Squeeze film lubrication during high load events

This combination of behavior results from the structure of the joint and from peculiarities in the nature of the lubricant, synovial fluid. As previously noted (Table 7.2), normal synovial fluid resembles serum in inorganic species but contains 30 to 50% of the amount of protein and lipids, a higher albumin to globulin ratio, and significantly more hyaluronate.

7.3.6 Types of Lubricant Behavior in Response to Shear

In general, lubricants display three types of relationships between apparent viscosity and shear rate (Dintenfass 1963) as shown in Figure 7.1. Conventional lubricants have a viscosity that is independent of shear rate. Thus, surface separation, h_c, as a function of relative velocity may be determined fairly easily, taking the lubricant properties as a constant (Hamrock and Dowson 1981). Under these conditions the lubrication process may remain

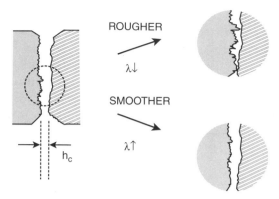

FIGURE 7.1
Effects of counterface roughness on γ.

constant over a wide range of velocities. For simple parallel geometries, as in concentric or parallel sliding interfaces *A* and *B*, one may then derive a dimensionless parameter, λ:

$$\lambda = h_c / (R^2_{rmsA} + R^2_{rmsB})^{1/2} \tag{7.2}$$

where R_{rmsA}, R_{rmsB} = root means square roughnesses of the opposing surfaces.

Thus, for λ < 1, one would expect predominantly boundary lubrication; for 1< λ< 3, one would expect mixed lubrication and for λ > 3 some form of fluid film lubrication would be expected.

If the lubricant and the relative surface velocity remain constant, the surface separation (h_c) remains nearly constant and the mode of lubrication is affected primarily by surface roughness. Here one can see graphically that, as the roughness of one of the counterfaces decreases, lubrication can transition from boundary to mixed to fluid film mode.

However, some lubricants are thixotropic; that is, they become reversibly less viscous as shear rates increase. An everyday example of such a fluid (although not a lubricant) is nondrip ceiling paint. This appears nearly solid in the can but becomes quite thin as it is brushed on the wall. The inverse of thixotropic is also possible; such a material would be called dilatant and would become reversibly more viscous with increasing shear rate. This material would not contribute to easy relative motion but might act to reduce wear at high relative velocities.

Thixotropic or dilatant lubricants can produce a change in lubrication mode as a function of relative velocity of the surfaces because h_c and thus λ now depend on actual viscosity, pressure, and relative velocity. For instance, a material pair with a thixotropic lubricant can display hydrodynamic lubrication at intermediate pressures and velocities and boundary lubrication at high pressures and velocities (Figure 7.2).

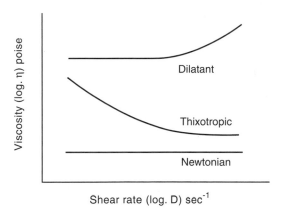

FIGURE 7.2
Types of lubricant behavior.

Synovial fluid, which is an ultrafiltrate of serum with the addition of a long chain polysaccharide complex, hyaluronic acid, is a highly thixotropic lubricant (Figure 7.3). Trauma resulting in joint effusion may reduce the osmolarity of synovial fluid, producing a generally less viscous but still thixotropic lubricant. However, in the presence of a persistent joint disease such as rheumatoid arthritis, the fluid thins and tends to lose its thixotropic property. This permits closer approach of the joint surfaces and may produce increased wear as a contributing factor to joint degeneration.

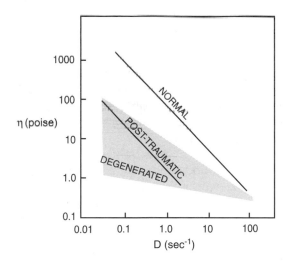

FIGURE 7.3
Viscosity–shear rate relationships for synovial fluid. (Adapted from Dintenfass, L., *J. Bone Joint Surg.*, 45A, 1241, 1963.)

7.4 Wear

7.4.1 Introduction

Wear is a more pronounced problem than frictional restraint for two reasons:

- Wear produces biologically "active" particles that can excite an inflammatory response (see Chapter 8).
- Wear produces shape changes that can affect function.

There are several mechanisms of wear. Probably the most important mechanism in biomedical applications is adhesive wear. This arises from the junction-making and -breaking process previously described. The rate of production of wear debris, expressed as a volume, is given most generally by:

$$V = \frac{kF_{\perp}x}{3p} \tag{7.3}$$

where
V = volume of wear debris
k = Archard's coefficient
$F_{\perp}$ = perpendicular force
p = surface hardness
x = total sliding distance

Figure 7.4 shows the range of k values of typical engineering situations. For the situation of a polymer on a metal *in vivo*, values for k should lie between 10^{-5} and 10^{-7} with conditions described by the lower right-hand corner of the diagram. Note that the ordinates are labeled differently. The left ordinate refers to transfer film formation (see Section 7.4.2) and the right refers to the production of loose particles.

It is interesting to note that, although values of μ_i and μ_s lie within a small range (between 0 and 1), k and thus wear rates vary over many orders of magnitude. This further reinforces the previous observation that friction forces and wear rates have little direct relationship.

7.4.2 The Transfer Film

Figure 7.4 suggests that two major wear processes are possible for any combination of materials: particle production as described previously, or the formation of a transfer film. This film is produced when a hard material, such as a metal, moves on a softer material (for instance, a polymer) and shears off and picks up a coating of polymer, as shown in Figure 7.5. This

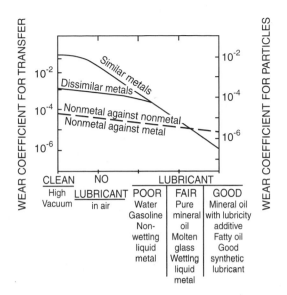

FIGURE 7.4
Variation of Archard's constant, k, with wear and lubrication conditions. (Adapted from Rabinowicz, E., *Mater. Sci. Eng.*, 25, 23, 1976.)

film bridges across the asperities on the surface of the metal, replacing metal–polymer contact with polymer–polymer contact; by increasing the actual contact area (as a function of the apparent contact area), it reduces local stresses.

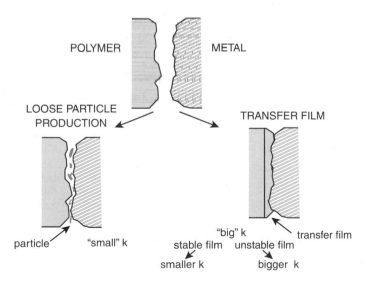

FIGURE 7.5
Transfer film vs. particle production.

The formation of a transfer film may lead to one of two circumstances:

- If the film is stable, wear rates may be reduced after an initial high-wear interval during film formation.

- If the film is unstable, it may peel and result in increased wear by abrasive or "three-body" wear.

McKellop et al. (1978) reported some interesting results involving transfer films (Table 7.3). The material pair is F138 type steel (316L [vacuum melted]) and ultrahigh molecular weight polyethylene (UHMWPE), with serum, distilled water, or saline as lubricants. Wear rates are reported as a calculated linear recession of the UHMWPE surface, based upon measurement of the volume of wear debris. Thus, the wear rate does not include a creep component. Distilled water apparently permitted the formation of a transfer film and produced the lowest wear rate. Wear in saline was some 65 times greater (than in distilled water) and was apparently accompanied by crevice corrosion of the stainless steel in the interface between substrate and transfer film as indicated by orange discoloration. This leads to occasional release of the film and very high wear rates — apparently case 2 cited earlier.

TABLE 7.3

Wear of UHMWPE[a] in Different Lubricants *in Vitro*

Lubricant	No. Specimens	Average Wear Rate (μm/10^6 cycles) (range)	Observations (μ_s= dynamic coefficient of friction)
Serum (bovine)	4	0.65 (±17%)	μ_s = 0.07–0.12 normally; μ_s = 0.35 during temporary high friction. Polymer transfer onto metal counterfaces occurred only during high-friction phase.
Distilled water	3	0.08 (±60%)	μ_s = 0.07–0.13 at start. A heavy polymer transfer layer formed by 3×10^5 cycles; μ_s then ranged from 0.14 to 0.18. The transfer layer remained intact for the duration of the test.[b]
0.9% saline (Ringer's solution)	3	5.2 (±17%)	μ_s = 0.07–0.10 at start. Heavy, orange-colored transfer layers formed as μ_s increased to 0.27. These layers occasionally broke up and μ_s dropped to the initial level.

[a] Against 316L (VM) stainless steel counterface at 3.45 MPa (500 psi) nominal contact stress, 10^6 sliding cycles @ 60 cpm (travel; 5×10^4 m [est.]).

[b] McKellop et al. (1978) also report transfer layer to be unstable at 6.90 Mpa.

Source: Adapted from McKellop, H. et al., *J. Biomed. Mater. Res.*, 12, 895, 1978.

Serum produced an intermediate wear rate with only occasional transfer. This suggests that, although serum does not completely reproduce synovial fluid, active molecules present *in vivo*, other than surfactants, can coat metal surfaces in metal/polymer wear combinations and, although preventing the formation of stable transfer films, the molecules reduce wear through surface lubrication.

Surface roughness, which plays a role in lubrication, also affects wear. Early polishing of rough surfaces may produce elevated wear rates that decline significantly after an initial "wearing in" period. However, a persistently rough hard surface bearing against a softer counterface can be expected to produce wear rates above those predicted by Equation 7.3 (Kurtz et al. 2000). Finally, surface roughness may change adversely *in vivo* through mechanical damage by third bodies or secondarily to intrinsic materials property changes, such as phase transformations in ceramic surfaces (Haraguchi et al. 2001).

7.4.3   Other Wear Mechanisms

Three other mechanisms of wear are of concern in this chapter. The first is abrasive wear — wear of a soft surface produced by a "plowing" of the surface by large asperities in the harder countersurface. Although this is a general mechanism in deliberately articulating interfaces, it may also play a role in supposedly fixed interfaces in modular devices. In this case, such wear is referred to as fretting and, in the case of metals, may have a corrosive component. Abrasive wear clearly occurs *in vivo*, as will be seen in the later discussion of the size of wear debris.

Corrosive wear of metals occurs secondarily to the physical removal of a passive or protective surface layer. The exposed surface may be more susceptible to wear, perhaps being softer and/or more chemically reactive, or wear may be accelerated by the repetition of cycles of passive film formation and mechanical removal. Figure 7.6 suggests this possibility graphically. In this experiment, a rod of passivated F-75 cobalt-base alloy was pressed against a dimple in a block of UHMWPE (Jablonski et al. 1986). After the equilibrium potential has been established (in an aerated 0.9% saline solution, reference: standard calomel electrode [S.C.E.]), a half sinusoidal stress, with a peak value of 3.4 MPa, was applied during 40% of a 60° back-and-forth rocking cycle, at 36 cpm (cycles per minute). These conditions replicate those thought to exist in the human hip joint prosthesis during slow walking. The potential (vs. S.C.E.) became more negative, indicative of the flow of an increased corrosion current. When motion ceased, the potential became less negative, paralleling the (presumed) re-establishment of the passive layer. The time to 50% of the maximum potential change ($t_{1/2}$max) decreased as the peak stress and the rate of rocking were increased. Similar results have been reported in all metal total joint replacement prostheses (Thull 1977).

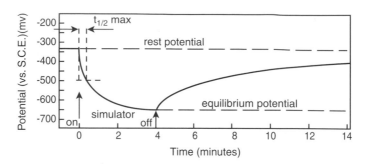

FIGURE 7.6
Effect of articulation on corrosive wear. (From Stone [Jablonski, J.E. et al., *Trans. SFB*, 9, 196, 1986], unpublished data.)

The third and final type of wear to be considered is a surface fracture or fatigue wear. Three routes lead to this process:

- Stresses produced by asperities may not exceed yield stress but may exceed the endurance limit for the softer of the material pair (generally a polymer in biomedical applications). This will lead to local fatigue failure of the softer surface and local fracture, "mud-caking," or spalling. This process may be accelerated by diffusion and internal reaction of chemical species, such as oxygen, with polymers such as UHMWPE.

- Design of devices may produce a rigid support to the soft component. If this component is too thin in comparison to the magnitude of the contact stress and its apparent contact area, local stress elevation occurs (Bartel et al. 1985), contributing to fatigue failure, as observed previously. Although suggesting alternative mechanisms, Dowling et al. (1978) were some of the first workers to observe such polymer surface failure in UHMWPE/metal hip prostheses after 8 years or more of implantation.

- Free particles, perhaps adventitial (e.g., bone or PMMA fragments), or fragments of incomplete or shed transfer films may roll between the moving surfaces. If these particles are relatively undeformable, they can easily generate stresses above the ultimate tensile strength of the surface, leading directly to surface cracking. As cracks join up, wear debris is released. This process is usually called "three-body" wear.

7.4.4   Evidence of Wear *In Vivo*

Wear is a considerable problem *in vivo*. Of the five heart valve poppets studied and reported in Table 3.2, four showed signs of wear as evidenced by strut grooves. These would be expected to have a profound effect on local hemodynamics and on valve closure. All 21 hip cups recovered after periods of 14 to 159 months and studied by Dowling et al. (1978) showed signs of adhesive (early) or fatigue (late) wear. Of these, nine showed evidence of the formation of a secondary socket or bearing area, with resultant theoretical effects on joint function (Dumbleton et al. 1984). As implant designs and materials have improved, wear rates *in vivo* have generally declined, but the majority of articulating components retrieved after service *in vivo* show signs of wear.

However, of more importance may be the formation of wear debris. Particulate materials usually elicit different host responses than bulk materials do. The observed cellular response is frequently different in nature (see Section 8.2.2) and far more vigorous than to comparable bulk materials.

7.4.5 Size of Wear Debris

Rabinowicz (1976) discussed a criterion for predicting the diameter of wear particles produced by adhesive wear processes:

$$d = \frac{6 \times 10^4 W_{12}}{p} \tag{7.4}$$

where

d	=	diameter of wear particle
W_{12}	=	surface energy of adhesion between materials 1 and 2
p	=	hardness of wearing surface

Similar relationships for abrasive wear and for stress concentration phenomena would suggest that hardness is the key parameter in determining typical wear debris particle size. Because the elastic modulus, E, is a good estimator of the hardness, p, one would expect particle diameter, d, to vary inversely with E.

Although Rabinowicz suggests that Equation 7.4 correlates well with observation (presumably in predominantly adhesive wear situations *in vitro*), broad ranges of wear debris particle sizes from submicron to hundreds of microns in principle dimension are seen in biomedical applications. Savio et al. (1994) conducted an extensive literature survey of debris associated with total joint replacements, comparing reports of findings at revision, at autopsy, during *in vitro* simulator testing, and, finally, during attempts to reproduce wear debris by other means for host response testing. Polymeric particles exhibit the largest absolute size as well as the largest size range; ceramic particles show much smaller sizes and quite small size ranges. Metals display an intermediate size range, with great differences in shape among different alloys and situations.

At the time of this literature study, it was not appreciated that very small particles below the resolving power of optical microscopy (≈0.25 µm) are present under many circumstances. Even *in vitro* wear and joint simulator studies failed to detect the presence of such ultrafine particles due to the extensive use of nuclear pore filters with a minimum pore size of 0.22 µm. More recently, it has come to be appreciated that such small particles may constitute a significant portion of the volume and the vast majority of the number of any species of wear debris.

Figure 7.7 compares polymeric wear debris, generated by cobalt-base alloy/UHMWPE wear pairs in a size range less than 2.0 µm in maximum dimension, extracted from capsular tissue recovered during total hip and total knee replacement revision surgery (Shanbhag et al. 1994). Note that, although essentially all THR-associated debris observed in this study are less than 2 µm in major dimension, only ~80% of TKR-associated debris is this small. Similarly, the median major dimension of THR debris is < that of TKR debris (0.45 vs. 1.10 µm). The differences in distribution may well reflect the differences in dominate wear mechanisms in the two types of devices, as well as differences in regional transport away from the two joints. Finally, comparison with the size distribution observed in a common resin precursor of polyethylene suggests that many of the very small particles (<0.25 µm) may be released by a fatigue mechanism rather than formed by adhesion or abrasion processes. Note that pre-1990 studies of wear debris tend to under-estimate the prevalence of submicron size particles due to the widespread use of 0.22-µm pore size filters.

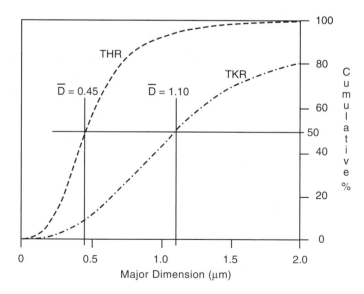

FIGURE 7.7
Cumulative percentile distributions of polymeric wear debris. (From Shanbhag, A.S. et al., *J. Bone Joint Surg.*, 76B, 60, 1994, and personal communication, A.S. Shanbhag.)

The finding of wear debris particles, in implant sites or in regional lymph nodes where they were deposited by phagocytosis and transport, during revision surgery or at autopsy, is quite variable. This suggests that several different wear processes are taking place simultaneously and that the mechanical and environmental details of each application influence the types of particles produced.

Finally, it should be pointed out that no animal or clinical study to date has shown a good correlation between wear loss of an articulating implant component and a volumetric estimate of wear debris in the tissues of the experimental subject. This is due to a number of factors:

- Systemic distribution of particles (previously referred to)
- Dissolution of metallic debris
- Deformational changes in polymeric components (creep, fluid absorption, etc.)

Thus, estimates of wear from examination of implants probably provide only upper bounds, and examination of tissues provides unrealistic lower bounds on wear rates. Carefully conducted *in vitro* wear testing with appropriate mechanical conditions and lubricants is required to measure actual wear rates with any degree of certainty.

7.4.6   Anomalous Wear

One final comment is in order. One normally thinks of wear in terms of a harder material wearing away a softer material. However, ample evidence suggests that the reverse can occur. In natural tissues, it is observed that soft tissues, such as tendons, moving over bone will rapidly form grooves while appearing unchanged. This may reflect dynamic remodeling but may also involve a direct wear process of the harder bone by the softer tendon. Gent and Pulford (1979) have shown a similar situation in the wear, *in vitro*, of steel and bronze alloys by a variety of elastomers. Obviously, no dynamic remodeling is possible here. The mechanism proposed is the formation of active radicals on the elastomer surface by mechanical cleavage, followed by chemical attack of the metal surface by these active sites. The enhancement of the effect by the exclusion of oxygen seems to support such a mechanism. The evidence discussed in Section 4.10 for the participation of amino acids in corrosion processes certainly suggests that one should consider the possibility of such anomalous wear processes when implant materials move in contact with biological materials.

7.5 Conclusions

Frictional restraint to relative motion of device components and the associated wear, releasing particulate debris, are inherent in the nature of materials. Careful material selection and component design can minimize but not eliminate these phenomena in biomedical devices fabricated from present biomaterials. Increased knowledge of the mechanistic details of friction and wear phenomena in these applications can be expected to produce improved performance. However, it may be the case that accumulation of wear debris and the host response to such accumulation will prove to be the ultimate limitation on the useful lifetime of articulating biomedical devices, such as total joint replacements. With this in mind, the next section of this book considers host response to biomaterials and their degradation products.

References

Bartel, D.L. et al., The effect of conformity and plastic thickness on contact stresses in metal-backed plastic implants, *J. Biomech. Eng.*, 107, 193, 1985.

Dintenfass, L., Lubrication in synovial joints: a theoretical analysis, *J. Bone Joint Surg.*, 45A, 1241, 1963.

Dörre, E., Beutler, H. and Geduldig, D., The properties required of bioceramics for artificial joints (author's transl.), *Arch. Orthop. Unfall.-Chir.*, 83, 269, 1975.

Dowling, J.M. et al., The characteristics of acetabular cups worn in the human body, *J. Bone Joint Surg.*, 60B, 375, 1978.

Dumbleton, J.H. and Black, J., Some long-term complications, in *Complications of Total Hip Replacement*, Ling, R.S.M. (Ed.), Churchill Livingstone, Edinburgh, 1984, 212.

Galante, J.O. and Rostoker, W., Wear in total hip prostheses. An experimental evaluation of candidate materials, *Acta Orthop. Scand.* (Suppl. 145), 1973.

Gent, A.N. and Pulford, C.T.R., Wear of metal by rubber, *J. Mater. Sci.*, 14, 1301, 1979.

Hamrock, B.J. and Dowson, D., *Ball Bearing Lubrication. The Elastohydrodynamics of Elliptical Contacts*, John Wiley & Sons, Inc., New York, 1981.

Haraguchi, K. et al., Phase transformation of a zirconia ceramic head after total hip arthroplasty, *J. Bone Joint Surg.*, [Br.] 83B, 996, 2001.

Hills, B.A. and Butler, B.D., Surfactants identified in synovial fluid and their ability to act as boundary lubricants, *Ann. Rheu. Dis.*, 43, 641, 1984.

Jablonski, J.E., Stone, J. and Black, J., The effect of articulation on the corrosion potential of cobalt–chromium alloy *in vitro*, *Trans. SFB*, 9, 196, 1986.

Kurtz, S.M., Muhlstein, C.L. and Edidin, A.A., Surface morphology and wear mechanisms of four clinically relevant biomaterials after hip simulator testing, *J. Biomed. Mater. Res.*, 52, 447, 2000.

Lentner, C. (Ed.), *Geigy Scientific Tables*, Vol. 1, Ciba–Geigy, Basle, 1981.

Levick, J.R., Synovial fluid and trans-synovial flow in stationary and moving normal joints, in *Joint Loading*, Helminen, H.J., Kiviranta, I.A., Säämänen, -M., Tammi, M., Paukkonen, K. and Jurvelin, J. (Eds.), Wright, Bristol, 1987, 149.

McKellop, H. et al., Wear characteristics of UHMW polyethylene: a method for accurately measuring extremely low wear rates, *J. Biomed. Mater. Res.*, 12, 895, 1978.

Rabinowicz, E., Wear, *Mater. Sci. Eng.*, 25, 23, 1976.

Savio, J.A., III, Overcamp, L.M. and Black, J., Size and shape of wear debris, *Clin. Mater.*, 15, 101, 1994.

Shanbhag, A.S. et al., Composition and morphology of wear debris in failed uncemented total hip replacement arthroplasty, *J. Bone Joint Surg.*, 76B, 60, 1994.

Thull, R., The long-term stability of metallic materials for use in joint endoprostheses, *Med. Prog. Tech.*, 5, 103, 1977.

Wang, A., Essner, A. and Schmidig, G., The effects of lubricant composition on *in vitro* wear testing of polymeric acetabular components, *J. Biomed. Mater. Res. Part B: Appl. Biomater.*, 68B, 45, 2004.

Weightman, B. et al., Lubrication mechanism of hip joint replacement prostheses, *J. Lubric. Tech.*, 94, 131, 1972.

Woodman, J.L. et al., Isolation of lubricating fraction from human synovial fluid after total-hip implantation, *Trans. ORS*, 2, 13, 1977.

Wright, V. (Ed.), *Lubrication and Wear in Joints*, J.B. Lippincott Company, Philadelphia, 1969.

Bibliography

Affatato, S. et al., Wear behavior of cross-linked polyethylene assessed *in vitro* under severe conditions, *Biomaterials*, 20, 3259, 2005.

Bartel, D.L., Bicknell, V.L. and Wright, T.M., The effect of conformity, thickness, and material on stresses in ultrahigh molecular weight components for total joint replacement, *J. Bone Joint Surg.*, 68A, 1041, 1986.

Bayer, R.G., *Engineering Design for Wear*, Marcel Dekker, New York, 2004.

Bayer, R.G. and Ruff, A.W. (Eds.), *Tribology. Wear Test Design and Application, STP 1247*, American Society for Testing and Materials, Philadelphia, 1993.

Bowden, F.P. and Tabor, D., *The Friction and Lubrication of Solids*, Oxford University Press, Oxford, 2001.

Bradgon, C.R. et al., Third-body wear of highly cross-linked polyethylene in a hip simulator, *J. Arthrop.*, 18(5), 553, 2003.

Davies, D.V., Synovial fluid as a lubricant, *Fed. Proc.*, 25, 1069, 1966.

Divakar, R. and Blau, P.J., (Eds.), *Wear Testing of Advanced Materials, STP 1167*, American Society for Testing and Materials, Philadelphia, 1992.

Dumbleton, J.H., *Tribology of Natural and Artificial Joints*, Elsevier, Amsterdam, 1981.

Freeman, M.A.R., Swanson, S.A.V. and Heath, J.C., Study of the wear particles produced from cobalt-chromium-molybdenum-manganese total joint replacement prostheses, *Ann. Rheum. Dis.* (Suppl.), 28, 29, 1969.

Good, V.D., Clarke, I.C. and Anissian, A., Water and bovine serum lubrication compared in simulator PTFE/CoCr wear model, *J. Biomed. Mater. Res.*, 33, 275, 1996.

Hall, R.M. and Unsworth, A., Friction in hip prostheses, *Biomaterials*, 18, 1017, 1997.

Heisel, C., Silva, M., and Schmalzried, T.P., Bearing surface options for total hip replacement in young patients, *AAOS Instruct. Course Lecs.*, 53, 49, 2004.

Hutchins, I.M., *Tribology. Friction and Wear of Engineering Materials*, CRC Press, Boca Raton, FL, 1992.

Howell, J.R. et al., *In vivo* surface wear mechanisms of femoral components of cemented total hip arthroplasties, *J. Arthroplast.*, 19, 88, 2004.

Jacobs, J.J. and Craig, T.L. (Eds.), *Alternate Bearing Surfaces in Total Joint Replacement*, ASTM STP 1346, ASTM, West Conshohocken, PA, 1998.

Lazennec, J.-Y. and Dietrich, M., (Eds.), *Bioceramics in Joint Arthroplasty, 9th BIOLOX® Symp. Proc.*, Steinkopf, Darmstadt, 2004.

Lee, L.-H. (Ed.), *Polymer Wear and Its Control.* ACS Symposium Series 287, American Chemical Society, Washington, D.C., 1985.

Ludema, K.C., *Friction, Wear, and Lubrication*, CRC Press, Boca Raton, FL, 1996.

Mears, D.C. et al., Ferrographic analysis of wear particles in arthroplastic joints, *J. Biomed. Mater. Res.*, 12, 867, 1978.

McCutcheon, C.W., Lubrication of joints, in *The Joints and Synovial Fluid*, Vol. I., Sokoloff, L. (Ed.), Academic Press, New York, 1978, 437.

McKellop. H.A., Bearing surfaces in total hip replacements: state of the art and future developments, *AAOS Instruc. Course Lec.*, 50, 165, 2001.

Rieker, C., Oberholzer, S. and Wyss, U. (Eds.), *World Tribology Forum in Arthroplasty*, Hans Huber, Bern, SW, 2001.

Schmalzried, T.P., Dorey, F.J. and McKellop, H. The multifactorial nature of polyethylene wear *in vivo*, *J. Bone Joint Surg.*, 80A, 1234, 1998.

Semlitsch, M. and Willert, H.-G., Implant materials for hip endoprostheses: old proofs and new trends, *Arch. Orthop. Trauma Surg.*, 114, 61, 1995.

Streichler, R.M. et al., Metal-on-metal articulation for artificial hip joints: laboratory study and clinical results, *Proc. Instn. Mech. Engs.*, 210, 223, 1996.

Torrance, A.A., A method for calculating boundary friction and wear, *Wear*, 258, 924, 2005.

Walker, P.S. and Bullough, P.G., The effects of friction and wear in artificial joints, *Ortho. Clin. N. Am.*, 4(2), 275, 1973.

Weightman, B., Frication, lubrication, and wear, in *The Scientific Basis of Joint Replacement*, Swanson, S.A.V. and Freeman, M.A.R. (Eds.), John Wiley & Sons, New York, 1977, 46.

Wright, T.M. and Goodman, S.B. (Eds.), *Implant Wear: The Future of Total Joint Replacement*, American Academy of Orthopedic Surgeons, Oakbrook, 1996.

Yust, C.S. and Bayer, R.G. (Eds.), *Selection and Use of Wear Tests for Ceramics, STP 1010*, American Society for Testing and Materials, Philadelphia, 1988.

Interpart 1

Implant Materials: Properties

I1.1 Introduction

The preceding discussions concerning material response have necessarily been generic; that is, they have largely treated biomaterials by classes related to their predominant chemical bond type (and resulting physical properties) rather than dealing with the response of a particular, specific composition of material to the biological environment. This is how it should be because the details of such response depend upon the composition (including impurities) of the specific material, the methods by which it is fabricated and finished, the device application in which it is used, the animal and/or clinical model in which it is evaluated, etc. The professional literature on material response is broad, so much of the information needed to make a preliminary selection based upon material response is usually available.

However, before such a selection may be made, a more fundamental question must be answered: does the material meet the physical requirements of the design? Again, this is a complex problem, requiring a well-structured design process for successful solution. This and related issues of design are dealt with in Chapter 21. In this interpart, tables of basic materials' properties are provided as an introduction to the broader issue of materials selection.

The reader must be warned that most properties tabulated here are nominal or typical properties. Materials specifications, whatever their source, usually permit a range of compositions and processing conditions; in addition, the choice of starting materials (feed stocks, master blends, etc.) may also affect final properties, particularly of polymers, fibers, and composites. Therefore, reference should be made to original sources (as provided in the reference and bibliography sections or elsewhere) for exact details of composition, fabrication, and test conditions producing the values or ranges cited.

The properties tabulated are density and typical hardness, when reported, and those mechanical parameters that may be obtained from a conventional stress–strain curve. Standards, such as those produced by the ASTM International (American Society for Testing and Materials), BSI (British Standards

Institute), ANSI (American National Standards Institute), and ISO (International Standards Organization) are cited when relevant.* However, whether they are consensus or regulatory in nature, standards most often describe minimum requirements; properties of actual manufactured materials frequently exceed these values in general and in the case of specific production lots. Other properties, such as fatigue endurance limit, coefficients of friction (for material pairs), workability parameters, etc., may be of equal or greater importance in material selection and should be sought out during the design process.

It should be remembered that high performance requirement materials applications, such as medical and surgical devices and implants, require a high degree of confidence in design and performance parameters. Thus, some form of intrinsic property verification up to and, in some cases, including 100% nondestructive preuse "proof" testing is often required to assure safe and effective material response in medical and surgical applications.

Finally, researchers and designers should remember that when a biomaterial is used in a new design and/or for a new medical indication, it should regain its status as a candidate material. That is, although successful performance under one set of conditions in one design provides useful knowledge, it does not produce any guarantee of success in another situation. Therefore, nothing in this interpart should be construed as qualifying or otherwise recommending any material as safe and/or effective for use in any specific medical or surgical instrument, implant, or device.

I1.2 Metals

Metallic biomaterials in common use are drawn from the stainless steels (Table I.1), the cobalt-base "superalloys" (Table I.2), and the titanium/titanium-base alloy system (Table I.3). Several refractory and precious metals that have seen limited use in biomedical applications are covered in Table I.4.

---

* Where feasible and relevant, the most recent revision of the standard has been cited in footnotes to the tables. However, some values may have appeared in earlier versions and then been deleted in revision.

TABLE I.1

Stainless Steels

Material:	F138 type 2	F138 type 2	F138 type 2	F745	F1314	F1314	F1586 High N$_2$	F1586 High N$_2$
Condition:	AN	HF	CW		An	CW	AN	CW
Source:	[1,2]	[1,2]	[1,2]	[3]	[1,4]	[4]	[5]	[1,5]
Density(g/cm³):	7.9	7.98	7.9	—	7.98	—	—	—
E (tensile) (GPa):	200	200	200	—	200	—	—	200
Hardness (Hv):	—	—	350	—	205	—	—	~365
$\sigma_{0.2\%}$ (MPa):	190	240	690	207	380	862	430	1000
σ_{UTS} (MPa):	490	550	860	483	690	1035	740	1100
Elong. (min.%):	40	55	12	30	35	12	35	10

Notes: AN: annealed; CW: cold worked; HF: hot forged.

Sources: [1]: BSI 3531 (Part 2, Sec.2) (Amend. 2, 1983); [2]: ASTM F138-03; [3]: ASTM F745-00; [4]: ASTM F1314-01; [5]: ASTM F 1586-02.

TABLE I.2

Cobalt-Base Alloys

Material:	Cast CoCrMo	Wrought CoCrMo	Wrought CoNiCr Mo	Wrought CoNiCr MoWFe	Wrought CoCrMo	Wrought CoNiCr Mo	Wrought CoNiCr MoWFe
Condition:	AN	AN	AN	AN	CW	CWA	CW
Source:	[1,2]	[1,3]	[4]	[5]	[1,3]	[4]	[5]
Density(g/cm³):	7.8	9.15	—	—	9.15	—	—
E (tensile) (GPa):	200	230	—	—	230	—	—
Hardness (Hv):	300	240	—	—	450	—	—
$\sigma_{0.2\%}$ (MPa):	455	310	241–449	275	1000	1585	1310
σ_{UTS} (MPa):	665	860	793–1000	600	1500	1795	1172
Elong. (min.%):	8	30	50	50	9	8	12

Material:	Wrought CoCrNiMoFe MoFe grade 2	Wrought CoCrNi MoFe grade 2	Wrought CoCrMo	Wrought CoCrMo
Condition:	CW	CWA	AN	HW
Source:	[6]	[6]	[7]	[7]
Density(g/cm³):	—	—	—	—
E (tensile) (GPa):	—	—	—	—
Hardness (Hc):	—	—	25	28
$\sigma_{0.2\%}$ (MPa):	—	1240–1450	517	700
σ_{UTS} (MPa):	1515–1795	1860–2275	897	1000
Elong. (min.%):	—	1–17	20	12

Notes: AN: annealed; CW: cold worked; CWA: cold worked, aged; HW: hot worked; Hv: Vickers hardness; Hc: Rockwell C hardness.

Sources: [1]: BSI 3531 (Part 2, Sec.4–5) (Amend. 2, 1983); [2]: ASTM F75-01; [3]: ASTM F90-86-01; [4]: ASTM F562-02; [5]: ASTM F563-00; [6]: ASTM F1058-02; [7]: ASTM F1537-00.

TABLE I.3

Titanium α–β and β Titanium-Base Alloys

Material:	Ti grade 1	Ti grade 4	Ti3Al2.5V	Ti6Al4V	Ti6Al7Nb	Ti6Al4V	Ti5Al2.5 Fe
Type:	—	—	α–β	α–β	α–β	α–β	α–β
Condition:	An	AN	AN	AN	HF	HF	AN
Source:	[1,2]	[1,2]	[3,4]	[1,5]	[6,7]	[8]	[9]
Density(g/cm^3):	4.5	4.5	4.51	4.4	4.52	4.4	4.45
E (tensile) (GPa):	127	127	105–120	127	105	127	—
Hardness (Hv):	—	240–280	—	310–350	400	—	—
$\sigma_{0.2\%}$ (MPa):	170	483	517–560	760–795	800	825–869	815
σ_{UTS} (MPa):	240	550	621–650	825–860	900	895–930	965
Elong. (min.%):	24	15	15	8	10	6–10	16

Material:	Ti5Al2.5 Fe	Ti12Mo 6Zr2Fe	Ti13Nb 13Zr	Ti13Nb 13Zr	Ti15Mo	Ti15Mo 3Nb0.3O$_2$	Ti35Nb 5Ta7Zr
Type:	α–β	β	β	β	β	β	β
Condition:	HF	AN	AN	QA	AN	AN	AN
Source:	[9]	[10,11]	[12,13]	[12–14]	[15]	[16]	[17]
Density(g/cm^3):	4.45	5.0	—	—	—	4.94	—
E (tensile) (GPa):	—	74–85	79	77	—	82	55
Hardness (Hv):	—	34–35*	26*	28*	—	—	—
$\sigma_{0.2\%}$ (MPa):	900	897–1000	900	725	483–552	1020	547
σ_{UTS} (MPa):	985	931–1060	1030	860	690–724	1020	597
Elong. (min.%):	13	12–22	15	8	12–20	—	19

Notes: *: Rockwell C; AN: annealed; HF: hot forged; QA: Water quenched, aged.

Sources: [1]: BSI 3531 (Part 2, Sec.6) (Amend. 2,1983); [2]: ASTM F67-00; [3]: ASTM F2146-01; [4]: TIMET, Inc.; [5]: ASTM F136-96; [6]: IMI Titanium Ltd, 1989; [7]: ASTM F1295-01; [8]: ASTM F1472-93; [9]: Borowy, K.-H. and Kramer, K.-H., in *Titanium Science and Technology,* Vol. 2, Luterjering, G., Zwicker, U. and Bunk, W. (Eds.), Deutsche Gesell. f. Metallkunde e. V., Oburereset, 1985, 1381; [10]: Wang, K. et al., in *Beta Titanium Alloys in the 1990s,* Eylon, D., Boyer, R.R. and Koss, D.A. (Eds.), Min. Met. and Materials Society, New York, 1993, 49; [11]: ASTM F1813-01; [12]: U.S. Patent 5,169,597; [13]: Davidson, J.A. et al., *Bio-Med. Mater. Eng.,* 4(3), 231, 1994; [14]: ASTM 1713-03; [15]: ASTM F2060-01; [16]: Long, M. and Rack, H.J., *Biomaterials,* 19, 1621, 1998; [17]: Ahmed, T. et al., *Proc. Inst. Metal. 8th World Titanium Conf.,* 1996, 742.

TABLE I.4

Other Metals and Alloys

Material:	TaP	TaP	Ti54.5 NiMA	Ti55.8 NiMA	PtP	Pt10 RhTC	Pt10 RhTC 75%	WP	Zr-2.5 Nb α–β
Condition:	An	CW	AN	AN	AN	AN	CW	SN	CW/AN
Source:	[1,2]	[1,2]	[3,4]	[3,4]	[1]	[1]	[1]	[1]	[5]
Density(g/cm^3):	16.6	16.6	6.5	6.5	21.5	20	20	19.3	6.64
E (tensile) (GPa):	186	186	28–41	41–75	147	—	—	345	99
Hardness (Hv):	—	—	—	—	38–40	90*	165*	225	—
σ_y (MPa):	140	345	—	—	—	—	—	—	379
σ_{UTS} (MPa):	205	515	1100	1070	135–165	310	620	125–140	552
Elong. (min.%):	20–30	2	10	10	35–40	35	2	~0	16

Notes: AN: annealed; CW: cold worked; MA: memory alloy; P: pure (elemental); SN: sintered bar; TC: thermocouple alloy; *: Brinell hardness.

Sources: [1]: *Metals Handbook*, 8th ed., Vol. 1 (ASM, Metals Park, 1961); [2]: ASTM F 560-04; [3]: ASTM F 2063-00; [4]: National Devices & Components, Inc.; [5] Wah Chang (Zircadyne 705 [contains Hf]); see ASTM B 351, F- standard pending.

I1.3 Polymers

The cautionary note previously sounded concerning the reliability of tabulated materials' properties applies especially to polymers. In the case of this material class, four additional problems interfere with interpretation of data:

- All polymers are viscoelastic; therefore, mechanical property measurements depend upon the strain *rate* used in evaluation. Because viscoelastic materials generally become stiffer and less ductile as strain rates increase, testing rates should equal or exceed those expected to be encountered in service.

- Properties of engineering polymers are closely related to average molecular weight and molecular weight distribution as well as to curing conditions and time (thermosets) and fabrication temperatures and postfabrication heat treatment (thermoplastics).

- Postsynthesis processing and/or sterilization, especially by ^{60}Co γ or electron beam irradiation, may alter final properties of some materials. This is particularly true for ultra high molecular weight polyethylene, for which more than a dozen commercial grades with varying amounts of irradiation and postirradiation heat treatment are now available (Kurtz 2004).

- Many polymers are subject to possible oxidation during room temperature storage; therefore, the chronology of production of the material and of the device may affect final properties in clinical use.

The data are presented in two tables: Table I.5 for thermosets and Table I.6 for thermoplastics. Both types of polymers have important roles as biomaterials, although thermoplastics tend to be preferred due to the relatively greater ease in fabricating them without low molecular weight leachable components.

Finally, fatigue behavior of biomedical polymers, especially of PMMA-type "bone-cements," is a sufficiently controversial subject that no data are provided here. The reader is referred to the professional literature.

TABLE I.5

Thermoset Resins

Material:	EP	PMMA 10BaSO$_4$	PMMA;	PEU	PSU	SR	SR (HP)
Condition:	CR	24 h CR	24 h CR	CR	CR	HV	HV
Source:	[1]	[2,3]	[3]	[4]	[5]	[5,6]	[6]
Density(g/cm^3):	1.11–1.40	1.183	1.088	1.1	1.2	1.12–1.23	1.15
E (tensile) (GPa):	2.4	1.31	2.4–3.1	5.9*	3.7*	<1.4*	2.4*
Hardness (Sh. A):	—	—	—	75	88	25–75	52
$\sigma_{y(C)}$ (MPa):	—	—	15.8	—	—	—	—
σ_{UCS} (MPa):	100–170	70	69–125	—	—	—	—
σ_{UTS} (MPa):	28–90	28–46	9.7–32	45	40	5.9–8.3	8.3–10.3
Elong. (min.%):	3–6	4.6	2.4–5.4	750	540	350–600	700

Notes: CR: room temperature cured; EP: epoxy; HV: heat vulcanized; PMMA: polymethyl methacrylate; SR: silicone rubber; HP: high performance; *: MPa.

Sources: [1]: *Modern Plastics Encyclopedia*, McGraw–Hill, New York, 1990; note: typical values; not specific medical grades; [2]: ASTM F 451-99a; [3]: Lautenschlager, E.P. et al., in *Functional Behavior of Orthopedic Biomaterials*, Vol. II, Ducheyne, P. and Hastings, G.W. (Eds.), CRC Press, Boca Raton, FL, 1984, 87; [4]: Boretos, J.W. and Pierce, W.S., *J. Biomed. Mater. Res.*, 2, 121, 1968; [5]: Braley, S., *J. Macromol. Sci.-Chem.*, A4(3), 529, 1970; see also ASTM F604-94 (withdrawn); [6]: Frisch, E.E., in *Polymeric Materials and Artificial Organs*, ACS Symp. 256, C.G. Gebelein (Ed.), American Chemical Society, Washington, D.C., 1984, 63.

TABLE I.6

Thermoplastic Resins

Material:	PE (UHMW)	PE (UHMW)	PE (UHMW)	PE (UHMW)	PLA (STCP)	PMMA	PSF	PEEK
Condition:	MM	EX	CM	HC	CM	CM	IM	IM
Source:	[1]	[1,2]	[1–3]	[3]	[4]	[5]	[6,7]	[8]
Density(g/cm³):	0.927–0.944	0.927–0.944	0.93–0.944	—	—	1.186	1.23-1.25	1.28–1.32
E (tensile) (GPa):	—	1.24	1.36	2.17	4–5	2.6-3.2	2.3–2.48	3-8.3*
Hardness (Sh. D):	60	60	62	66	—	—	—	—
σ_y (MPa):	19–21	19–28	19–29	28	—	—	65–96	70
σ_{UCS} (MPa):	—	—	—	—	—	80–125	—	—
σ_{UTS} (MPa):	27–35	37–47	27–40	—	50–60	50–75	106*	90–152
Elong. (min.%):	300	250–300	350	230	2–3	2–10	20–75	4.9**

Notes: IM: injection molded; MM: molded, machined; EX: extruded; CM: compression molded; HC: high crystallinity; PE (UHMW): ultra high molecular weight polyethylene; PLA (STCP): polylactic acid stereo copolymer; PMMA: polymethyl methacrylate; PSF: polysulfone; *: flexural; **: at yield.

Sources: [1]: ASTM 648-00; [2]: Roe, R.-J. et al., *J. Biomed. Mater. Res.*, 15, 209, 1981; [3]: Depuy (1989); [4]: Christel, P. et al., in *Proceedings of the 1st International Conference on Composites in Biomedical Engineering*, November 19–20, London. Imprint of Luton, Luton, 1985, p. 11/1; note: resorbable; properties depend upon L/D ratio; [5]: Lautenschlager, E.P. et al., in *Functional Behavior of Orthopedic Biomaterials*, Vol. II, Ducheyne, P. and Hastings, G.W. (Eds.), CRC Press, Boca Raton, FL, 1984, 87; [6]: Dunkle, S.R., in *Engineered Materials Handbook*, Vol. 2: *Engineering Plastics*, Dostal, C.A. (Ed.), American Society for Metals Int., Metals Park, 1988, 200; [7]: ASTM F 702-98a; [8]: Lewis (1990); see also ASTM F 2026-02.

I1.4 Ceramics

At room and body temperature, ceramic materials suitable for biomedical applications possess negligible ductility; thus, no tensile or elongation data are included in Table I.7. Note that strength of ceramics depends very strongly on density (as percent of ultimate) and grain size, so data on actual commercial formulations must be sought for engineering use. Data are provided only for some of the most common structural ceramics; no information is provided on resorbable or so-called bioactive ceramics due to their variety and complexity. (See deGroot, 1983; Hench and Wilson, 1984; and Manley, 1993.)

TABLE I.7

Ceramic Materials

Material: Condition: Source:	Al_2O_3 HP [1,2]	C LTI [3]	C VT [3]	C ULTI [3]	ZrO_2 SHP [4,5]
Density (g/cm³):	3.98	1.7–2.2	1.4–1.6	1.5–2.2	6.1
Grain size(μm):	1.8–4	30–40*	10–40*	8–15*	<0.5
E (tensile) (GPa):	400–580	18–28	24–31	14–21	200
Hardness (Hv):	2300	150–250	150–200	150–250	1300
σ_{UFS} (MPa):	550	280–560	70–210	350–700	1200
σ_{UCS} (MPa):	4500	—	—	—	—

Notes: HP: high purity; LTI: low-temperature isotropic; SHP: sintered, hot isostatic pressed (5% Y_2O_3 stabilized); ULTI: ultra low temperature isotropic; VT: vitreous (glassy); *: angstroms.

Sources: [1]: CeramTec; [2]: ASTM F603-00; ISO 6474; [3]: various; compilation by Intermedics Orthopedics (1983); [4]: Christel, P. et al., *J. Biomed. Mater. Res.*, 23, 45, 1989; [5]: Norton Demarquest; 6ASTM F 2393-04.

I1.5 Composites

Composites, or more properly composite materials, is a term that has come to describe a wide range of engineered or designed materials. Mechanical properties of composite materials depend upon the properties of the phases (matrix and strengthening, or reinforcing, phase or phases) as well as on the nature of the phase interfaces, their volume fractions, net porosity, and the local and global arrangement of the reinforcing phases. This complexity dictates an economy of action here because an entire volume could be (and has frequently been) devoted to the subject. Thus, as a brief guide, Table I.8 presents properties of some more common reinforcing phases useful in composite biomaterials design, and Table I.9 presents properties of a few representative composites that have been evaluated to some degree as biomaterials.

TABLE I.8

Reinforcing Phases

Material:	E-glass	S-glass	C-glass	C* (low E)	C* (High E)	PA (K29)+	PA (K49)+	PA (K149)+
Condition:	AN, CF	AN, CF	AN, CF	HT, CF	HT, CF	CF	CF	CF
Source:	[1,2]	[1,2]	[1,2]	[1]	[1]	[1]	[1]	[1]
Density (g/cm³):	2.62	2.50	2.56	1.76	1.9	1.44	1.44	1.47
Diameter(μm):	3–20	3–20	3–20	7–8	7	12	12	12
E (tensile) (GPa):	72–81	85–89	69	230	390	83	131	286
σ_{UTS} (MPa):	3450	4580	3000–5300	3300	2400	2800–3600	3600–4100	3400
Elong. (min.%):	4.9	5.7	4.8	1.4	0.6	4.0	2.8	2.0

Material:	Al_2O_3	Al_2O_3– 48SiO_2	SiO_2	βSiC	αSiC	βSiC	BN	B_4C
Condition:	CF	DF	CF	CF	WH	WH	CF	WH
Source:	[1]	[1]	[1]	[1]	[1]	[1]	[3]	[3]
Density (g/cm³):	3.95	2.73	2.2	2.55	3.2	3.19	1.91	2.52
Diameter(μm):	20	2–3	9	10–15	0.6	0.1–0.5	7	—
E (tensile) (GPa):	379	100	69	180–200	690	400–700	90	483
σ_{UTS} (MPa):	1380	1900	3450	2500–3200	6900	3000–14000	1380	13800

Notes: AN: annealed; CF: continuous fiber; DF: discontinuous fiber; WH: whisker; HT: heat treated; *: polyacrylonitrile (PAN) precursor; +: Kevlar™ (DuPont).

Sources: [1]: *Composites, Engineered Materials Handbook*, Vol. 1, ASM International, Metals Park, 1987; [2]: Lubin, G. (Ed.), *Handbook of Composites*, Van Nostrand, New York, 1982; [3]: Schwartz, M.M., *Composite Materials Handbook*, McGraw–Hill, New York, 1984.

TABLE I.9

Composite Materials

Material:	PMMA- 2C	C60SiC	C60SiC (5% por.)	CFRC	CFRC (7% por.)	EP- 12.5C	CFPSU	PE (UHMW)- 10C
Condition:	RT					ET		
Source:	[1]	[2]	[3]	[2]	[3]	[4]	[5]	[6]
Density (g/cm³):	—	2.6	2.4	1.7	1.78	—	—	0.98
E (tensile) (GPa):	5.52	100	80–90	140	40–58	14	110	1.94**
σ_{UCS}(MPa):	—	1000	250–370	800	230–320	—	—	14.2
σ_{UTS} (MPa):	38	220*	220–360*	800*	350–600	200*	1600*	22
Elong. (min.%):	0.7	<1	—	>4	—	—	1.3	150

Notes: PMMA: polymethyl methacrylate; RT: room temperature cured; ET: 70°C cured; CFRC: carbon fiber-reinforced carbon; CFPSU: continuous fiber carbon reinforced polysulfone; EP: epoxy; por.: open porosity; *: flexural strength; **: estimated.

Sources: [1]: Pilliar, R.M. et al., *J. Biomed. Mater. Res.*, 10, 893, 1976; [2]: Brückmann, H. and Hüttinger, K.J., *Biomaterials*, 1, 67, 1980; [3]: Christel, P. et al., *J. Biomed. Mater. Res, Appl. Biomater.*, 21(A2), 191, 1987; [4]: Hastings, G.W., *Composites*, 7, 193, 1978; [5]: Claes, L. et al., in *Biological and Biomechanical Performance of Biomaterials*, Christel, P., Meunier, A. and Lee, A.J.C. (Eds.), Elsevier, Amsterdam, 1986, 81; [6]: Zimmer, 1978.

References

Ahmed, T. et al., A new low-modulus, biocompatibile titanium alloy, *Proc. Inst. Metal. 8th World Titanium Conf.*, 1996, 742.

Boretos, J.W. and Pierce, W.S., Segmented polyurethane: a polyether polymer, *J. Biomed. Mater. Res.*, 2, 121, 1968.

Borowy, K.-H. and Kramer, K.-H., On the properties of a new titanium alloy (TiAl5Fe2.5) as implant material, in *Titanium Science and Technology*, Vol. 2, Luterjering, G., Zwicker, U. and Bunk, W. (Eds.), Deutsche Gesell. f. Metallkunde e. V., Oburoresel, 1985, 1381.

Braley, S., The chemistry and properties of the medical-grade silicones, *J. Macromol. Sci.-Chem.*, A4(3), 529, 1970.

Brückmann, H. and Hüttinger, K.J., Carbon, a promising material in endoprosthetics. Part 1: the carbon materials and their mechanical properties, *Biomaterials*, 1, 67, 1980.

Christel, P. et al., Mechanical properties and short-term *in-vivo* evaluation of yttrium–oxide partially stabilized zirconia, *J. Biomed. Mater. Res.*, 23, 45, 1989.

Christel, P. et al., Development of a carbon–carbon hip prosthesis, *J. Biomed. Mater. Res, Appl. Biomater.*, 21(A2), 191, 1987.

Christel, P. et al., PGA (polyglycolic acid)-fiber-reinforced-PLA (polylactic acid) as an implant material for bone surgery, in *Proceedings of the 1st International Conference on Composites in Biomedical Engineering*, November 19–20, London. Imprint of Luton, Luton, 1985, p. 11/1.

Claes, L., Hüttner, W. and Weiss, R., Mechanical properties of carbon-fiber reinforced polysulfone plates for internal fracture hardware, in *Biological and Biomechanical Performance of Biomaterials*, Christel, P., Meunier, A. and Lee, A.J.C. (Eds.), Elsevier, Amsterdam, 1986, 81.

Composites, Engineered Materials Handbook, Vol. 1, ASM International, Metals Park, OH, 1987.

deGroot, K. (Ed.), *Bioceramics of Calcium Phosphate*, CRC Press, Boca Raton, FL, 1983.

Davidson, J.A. et al., New surface-hardened, low modulus, corrosion-resistant Ti-13Nb-13Zr alloy for total hip arthroplasty, *Bio-Med. Mater. Eng.*, 4(3), 231, 1994.

Depuy, Warsaw, IN, 1989.

Dunkle, S.R., Polysulfones (PSU), in *Engineered Materials Handbook*, Vol. 2: *Engineering Plastics*, Dostal, C.A. (Ed.), American Society for Metals Int., Metals Park, 1988, 200.

Frisch, E.E., Silicones in artificial organs, in *Polymeric Materials and Artificial Organs*, ACS Symp. 256, Gebelein, C.G. (Ed.), American Chemical Society, Washington, D.C., 1984, 63.

Metals Handbook, 8th ed., Vol. 1, ASM, Metals Park, OH, 1961.

Hastings, G.W., Carbon fiber composites for orthopedic implants, *Composites*, 7, 193, 1978.

Hench, L.L. and Wilson, J., Surface-active biomaterials, *Science*, 226, 630, 1984.

Kurtz, S.M., *The UHMWPE Handbook: Ultra-High Molecular Weight Polyethylene in Total Joint Replacement*, Academic Press (Elsevier), New York, 2004.

Lautenschlager, E.P., Stupp, S.I. and Keller, J.C., Structure and properties of acrylic bone cement, in *Functional Behavior of Orthopedic Biomaterials*, Vol. II, Ducheyne, P. and Hastings, G.W. (Eds.), CRC Press, Boca Raton, FL, 1984, 87.

Lewis, G., *Selection of Engineering Materials*, Prentice Hall, Englewood Cliffs, NJ, 1989.
Long, M. and Rack, H.J., Titanium alloys in total joint replacement — a materials science perspective, *Biomaterials*, 19, 1621, 1998.
Lubin, G. (Ed.), *Handbook of Composites*, Van Nostrand, New York, 1982.
Manley, M.T., Introduction, in *Hydroxyapatite Coatings in Orthopedic Surgery*, Geesink, R.G.T. and Manley, M.T. (Eds.), Raven Press, New York, 1993, 1.
Modern Plastics Encylopedia, McGraw–Hill, New York, 1995.
Pilliar, R.M. et al., Carbon fiber-reinforced bone cement in orthopedic surgery, *J. Biomed. Mater. Res.*, 10, 893, 1976.
Roe, R.-J. et al., Effect of radiation sterilization and aging on ultrahigh molecular weight polyethylene, *J. Biomed. Mater. Res.*, 15, 209, 1981.
Schwartz, M.M., *Composite Materials Handbook*, McGraw–Hill, New York, 1984.
Wang, K., Gustavson, L. and Dumbleton, J., The characterization of Ti-12Mo-6Zr-2Fe — a new biocompatible titanium alloy developed for surgical implants, in *Beta Titanium Alloys in the 1990s*, Eylon, D., Boyer, R.R. and Koss, D.A. (Eds.), Min. Met. and Materials Society, New York, 1993, 49.
Zimmer, Nonauthored technical material, Warsaw, IN, 1978.

Bibliography

2004 Annual Book of ASTM Standards, Vol. 13.01, *Medical Devices*, ASTM International, West Conshohocken, PA, 2004.
Ashby, M., *Materials Selection in Mechanical Design*, 2nd ed., Butterworth–Heinemann, London, 1999.
Ashby, M. and Johnson, K., *Materials and Design: The Art and Science of Material Selection in Product Design*, Butterworth–Heinemann, London, 2002.
Black, J. and Hastings, G. (Eds.), *Handbook of Biomaterial Properties*, Chapman & Hall, London, 1998.
Boretos, J.W., *Concise Guide to Biomedical Polymers*, Charles C Thomas, Springfield, IL, 1973.
Boutin, P. et al., The use of dense alumina–alumina ceramic combination in total hip replacement, *J. Biomed. Mater. Res.*, 22, 1203, 1988.
Brown, S.A. and Lemons, J.A. (Eds.), *Medical Applications of Titanium and its Alloys*, STP 1272. ASTM, West Conshohocken, PA, 1992
Bush, R.B., A bibliography of monographic works on biomaterials and biocompatibility, *J. Appl. Biomater.*, 4, 195, 1993.
Catledge, S.A. et al., Nanostructured ceramics for biomedical implants, *J. Nanosci. Nanotechnol.*, 2(3–4), 293, 2002.
Cowin, S.C., *Bone Mechanics Handbook*, 2nd ed., CRC Press, Boca Raton, 2002.
Disegi, J.A., Kennedy, R.L. and Pilliar, R. (Eds.), *Cobalt-Base Alloys for Biomedical Applications*, STP 1365, ASTM, West Conshohocken, PA, 1999.
Donachie, M.J., Jr. (Ed.), *Superalloys Source Book*, ASM Int., Metals Park, 1984.
Donachie, M.J., Jr. (Ed.), *Titanium: A Technical Guide*, ASM Int., Metals Park, 1984.
Epinette, J.-L. and Manley, M.T. (Eds.), *Fifteen Years of Clinical Experience with Hydroxyapatite Coatings in Joint Arthroplasty*, Springer–Verlag, Paris, 2004.
Fisher, L.W., *Selection of Engineering Materials and Adhesives*, Taylor & Francis, Boca Raton, FL, 2005.

Ito, A. et al., *In vitro* biocompatibility, mechanical properties, and corrosion resistance of Ti-Zr-NB-TA-PD and Ti-Sn-Nb-Ta-Pd alloys, *J. Biomed. Mater. Res.*, 29, 893, 1995.

Kingery, W.D., *Introduction to Ceramics*, 2nd ed., John Wiley & Sons, New York, 1976.

Kokubo T. et al., Bioactive metals: preparation and properties, *J. Mater. Sci. Mater. Med.*, 15(2), 99, 2004.

Lambda, N.M.K., Woodhouse, K.A. and Cooper, S.L. (Eds.), *Polyurethanes in Biomedical Applications*. CRC Press, Boca Raton, FL, 1997.

Mishra, A.K. et al., Ti13Nb13Zr: A new low modulus, high strength, corrosion resistant, near beta alloy for orthopaedic implants. In: Eylon, D., Boyer, R.R. and Koss, D.A., (Eds.), *Beta Titanium Alloys in the 1990's*. Warrendale, PA: The Minerals, Metals and Materials Society, 1993, 61.

Pelton, A.R., Stoeckel, D. and Duerig, T.W., Medical uses of nitinol, *Mater. Sci. For.*, 327–328, 63, 2000.

Portnoy, R.C. (Ed.), *Medical Plastics: Degradation, Resistance, and Failure Analysis*, Plastics Design Library, Norwich, CT, 1998.

Ratner, B.D. and Bryant, S.J., Biomaterials: where we have been and where we are going, *Annu. Rev. Biomed. Eng.*, 6, 41, 2004.

Ravglioli, A. and Karjewski, A. *Bioceramics and the Human Body*, Kluwer Academic, London, 1992.

Santavirta S. et al., Alternative materials to improve total hip replacement tribology, *Acta Orthop. Scand.*, 74(4), 380, 2003.

Semlitsch, M., Staub, F. and Weber, H., Titanium–aluminium–niobium alloy development for high-strength surgical implants, *Biomed. Technik*, 30, 334, 1985.

Shackelford, J.F., Alexander, W. and Park, J.S. (Eds.), *CRC Practical Handbook of Materials Selection*, CRC Press, Boca Raton, FL, 1995.

Szycher, M. (Ed.), *Biocompatible Polymers, Metals, and Composites*, Technomic, Lancaster, PA, 1983.

Toni, A. et al., Ceramics in total hip arthroplasty, in *Encyclopedic Handbook of Biomaterials and Bioengineering*, Part A, Vol. 1, Wise, D.L. et al. (Eds.), Marcel Dekker, New York, 1995, 1501.

Willert, H.-G., Buchorn, G.H. and Eyerer, P. (Eds.), *Ultra-High Molecular Weight Polyethylene as a Biomaterial in Orthopedic Surgery*, Hogrefe & Huber, Toronto, 1990.

Part III

Host Response: Biological Effects of Implants

8

The Inflammatory Process

8.1 Introduction

Inflammation is a nonspecific physiological response to tissue damage in animal systems. It arises as a response to trauma, infection, intrusion of foreign materials, or local cell death, or as an adjunct to immune or neoplastic responses. If the initiating agent causes damage to or frank rupture of vascular tissue, blood coagulation, which is related, may be superimposed on the inflammatory response. The general inflammatory response will be considered in this chapter. Coagulation is dealt with in Chapter 9, immune, or specific, responses are dealt with in Chapter 12, and neoplastic transformation, whether chemically or mechanically mediated, is the subject of Chapter 13.

8.2 The Inflammatory Response

8.2.1 Introduction

The four classical clinical signs of inflammation in animals and humans are redness (*rubor*), swelling (*tumor*), pain (*dolor*), and heat (*calor*). The magnitude of these signs is related to the intensity and extent of the inflammatory process. The presence of an implant does not produce additional signs or symptoms but may alter their severity and duration.

8.2.2 Initial Events

The first events that occur in response to an inflammatory stimulus are rapid dilation of the local capillaries and an increase in the permeability of their endothelial cell linings. The dilation (vasodilation) arises from the activation of a coagulation factor, factor XII (the Hageman factor), most probably by contact with collagen or a foreign protein or material. Through the intermediate activation of a polypeptide, kallikrein, this leads to conversion of a group of additional molecules to kinins. The kinins are strong mediators of vasodilation and endothelial permeation.

The vasodilation leads to an increase in blood entry into the capillary beds. Local aspect ratio changes in the capillaries, combined with loss of plasma through the capillary walls and a tendency for the platelets and erythrocytes to become "sticky," lead to slower flow and sludging. This results in the first clinical sign, redness (erythema), simply reflecting a higher local concentration of erythrocytes.

The increased permeability of the capillary endothelium allows fluid to move into the surrounding tissue bed. Under normal conditions there is a 10 to 15 mmHg positive pressure differential between the arteriole end of a capillary and the external tissue bed. However, the endothelium is tight and permits only a very slow flow of water and small molecules into the surrounding tissue. This fluid is normally drained away by local lymphatic vessels maintaining a constant tissue volume. As permeability increases, water and larger molecules, including normal plasma proteins and locally activated kinins, move into the tissue. The increased fluid influx, if not promptly balanced by increased lymphatic drainage, distends or swells the tissue. The local lymphatics may be constricted or blocked due to the original trauma, occlusion by cell fragments, or hydraulic compression. Additionally, the presence of plasma fractions raises the local osmotic pressure and tends to hold fluid in place. Thus, swelling (edema), the second clinical sign, is a usual early concomitant of inflammation. In the extreme case, all inflow and outflow of fluid may be prevented, leading to the so-called "compartment syndrome" that, if not promptly relieved, results in cell death and tissue necrosis.

Pain, the third clinical sign, results from at least two causes. First, edema may activate local deep pain receptors. In patients, this is felt as a throbbing pain as it peaks repetitively with peak systolic pressure. Second, the kinins act directly on nerve ends to produce pain sensation. The familiar acute pain of a bee sting is associated with the activation of a kinin called bradykinin in bee venom.

The origin of the local heating effect, the fourth sign, is unclear. In the general case, it may be associated with local disturbances of fluid flow in the presence of increased cellular metabolic activity (and resulting heat production). Although not yet shown conclusively, a group of contaminants termed pyrogens, which are known to cause systemic fever, may be generated locally by tissue necrosis or, in the presence of infection, as a result of activation by bacterial or viral toxins, especially endotoxin. Fine particles or bacterial fragments left on implants that are sterilized after inadequate cleaning may also be pyrogenic. The presence of such pyrogens or other surface contaminants may mask the intrinsic local host response.

These early events of inflammation are largely chemical in origin and effect. Shortly after initiation, however, a series of cellular invasions take place. These cells are responsible for the removal of dead tissue and the repair of the resulting defect.

8.2.3   Cellular Invasion

The first new cells to appear at the site of injury are neutrophils. They are the most common of the granulocytes, also termed polymorphonuclear leukocytes (PMNs) due to their horseshoe-shaped, multilobed nuclei. Because their granules are readily stainable by neutral dyes, they can be distinguished from related cell types, basophils and acidophils.*

At the earliest stages of the inflammatory response, the neutrophils become sticky. At first they stick momentarily to the capillary endothelium and then are released. More of them stick and remain for longer periods. Then, neutrophils begin to penetrate between the endothelial cells and move into the surrounding damaged tissue. Neutrophil emigration (diapedisis) begins minutes to hours after insult and may continue for as long as 24 hours. The time course varies with the nature and severity of the insult. Although following an initial but transient episode of increased vascular permeability, this emigration is accompanied by longer sustained endothelial permeability. This second phase of permeability parallels the maturation of edema and erythema and subsides as neutrophil emigration draws to a halt.

The primary role of the neutrophil is phagocytosis. This process, the engulfing and degradation or digestion of fragments of tissue or material, is common to this and several other cell types. What distinguishes each cell type in regard to its phagocytic function is the nature and amount of the degradative enzymes (lysozymes) that each has available. Lysozymes are stored as cytoplasmic granules, perhaps 200 per neutrophil that are readily seen in the electron microscope. Before encountering foreign particles, phagocytic cells are inactive; after such contact, they become activated. Activation is characterized by a change in metabolic activity, especially an increase in oxygen consumption (the "respiratory burst"), a change in cell shape, and an internal degranulation as lysozymes are released into vacuoles, termed phagosomes, or more particularly, primary lysozomes.

Phagocytosis proceeds from an initial contact between the cell membrane and a foreign material (inorganic or organic). Neutrophils are specialized to find and phagocytize bacteria; how they find the foreign material particles, such as splinters or wear debris, is poorly understood, but there appear to be several mechanisms. The neutrophil may be attracted by a particular chemical composition (chemotaxis), by local pH differences, or by electrochemical factors associated with the foreign particle and its surroundings. In addition, a group of native molecules, opsonins, coat foreign surfaces (opsonization), thus rendering them chemoattractive. Opsonins are small molecules excreted by a variety of cells and include the activated form of

---

* So called because of their granule stainability by, respectively, basic and acidic histological dyes.

complement factor five (C5a). When in contact with and recognizing a foreign material through antigen (opsonin)-membrane receptor binding, a dimple develops in the cell wall (invagination) of the phagocyte. The particle is drawn in and the dimple closes, often breaking off to form a vacuole, termed a secondary lysozome, which leaves the particle inside the cell and surrounded by an everted unit membrane. This vacuole merges with primary lysosomes, whose contents are then released into the vacuole and attack foreign or denatured proteins. This process of degranulation, as previously noted, is accompanied by a respiratory burst involving production of hydrogen peroxide and superoxide anions, which act nonspecifically to digest nonproteinaceous foreign materials that are not attacked by lysozymes. The vacuole may clear and be absorbed, or its contents, presumably altered to be less objectionable, may be released outside the cell.

The complement system, of which factor C5 is an element, is a complex series of glycoproteins and protein inhibitors present in the circulating and interstitial fluids of mammals. It constitutes a powerful, noncellular part of the biological defense system against foreign materials. It can be activated by contact with antigen–antibody complexes (see Chapter 12), bacterial proteins and polysaccharides, endotoxins, and many polymers, of natural or synthetic origin. Once activation is initiated, it proceeds along two pathways through a series of enzymatic cascade amplifying steps, much like the blood coagulation cascade (see Chapter 9). The end products are activated complement factors, which can mediate membrane damage directly, or molecular fragments that can influence inflammatory and immune processes (Anderson and Miller 1984; Frank 1979).*

Accompanying the neutrophils is a far smaller number of another type of leukocyte, the eosinophil. These are similar in structure to the neutrophils and, although they perform a similar phagocytic function, they can also phagocytize antigen–antibody complexes (see Section 12.2.1). Their name stems from the observation that, unlike the neutrophils, their granules can be stained by eosin, an acidic dye. They contain a different distribution of enzymes and are usually only present in significant numbers in association with immune responses.

The neutrophils and eosinophils serve as the first active line of defense against foreign material in tissue. Leukocytes have a life span of only hours in blood and a few days in tissue. They are end-state cells and cannot replicate by division (mitosis). Although capable of oxidative phosphorylation, they obtain their energy primarily from the anaerobic metabolism of stored glycogen, so they can persist in areas with highly disturbed metabolic states. After fulfilling their function, they die rapidly. Normally, they constitute an "emergency squad" whose duties are later supplanted by another cell, the monocyte. Thus, the presence of extensive numbers of live neutrophils in tissue may be interpreted as evidence of continued inflammatory challenge.

---

* The complement system is discussed at greater length in Section 12.2.2.

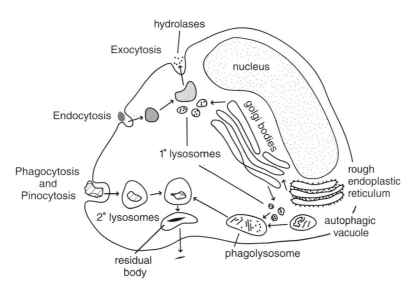

FIGURE 8.1
Phagocytic cell functions.

The monocyte is the largest of the freely circulating leukocytes, extending to perhaps 15 μm in diameter. It is distinguished from the neutrophil by its larger size and its single, centrally located large nucleus. Once in tissue, it becomes a macrophage or mononuclear phagocyte (MNP) (Figure 8.1). In addition to circulating monocytes, a resident population of monocytes in tissue can also rapidly become macrophages and migrate to the site of injury. From whatever source, macrophages arrive at the site of inflammation after the neutrophilic invasion has begun to subside and concentrate in appreciably smaller numbers. Their role is similar to that of the neutrophil in that they can actively phagocytize materials and digest them. They also possess specialized membrane sites that mediate specific reactions. When activated by a suitable challenge, the macrophage possesses a number of functional capabilities, as seen in Figure 8.1.

The activated macrophage is not an end state cell; it has an active aerobic glycolysis cycle and can undergo a number of transformations. In addition to releasing lysozymes, both internally and externally, related to attempts to digest foreign materials, activated macrophages synthesize and release a wide range of biochemical factors which can mediate the activity of many other cells including lymphocytes, fibroblasts, osteoblasts, osteoclasts, and foreign body giant cells (Ziats et al. 1988).

Macrophages may multiply by mitosis (Figure 8.2). By fusion, the macrophage is the progenitor of the next major cell type seen, the multinuclear foreign body giant cell (FBGC). This cell is up to 80 μm in diameter, is found primarily in foreign body or implant sites, and can be more aggressive and active than the neutrophil, eosinophil, or macrophage. Because of its larger size, it can phagocytize still larger particles. It has a relatively short life span

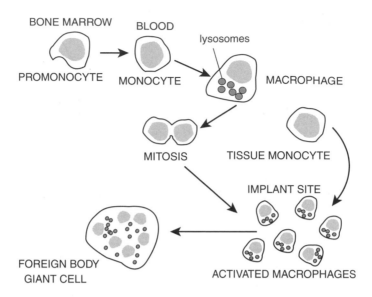

FIGURE 8.2
Development of the foreign body giant cell. Key: I = insult; CP = cellular proliferation; R = reorganization; C = chronic host response.

that is on the order of days. Thus, the presence of multinuclear giant cells long after implantation would suggest the presence of a chronic FB reaction. It is possible that macrophage fusion to form multinuclear giant cells is specifically stimulated by foreign bodies (Mariano and Spector 1974; Chambers 1977).

The presence and activity of phagocytic cells is particularly related to the presence of "small" particles. The relationship between size and stimulus is not understood, except in a general way. Maximum stimulus seems to occur when the average particle size is in the 0.1- to 1.0-µm range. Particles bigger than 50 µm do not excite a reaction greater than bulk materials, unless they possess a dimension in the size range previously indicated (for instance, long slender fibers). Large particles or even bulk implants may still activate phagocytic cells, resulting in external release of lysozymes and oxidative products. This process is often termed frustrated phagocytosis and may prevent the phagocytes from performing their normal functions. Smaller particles, especially less than 0.1 µm (<100 nm) in major dimension (variously termed microparticles or nanoparticles), tend to be phagocytozed in clumps or clusters in a manner termed pinocytosis by which immiscible liquids are taken up by phagocytic cells.

Although the intrinsic chemical activity* of phagocytozable particles does not seem to be primarily responsible for their cellular stimulatory effect, the

---

* Care must be taken in *in vitro* studies to avoid drawing erroneous conclusions due to particle surface contamination by endotoxin (Brooks et al. 2002) or other foreign materials that may affect behavior of phagocytes.

cellular response depends indirectly upon ease of degradation. If the particle is toxic to the ingesting cell and/or is expelled unchanged, the result may be massive accumulations of dying and dead neutrophils and macrophages. The resulting "pus" or cellular debris accumulation (caseation) resembles that which accompanies massive bacterial infection. Unsuccessful or successful phagocytosis is a mechanism for moving foreign particulate material away from the implant sites. Cells and cell fragments pass into the local lymphatic drainage system and may accumulate in local and regional lymph nodes. Small particles may accumulate in such nodes, as well as in remote organs such as liver and spleen (Urban et al. 2000), or be cleared into the lungs via the lymphatics and exhaled or swallowed (Styles and Wilson 1976).

In numbers and in temporal displacement of cell types, the progression described here reflects the increased threat that the intrusive agent represents. In parallel with this progression, an invasion of blood-borne lymphocytes occurs. These cells, which normally pass directly through the endothelial lining and are taken up by the lymphatic processes, will pass through the lymphatic nodes and eventually return to arterial circulation. Their function in inflammation is not well understood, and they are associated primarily with immunologic response (see Chapter 12). Their numbers do increase in areas of inflammation, and they are found associated with neutrophils and foreign particles in regional lymph nodes. It is possible that they respond to foreign proteins or to proteins denatured by foreign contact and have some ability to phagocytize particles. They may participate in fibroplasia, the final stage of inflammation.

8.2.4   Remodeling

Successful response to an inflammatory challenge will result in a locally decreased tissue mass. Dead cells have been phagocytized and removed by neutrophils and macrophages. Cells will be produced *in situ* by mitosis of the cell types present or by maturation of more primitive precursor or stem cells. This newly forming tissue is termed granulation tissue because of the pebbly specular appearance it has when seen growing at a free surface. The "pebbles" are vascular "buds" — capillary and arteriole loops that grow rapidly out from stable tissue into the disturbed area. They "burrow" through, bringing the benefits of improved circulation and stimulating cellular activity.

In addition, large amounts of muccopolysaccharides and collagen will be synthesized. The resulting tissue expansion is termed fibroplasia. These new tissue elements, forming the familiar scar, create a scaffold for cellular reconstruction and remodeling of the damaged area. The primary mediators of fibroplasia are fibroblasts, although *in vitro* studies suggest that a wide variety of cells can be stimulated to produce collagen and, to a lesser degree, muccopolysaccharides.

The remodeling of granulation tissue proceeds differently in different tissues. In skin, the reformation of tissue may be nearly complete, except for a possible absence of hair follicles and a small residual collageneous scar representing the collapsed remnant of the capsule that formed around the injury site. Bone has the ability to remodel completely to such a degree that it is said to regenerate. At the other extreme, articular (hyaline) cartilage never remodels but is repaired or replaced by formation of a loose tissue called fibrocartilage, which is different from normal cartilage in composition and structure and eventually deteriorates under repeated mechanical stress. Remodeling is also the primary mechanism involved in tissue adaptation (see Chapter 10).

8.2.5   Capsule Formation

The maturation of the scar tissue (in soft-tissue sites) marks the end of the process termed inflammation. The continuing presence of an implant prevents the collapse of the capsule that forms around the injured tissue and its maturation into a scar. The degree of scarring or capsule formation seen at later times depends upon the degree of original insult, the amount of subsequent cell death, and the location of the site.

Grading the host response at the implant site by a method such as that described in Appendix 1 and Appendix 2 in Chapter 18 actually evaluates the sum of two responses: the intrinsic inflammatory response to trauma and the host response to the implant. The response to trauma is relatively brief, passing through phases of insult, cellular proliferation, and reorganization in 1 to 2 weeks, as seen in the lower left of Figure 8.3. The host response to an implant is similar in its early phases, but then enters a chronic phase. The time required to enter the chronic phase or, in other words, achieve steady state, varies with the degree of host response elicited. Thus, although it may be safe to evaluate a low-reactivity implant after 3 to 4 weeks, one may not gain a true picture of the host response to a high-reactivity implant unless studies are extended to 6 or even 8 weeks after implantation.

Explorations of an implant site 4 or more weeks after implantation will usually reveal a relatively acellular fibrous capsule. This capsule is maintained by the continuing presence of the implant. In the absence of an implant (or after its removal or resorption), the capsule may contract or collapse into a residual scar or be completely remodeled, as described earlier. Spindle-shaped fibroblasts are usually associated with the capsule, and small numbers of macrophages may be found in the vicinity. The presence of neutrophils suggests the possibility of a continuing inflammatory challenge, including infection. Detection of multinuclear (foreign body) giant cells (FBGCs) suggests the production of small particles by corrosion, depolymerization, dissolution or wear, and a continuing general tissue response. Observation of large numbers of lymphocytes suggests the possibility of a specific immune response (see Chapter 12).

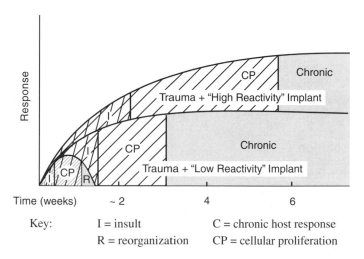

Time (weeks)   ~ 2   4   6

Key: I = insult   C = chronic host response
        R = reorganization   CP = cellular proliferation

FIGURE 8.3
Variations of local host response with implant "reactivity." Key: C = chemical mediation; M = mechanical mediation; E = electrical mediation; "?" = may be a mediating factor or may progress to resolution; ⊕ = enhances effect present without implant.

The thickness of the fibrous capsule is related to several factors. Materials that are chemically active, such as metals that corrode freely or polymers with leachable constituents, will mediate formation of a capsule whose thickness is directly proportional to the rate (and thus local concentration) of release of these small molecules. In addition to concentration, the chemical nature of the released material is important. It may be cytotoxic, inhibitory, or neutral. The combination of these factors may lead to specific capsular morphology at a histological and an ultrastructural level, which is characteristic of the particular material composition of the implant. These differences can only be fully appreciated when the responses to otherwise identical implants of different compositions are studied (McNamara and Williams 1982).

Mechanical factors are also important in mediating capsule formation. Capsule thickness is presumed to increase with increased relative motion between implant and tissue. In extreme cases, a fluid-filled bursa mimicking a synovial capsule may form; these bursae may be painful. The shape of the implant also affects the fibrous capsule thickness. The capsule will be thicker over edges and sharp changes in surface features. Thus, the capsule around a rectangular slab of reactive material will be dog-bone or club shaped. For this reason, the phenomenon is called clubbing (Wood et al. 1970).* Electrical currents, such as those emanating from an implanted stimulating electrode, also produce capsules whose thicknesses are related to current density. Because electrodes can also mediate changes in local pH and pO_2 as well as releasing corrosion products,** effects due to direct electrical (faradic) and indirect electrochemical (electrodic) stimulation may easily be confused.

---

* See Section 18.2.1 for a more complete discussion of this point.
** See Section 4.7.2 and Section 4.8.

In addition to depending upon tissue type, these general responses are species dependent and, in humans, may have age dependence. Furthermore, identification of intrinsic tissue response to an implant may be complicated by the presence of an overlying acute or chronic infection. Section 8.3 will take up the relationship between implants and infection as a special case of the inflammatory response to implant materials.

8.2.6   Resolution

When injury occurs to tissue, the overall aim of the process initiated is to produce a return to the status *quo ante,* a re-establishment of homeostasis. The presence of an implant in an operative site must, of necessity, prevent attainment of the original condition, but a steady state is possible in many cases. Reaching this condition is termed resolution. Figure 8.4 shows an overall schematic of the progression of the local host response from insult through resolution in the presence of an implant. The nature of the physical signals that mediate the local host response is still somewhat unclear; the symbols C, M, and E are used here to reflect the most likely situation. In particular circumstances, it is clear that these signals can interact in synergistic or antagonistic ways (Chesmel et al. 1995).

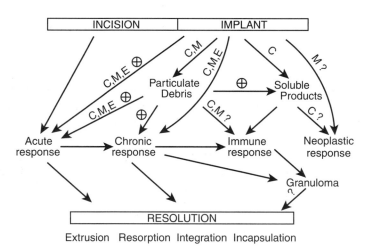

FIGURE 8.4
Schematic of development of local host response.

Four types of response are noted: acute, chronic, immune, and neoplastic. The first two usually reach resolution, the third may lead to a granuloma (a benign tumorous condition due to continued tissue elaboration without progressive remodeling), and the fourth does not resolve and always represents a failure of the implant. If resolution — that is, an achievement of a final state after which no more progressive biological changes occur — is a possibility, a distinction may be made among four possible outcomes:

- Extrusion: if the implant is in contact with epithelial tissue, the local host response will be the formation of a pocket or pouch continuous with the adjacent epithelial membrane. The process is termed marsupialization due to the similarity of the resulting structure to a kangaroo's pouch. In the case of the external epithelium (skin), this results in the effective externalization or extrusion of the implant from the host.

- Resorption: if the implant is resorbable, the implant site eventually resolves to a collapsed scar or, in the case of bone, may completely disappear.

- Integration: in a very limited number of cases, such as the implantation of pure titanium (Albrektsson et al. 1983) or tantalum (Aronson et al. 1977) in bone, a close, possibly adhesive, approximation of nearly normal host tissue to the implant is possible without an intervening capsule, although inflammatory cells may persist in small numbers. This special case of resolution is termed osseointegration (sometimes osteointegration).

- Incapsulization (the most usual response as previously described): if the implant is placed in a location where bone may form, such as within a medullary space, and integration does not take place, the capsule may become mineralized, in which case the structure is called a sequestrum.

In addition, it is possible with the passage of time for granulomas to resolve if the challenge presented by the implant changes or subsides.

Unlike the chronic granuloma and neoplastic transformation responses, whether each of these resolution outcomes represents success or failure of the implant depends on the circumstances — that is, upon the desired consequences of the insertion of the implant. This is the basic idea of biocompatibility, as discussed earlier: biological performance in a specific application that is judged suitable to that situation.

8.3   Infection

8.3.1   Types

A common phrase in research and clinical situations is "infected implant." This is a misnomer because the tissue surrounding the implant is infected rather than the implant. Infection is specifically the invasion and multiplication of microorganisms in tissue. However, the misuse of the term serves as a reminder of special problems that arise when bacterial infection is associated with an implant in animal experimentation or in human clinical practice. Immediate postoperative implant site infections were a considerable clinical problem in the 1960s and 1970s; incidence rates approached 5 to 10% in some series. Now, with a greater appreciation of the problem and better operating room techniques, rates are well below 1% for most permanent devices.

Three types of infection are associated with implants. The first, the superficial immediate infection, is due to the growth of organisms on the skin (or near it) in association with an implant. Examples of this include suture infections and growth of microorganisms under burn dressings. These infections can usually be traced to bacteria residing normally on human skin, such as *Staphylococcus aureus* or *Staphylococcus epidermidis,* or to airborne bacteria that are trapped and cultured in the moist conditions at the superficial site.

The second and third types are, collectively, deep infections. The second, the deep immediate infection, is the usual type of (now) low-frequency infection seen immediately after surgery. The bacteria responsible are usually skin-dwelling types, generally staphylococci, carried into the implant site during the surgical procedure. Less commonly, they are airborne types, and, even less frequently, bacteria already present, but relatively inactive, in the operative site. This last source reflects the physical disruption of tissue during surgery, resulting in the release of material in cysts or sequestered sites into areas where bacteria experience better growth conditions. Infections of this type, although extremely infrequent, may arise in patients with a previous history of infection in the operative site, such as a septic joint, or a systemic chronic infection. The common external origin of deep immediate infections is underlined by the well-known positive correlation between rate of infection and length of the surgical procedure.

Standard operating room environments contain 50 to 500 cfu/m^3 of bacteria (Antti–Poika et al. 1990). A colony-forming unit (cfu) is the minimum number of bacteria required to grow a cell cluster or colony on a suitable solid culture medium. Special precautions, including air-tight gowns and hoods for surgeons, body exhaust systems for operating room personnel, and control of air supply to cause laminar flow away from the patient, can reduce the level of airborne bacteria to as low as 1 to 5 cfu/m^3. Risk of clinical infection for similar operation duration is subsequently reduced.

The last of the three types, the late infection, has the most cryptic origin. This infection, of the nonsuperficial or deep type, may occur months to years after surgery in sites with no prior history of infection. Its cause is generally believed to be the transport and seeding of blood-borne bacteria from an established infection, such as a tooth-root abscess or a urinary tract infection, at a remote site. However, late infections that occur more than 1 month but less than 3 months after surgery are sometimes distinguished as delayed infections and ascribed to slow development of intraoperative bacterial contamination. Delayed and late infections represent a major problem in many procedures, such as total joint replacement or heart valve implantation. This is the case not because they are a frequent occurrence but because of the great difficulty encountered in treatment of the infection once it is established on and around the implant.

Whether infections become established in a site containing an implant has a great deal to do with the nature of the implant–tissue interface. Gristina (Gristina and Costerton 1984; Gristina 1987) has suggested that infection is a competition or "race for the surface" between bacteria and host cells, which, through encapzulization and resolution, produce the desired tissue integration. If the bacteria arrive first (before encapulization) or later, due to transient damage to the surrounding tissue, they can establish residence on the surface. Some bacteria, such as *Staphylococcus aureus* and *Staphylococcus epidermidis*, are said to be slime formers, in that they elaborate a muccoplysacchride film, termed glycocalyx, that protects them from outside influences such as phagocytic cells and diffusion of antibiotics.

Positive culture from carefully acquired specimens is proof of infection in an implant site in animals or patients. However, failure to obtain such positive results, even with multiple cultures, is not proof of the absence of infection because the culture conditions may have been inappropriate or each inoculum too small (containing less than 1 cfu). Even in the absence of clinical signs of frank infection, low-level or occult chronic infection may be present and unrecognized. In some cases, occult infection may be verified by the detection of bacterial DNA through the use of molecular multiplication techniques; however, such apparently positive results may be due to specimen contamination and should be interpreted with care.

8.3.2 Use of Antibiotic-Impregnated Implants

The advent of modern bacteriostatic and bactericidal antibiotics has suggested the possibility of utilizing them to suppress or prevent infection associated with implants. An obvious approach would be to design a diffusion-controlled delivery system that could be made part of the clinical implant or implanted as an adjunctive device.

A common form of late infection is that associated with the use of poly (methyl) methacrylate cements in total joint replacement; thus, a number of investigators have proposed that appropriate antibiotics could be mixed with

TABLE 8.1

Influence of Antibiotic in PMMA Cement on Immediate and Late
Infection in the Rat

			Results	
Group[a]	Number of Legs	Antibiotic (wt. %)	Infected (%)	Sterile (%)
A	60	—[b]	42 (70)	18 (30)
	42	1.25[b,c]	2 (5)	40 (95)
B	64	—[b]	11 (17)	53 (83)
	12	1.25[b,c]	1 (8)	11 (92)

[a] In group A, the injection (2.5×10^7 *Staphylococcus aureus*) was given 1/2 hour after closure of leg wound; in group B, it was delayed for 6 weeks. Plugs of cement and adjacent bone were cultured after 2 weeks.

[b] Palacos™ (Sulzer Bros., Bad Homberg, Germany).

[c] Gentamicin added (0.5 g/40 g PMMA).

Source: Adapted from Elson, R.A. et al., *J. Bone Joint Surg.*, 59B, 452, 1977.

the cement at insertion. Release by dissolution or diffusion could then be depended upon to maintain an inhibitory but decreasing antibiotic concentration in the vicinity of the joint replacement components and reduce the incidence of late infection. This technique has been used clinically for some time but can be criticized on three grounds:*

- It is difficult to be able to select the appropriate antibiotic because a range of bacteria with different sensitivities produces the late infection.

- The patient may develop an antibiotic sensitivity that would require the removal of the device to alleviate it.

- The antibiotic may not be able to penetrate all of the infectible tissue around the implant effectively.

Elson et al. (1977) performed an experiment that sheds some light on these concepts. Defects were created in rat tibiae; plugs of cement with and without antibiotic impregnation were inserted and allowed to cure in place before a bacterial inoculum was injected systematically within 1/2 hour of surgery (group A) or after a 6-week delay (group B) (Table 8.1).

The antibiotic-impregnated cement was highly effective ($\chi^2 = 48.55$, $p < 0.001$) in reducing immediate postoperative infection, but not to a statistically significantly extent by 6 weeks ($\chi^2 = 0.185$, n.s.). The latter comparison is complicated by the low incidence of infection in the animals receiving unimpregnated cement and the small size of the antibiotic-impregnated cement group at 6 weeks. Thus, the conclusion seems to be that the technique is effective if infection by a sensitive organism occurs immediately after the operation, but the effect on late infections is doubtful. This latter point is no

---

* PMMA bone cements with particular antibiotics added by the manufacturer are now widely available.

surprise because the diffusion release of antibiotic by cement must fall rapidly with time.*

Bone cement cured in place seems especially to permit local infection, but all implanted materials increase the risk of infection to some degree (Petty et al. 1985). The efficacy of antibiotic impregnation of bone cement in reducing or preventing immediate infection was verified in a more severe canine model using a direct infusion of *Staphylococcus aureus* into a bony site just before cement insertion (Petty et al. 1988). This principle has been extended to the use of precured antibiotic-impregnated PMMA "beads" (balls) (Blaha et al. 1990) or preforms in the shape of the removed device (Younger et al. 1997) as temporary implants to treat deep-seated infections. However, antibiotic-impregnated cement has clearly been seen to be a failure in preventing late infection in more realistic models such as a clinically functional total knee replacement in the rabbit subjected to a systemic bacteremia 6 to 8 weeks after implantation (Blomgren 1981).

This last point attracts attention to the question of associations between implants and infection. Bacterial growth in the presence of implants is tenacious and difficult to deal with. Some bacteria undergo a transformation of behavior and increase their activity and pathogenicity. Conventional treatments for bacterial infections that may be successful in nonsurgical cases often have reduced efficacy or fail in the presence of implants.

The difficulty of treatment often leads to the removal of the implant and the need to delay reimplantation until after the infection is successfully suppressed. This is possible in some cases as total hip replacement, but not in others as mitral (heart) valve replacement. Thus, "infection" constitutes a major source of implant "failure," despite the inability of an implant to become infected. A final concern is that the chronic use of antibiotics in treatment of patients and in decontamination of hospital facilities has led to the emergence of ever more resistant and virulent strains of microorganisms. Thus, although the incidence of implant infection can be expected to continue to fall, the problems raised by each case may well become more difficult, especially as the practice of combining antibiotics with implants to form combination products increases in popularity. More benign approaches may be introduction of molecular species that may interfere with bacterial adhesion and formation and/or properties of the glycocalyx (Trampuz et al. 2003).

8.3.3 Geometric Factors

Geometric factors are extremely important to the consideration of interactions between implants and infecting microorganisms. Initiation (seeding or colonization) and propagation of infection constitute a competitive process

---

* The result of studies such as Elson et al. (1977) has been the growing contemporary use of antibiotic-containing PMMA formulations in primary joint replacement procedures, even in the absence of known (proven) infection. The long-term consequences of such practice are still unknown.

pitting the ability of the invading bacteria to replicate against the ability of the host tissues and support cells to annihilate. This competition defines the size of the cfu for each microorganism. Therefore, the exposure of the bacteria to tissue and, especially, vascular processes is a critical factor in successful host defense against infection.

As has been shown, tissue immediately adjacent to an implant is relatively acellular at maturity. Bacteria that can grow within the capsular membrane will encounter little active opposition until they break out into the surrounding tissues. In addition to general and specific immune responses, the immediate response to infection is the inflammatory response. The cells that mediate the response are blood borne. Thus, the reduction of the solid angle of surrounding tissue near an implant takes on extreme importance; it reduces the accessibility of the infected tissue near an implant to neutrophils and macrophages.

The existence of a "dead space," a volume filled with cell-free fluid rather than tissue, represents a special hazard of the geometric type. Design and implantation practices should try to avoid such features because this fluid can act as an *in vivo* culture medium for bacteria. Even in the absence of an acellular membrane and/or a dead space, as previously noted, some bacteria can produce their geometric defense by forming a glycocalyx about them on the surface of the implant.

Although porous bodies represent no particular structural hazard when viewed from the aspect of carcinogenesis (see Chapter 13), they might be expected to present a geometric hazard in the initiation and/or support of infection. Kiechel et al. (1977) have studied the influence of porosity in poly(methyl) methacrylate implants in rabbits on the propagation of an aerobic infection by *Staphylococcus aureus* and its treatment by penicillin. Using a muscle site (corresponding to an immediate deep infection), they concluded that there was no effect on the inoculum size needed to initiate infection or on the response of established infection to penicillin. Whether the outcome would have been different in the case of a late infection or an infection due to an anaerobic bacterium cannot be determined from this experiment.

A somewhat more sophisticated repetition of this study (Merritt et al. 1979) reached a somewhat different set of conclusions. Using a variety of porous and dense implant materials, but the same microorganism, and comparing the effects of immediate (at implantation) injection of an inoculum to an inoculation after a 1-month delay, this later study concluded that porosity had an effect on infection rates. In the immediate injection (acute) group, the infection rate for porous materials was higher, and in the 1-month delay (chronic) group, the infection rate for dense materials was higher. The authors suggested that these findings support the hypothesis that bacteria can evade host defense mechanisms if they enter the pores of an implant before tissue invasion; but once the implant is invaded by host tissue, the bacteria are more exposed to cellular attack.

However, these conclusions are drawn from a comparison of porous polyethylene and dense alumina ceramic and devolve from relatively small experimental groups. Furthermore, as the authors advance it, the hypothesis can explain the acute results but not the chronic results. Thus, the question is still open to debate. Using a slightly different model, Cordero et al. (1994) reproduced this result for immediate (intraoperative) infection and further were able to distinguish CoCrMo implant sites as more easily infectable (requiring fewer cfus) by *Staphylococcus aureus* than sites with pure titanium implants of identical configuration, probably reflecting differences in corrosion products. A study of the outcome of porous percutaneous carbon implants in rabbits for up to 4 years (Krouskop et al. 1988) further supports the view that implant porosity, if not immediately colonized by bacteria, represents no long-term hazard for infection.

The clinical practice of removing the "infected implant" is based most directly on geometric arguments and on their physiological consequences. Two other types of arguments can be proposed: one based upon chemically mediated interactions between the implant and the bacterial infection and the other based upon chemical effects on the cell populations in the host that act against infection. Both of these are controversial today.

It is thought that if implants can provide metals valuable to metabolism (see Section 14.1) through the corrosion of metallic parts, then they can also be shown to participate in bacterial metabolism. Thus, the view is that metallic implantation is similar in effect to putting fertilizer on a garden. However, one metal — iron — occupies a special position. Iron levels in the body are evidently subject to active control and change rapidly in response to infection (see Chapter 14). It has been suggested that the interference of endogenous iron sources with this control system plays a role in the propagation of certain infections (Weinberg 1974).

8.4 Effects of Implant Degradation Products

8.4.1 Effects on Phagocytosis

One comes then to a consideration of the effects of implants, primarily metals, on the cellular elements of the host defense system. There are many possible mechanisms for such effects but this chapter will focus on one: alteration of phagocytic function. Phagocytic cells play key roles in inflammatory response, as previously discussed. Several studies that explore various aspects of reduction of phagocytic function through a variety of animal models will be considered.

Graham et al. (1975) were interested in determining whether the inhalation of metallic particles from industrial pollution would reduce the number or the activity of lung macrophages. They used cultured rabbit alveolar

TABLE 8.2

Effects of Trace Metals (as Ions) on Alveolar Macrophages

	VO_3^-	Cr^{+3}	Mn^{+3}	Ni^{+2}	Ni^{+2}	Ni^{+2}
Ion concentration (M) (ppm):	7×10^{-5}	3×10^{-3}	2×10^{-3}	5×10^{-4}	8×10^{-4}	1×10^{-3}
	6.9	156	110	29	47	59
Phagocytic index (%)	100	70	75	50	20	13
Cell survival (%)	79	84	69	92	85	76
Phagocytic efficiency (%)	79	59	52	46	17	10

Notes: The phagocytic index is the percentage of living cells that contain one or more latex spheres after a 1-hour exposure at a ratio of 120 spheres/cell. Phagocytic efficiency = phagocytic index × cell survival.

Source: Original data from Graham, J.A. et al., *Infect. Immunol.*, 11, 1278, 1975.

macrophages, which were challenged by a 1-day incubation in the presence of metallic salts of various types, and examined the ability of the survivors to phagocytize 1.1-μm-diameter latex spheres. For the metals of interest in implant applications, they obtained the data shown in Table 8.2.

Each of the metal ions in this table exhibited cytotoxic effects at the tested concentrations. All but vanadate also produced a reduction in phagocytotic behavior, generally independent of the cytotoxic effect. In the case of nickel, in which three concentrations were employed, the sign of both effects were the same, but the reduction of phagocytosis was more extreme. Note that the true *in vivo* effect would depend upon the product of the cell survival index and the phagocytic index, here called the phagocytic efficiency. Thus, for nickel, an increase of concentration by a factor of ~2 (from 29 to 58 ppm) produces a depression of macrophage effect of 78%.

The authors point out that the ion concentrations used were one to two orders of magnitude below those found in human lung tissue obtained in highly polluted industrial environments. However, this comment is based upon comparison to average tissue concentrations; in Chapter 14, it will be seen that concentrations immediately adjacent to corroding implants may be two to three orders of magnitude higher than average values. Thus, the concentrations used by Graham et al. are relevant. They also report a study showing a positive correlation between metal aerosol inhalation in mice and susceptibility to infection, as well as studies in human populations showing positive correlations between metal dust inhalation and respiratory infection rate.

Rae (1975) has pursued this issue further. He incubated mouse macrophages with finely divided implant alloys and pure metals and examined the activity of two enzyme systems:

- Lactic dehydrogenase (LDH) is an enzyme normally contained wholly within cells. Thus, its detection is a measure of the leakiness of, or damage to, cell membranes.

- Glucose-6-phosphate dehydrogenase (G6PD) is an enzyme required for synthetic processes and must be present for phagocytosis to take place. Thus, its reduction signals a reduction in the phagocytotic ability of cells.

Cobalt and nickel particles were found to be cytotoxic. At the concentrations obtained in this study, no cytotoxic effect was observed for chromium or molybdenum. Nickel, cobalt, and cobalt–chromium alloy particles were found to reduce the phagocytic ability of the surviving macrophages significantly (as measured by G6PD activity).

The mechanisms of these two effects, cell death and reduction of phagocytotic ability, are unclear. In particular, they interacted in Rae's experiment, and an effect of particle size was displayed; smaller particles were at the same time more frequently phagocytocized and more toxic.

A study by Ward et al. (1975) suggests that a wide variety of effects exist that are not closely related. This view supports the results of the previous two studies. The authors studied a wide variety of metallic salts and their effects on neutrophil chemotaxis and on the incorporation of amino acids into neutrophils and fibroblasts. Rabbit neutrophils, HeLa (a human cancer cell line), and human gingival fibroblasts were used. An *Escherichia coli* filtrate was used as a neutrophil challenge to study chemotaxis by neutrophils. Incorporation inhibition (a reduction in phagocytic efficiency) was shown for a variety of metal salts; however, the antichemotaxis results are of more interest here. An extract of the results of these studies is given in Table 8.3.

The authors discuss these chemical agents primarily as anti-inflammatory agents. It is interesting to note that these data do not support either of the two previous studies. This disagreement stems from several origins:

- Chemotaxis is only one factor in phagocytosis.
- Rae's study associated a small effect (reduction in phagocytic efficiency) of chromium and molybdenum with low solubility of metallic particles; this study bypassed the problem by using soluble salts.
- Graham's study utilized a passive challenge to the macrophage rather than one of biological origin.

TABLE 8.3

Chemotaxis Inhibition by Metallic Ions

		Cr^{+3}	Mn^{+3}	$Fe^{+2,+3}$	W^{+4}	Mo^{+4}	Co^{+2}
Ion concentration for 50%	M:	3×10^{-4}	5×10^{-3}	10^{-3}	10^{-3}	10^{-3}	10^{-3}
inhibition of chemotaxis	ppm:	16	27	56	18	96	59

Source: Data extracted from Ward, P.A. et al. *J. Reticuloendothel. Soc.*, 18, 313, 1975.

Using a bacterially derived chemoattractant with human neutrophils, Remes and Williams (1990) concluded that Cr^{+3} (2.5 ppm) (56% inhibition), Co^{+2} (≥20 ppm) (100%), and Ni^{+2} (≥30 ppm) (50%) all actively interfered with chemotaxis. The greater apparent sensitivity to chromium and cobalt than seen in Graham's study may reflect differences in experimental technique, challenge agent, and/or cell source and underline the difficulties inherent in such.

8.4.2   Effects of Phagocytosis

Section 8.2.3 considered the process of phagocytosis as carried forward by macrophages and foreign body giant cells. This is a normal process existing in all tissues, primarily for the removal of dead cells, cellular debris, and damaged tissue matrix, as well as to aid in defense against infection. In the majority of these situations, phagocytosis, digestion, and/or transport and excretion are successful. However, as previously noted, excessive amounts of foreign material or debris too large for phagocytosis or cytoxic materials result in abnormal cellular behavior.

Willert (Willert and Semlitsch 1977) was the first to suggest that abnormal response to small particles might play a role in the modification of interfaces between implants and surrounding tissue, particularly in the case of joint replacement components secured to bone with poly (methyl) methacrylate "bone cement." Patients with such devices often show a localized or progressive loss of bone adjacent to the bone–bone cement interface. This interface often contains wear debris with associated cells in a fibrous membrane, perhaps 100 μm in thickness; in some cases this may resemble the synovial membrane found in normal articular joints.

Willert suggested that although small amounts of indigestible debris could be stored locally or transported away through the lymphatic drainage, large amounts overwhelmed the normal process and produced a histiocytic granulation tissue with accompanying fibrosis, due to attempts to encapsulate and isolate the reaction. He suggested that these tissues interfere with motion of the joint and invade the interface between the implant and bone, producing progressive tissue loss through necrosis and attempts at remodeling.

This phenomenon — previously called cement disease or polyethylene disease, but now most generally small particle disease — is currently understood as shown in Figure 8.5. Macrophages and tissue monocytes ingest foreign particles and, in the process of being activated, release a variety of organic molecules collectively called cytokines (Masui et al. 2005). Cytokines are naturally occurring molecules used by cells to communicate with each other, particularly to regulate stages in processes in which many cell types are involved. For instance, the invasion of capillaries during formation of granulation tissue is stimulated by a group of cytokines called AGFs or angiogenic growth factors that are released by a variety of other cells.

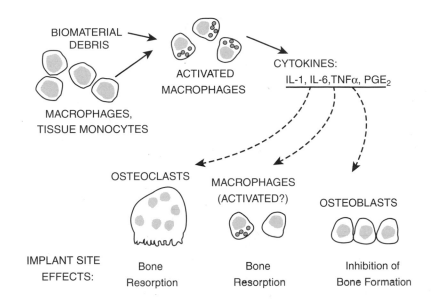

FIGURE 8.5

Small particle disease. (Adapted from Willert, H.-G. and Semlitsch, M., *J. Biomed. Mater. Res.*, 11, 157, 1977; Howie, D.W. et al., *Orthop. Clin. N. Am.*, 24(4), 571, 1993.)

Although more than 40 human cytokines are known, only a few have been so far implicated in small particle disease. Principal among these are several interleukins (IL-1 and IL-6), tumor necrosis factor (TNF), and prostaglandin E_2 (PGE$_2$). Each cytokine may have numerous effects on cell activity, depending upon the exact nature of the cytokine (many cytokines have variants, such as IL-1α, IL-1β, etc.), the concentration in tissue, the presence of other cytokines, and the nature of the target cell. Thus, research in this area, which is extremely active in the biomaterials field as well as the general medical and biological community, is remarkably complex and, to a great degree, opaque to nonspecialists.

The primary effect in the presence of small particles appears to be the production of one or more cytokines that stimulate large phagocytic cells called osteoclasts to resorb (remove) bone (Teitelbaum 2000). Osteoclasts are present on bone surfaces throughout the skeleton of mammals and the amount of bone present is due, in part, to the balance between bone resorption by osteoclasts and bone formation by osteoblasts. Increase in osteoclastic activity stimulated by cytokines released by phagocytes, without an accompanying increase in osteoblastic activity, results in overall bone loss, with subsequent loss of integrity of the implant–bone interface, loosening, pain, and the eventual need for surgical intervention. The actual process is far more complex: macrophages (which may not have been previously activated) may resorb bone directly; osteoblastic activity may be suppressed and cells at the bone–implant interface also produce and release cytokines, affecting each other's actions. Finally, because tissue necrosis may occur, depending on the nature and composition of the foreign material, the normal events of the inflammatory process (Section 8.2) may also occur, superimposed on the increased osteoclastic activity and its consequences.

As a result of these complex and inter-related effects, small particle disease is still poorly understood and efforts to prevent or treat it in animal models and patients are still in their very early stages (Goodman et al. 2005).

8.5   A Final Comment

In the first edition of this work, I emphasized that the effects of apparent chemical interactions between implant and bacteria and implant and host cells were at that time highly speculative and based almost completely on *in vitro* studies. Similar mistakes were being made in the study of the clinical consequences of particulate phagocytosis (small particle disease). *In vitro* studies lack the humeral, metabolic, catabolic, and excretory influences seen in whole-animal experiments. Most animal models are also incomplete, in that they fail to reproduce key aspects of actual clinical implant composition and structure and rely, in large part, on single or repeated (divided) doses, rather than on continual infusion or release. I had further pointed out that many critical experiments remained to be done before any of these supposed effects could be established or disproved.

Unfortunately, the situation remains much the same today, if not more confused due to the growing awareness of the role of physical and electrical factors mediating cell behavior. These chemical, physical, and electrical factors may act separately or in concert in synergistic or antagonistic manners. Until studies use appropriate animal models and forms of implant materials, as well as control chemical, physical, and electrical aspects of the biomaterials under study in single experiments, much smoke and heat will be produced but little light shed on key issues of local host response to implants in patients.

References

Albrektsson, T. et al., The interface zone of inorganic implants *in vivo*: titanium implants in bone, *Ann. Biomed. Eng.*, 11, 1, 1983.

Anderson, J.M. and Miller, K.M., Biomaterial biocompatibility and the macrophage, *Biomaterials*, 5, 5, 1984.

Antti–Poika, I. et al., Hip arthroplasty infection, *Acta Orthop. Scand.*, 61, 163, 1990.

Aronson, A.S., Hansson, L.I. and Selvik, G., Roentgen stereophotogrammetry for determination of bone growth. Comparison with the tetracycline method, *Acta Radiol. Diagn. (Stockh.)*, 18, 87, 1977.

Blaha, J.D. et al., The use of Septopal (polymethylmethacrylate beads with gentamicin) in the treatment of chronic osteomyelitis, *Instruct. Course Lect.*, 39, 509, 1990.

Blomgren, G., Hematogenous infection of total joint replacement, *Acta Orthop. Scand.*, 52(Suppl. 187), 1, 1981.

Brooks, R.A., Wimhurst, J.A. and Rushton, N., Endotoxin contamination of particles produces misleading inflammatory cytokine responses from macrophages *in vitro*, *J. Bone Joint Surg.*, 84B, 295, 2002.

Chambers, T.J., Fusion of macrophages following simultaneous attempted phagocytosis of glutaraldehyde-fixed red blood cells, *J. Pathol.*, 122, 71, 1977.

Chesmel, K.D. et al., Cellular response to chemical and morphological aspects of biomaterial surfaces: II. The biosynthetic and migratory response of bone cell populations, *J. Biomed. Mater. Res.*, 29, 1101, 1995.

Cordero, J., Munuera, L. and Folgueira, M.D., Influence of metal implants on infection, *J. Bone Joint Surg.*, 76B, 717, 1994.

Elson, R.A. et al., Bacterial infection and acrylic cement in the rat, *J. Bone Joint Surg.*, 59B, 452, 1977.

Frank, M.M., The complement system in host defense and inflammation, *Rev. Infect. Dis.*, 1, 483, 1979.

Goodman, S.B. et al., Pharmacologic modulation of periprosthetic osteolysis, *Clin. Orthop. Rel. Res.*, 430, 39, 2005.

Graham, J.A. et al., Effect of trace metals on phagocytosis by alveolar macrophages, *Infect. Immunol.*, 11, 1278, 1975.

Gristina, A.G., Adhesive colonization of biomaterials and antibiotic resistance, *Science*, 237, 1588, 1987.

Gristina, A.G. and Costerton, J.W., Bacterial adherence and the glycocalyx and their role in musculoskeletal infection, *Ortho. Clin. N. Am.*, 15, 517, 1984.

Howie, D.W. et al., The response to particulate debris, *Orthop. Clin. N. Am.*, 24(4), 571, 1993.

Kiechel, S.F. et al., The role of implant porosity on the development of infection, *Surg. Gynecol. Obstet.*, 144, 58, 1977.

Krouskop, T.A. et al., Bacterial challenge study of a porous carbon percutaneous implant, *Biomaterials*, 9, 398, 1988.

Mariano, M. and Spector, W.G., The formation and properties of macrophage polykaryons (inflammatory giant cells), *J. Pathol.*, 113, 1, 1974.

Masui, T., Expression of inflammatory cytokines, RANKL and OPG induced by titanium, cobalt–chromium and polyethylene particles, *Biomaterials*, 26, 1695, 2005.

McNamara, A. and Williams, D.F., Scanning electron microscopy of the metal-tissue interface. I. Fixation methods and interpretation of results, *Biomaterials*, 3, 160, 1982.

Merritt, K., Shafer, J.W. and Brown, S.A., Implant site infection rates with porous and dense materials, *J. Biomed. Mater. Res.*, 13, 101, 1979.

Petty, W. et al., The influence of skeletal implants on incidence of infection, *J. Bone Joint Surg.*, 67A, 1236, 1985.

Petty, W., Spanier, S. and Shuster, J.J., Prevention of infection after total joint replacement, *J. Bone Joint Surg.*, 70A, 536, 1988.

Rae, T., A study on the effects of particulate metals of orthopedic interest on murine macrophages *in vitro*, *J. Bone Joint Surg.*, 57B, 444, 1975.

Remes, A. and Williams, D.F., Chemotaxis and the inhibition of chemotaxis of human neutrophils in response to metal ions, *J. Mater. Sci.: Mater. Med.*, 1, 26, 1990.

Styles, J.A. and Wilson, J., Comparison between *in vitro* toxicity of two novel fibrous mineral dusts and their tissue reactions *in vivo*, *Ann. Occup. Hyg.*, 19, 63, 1976.

Teitelbaum, S.L., Bone resorption by osteoclasts, *Science*, 289, 1504, 2000.

Trampuz, A. et al., Molecular and antibiofilm approaches to prosthetic joint infection, *Clin. Orthop. Rel. Res.*, 414, 69, 2003.

Urban, R.M. et al., Dissemination of wear particles to the liver, spleen, and abdominal lymph nodes of patients with hip or knee replacement, *J. Bone Joint Surg.*, 82(4), 457, 2000.

Ward, P.A., Goldschmidt, P. and Greene, N.D., Suppressive effects of metal salts on leukocyte and fibroblastic function, *J. Reticuloendothel. Soc.*, 18, 313, 1975.

Weinberg, E.D., Iron and susceptibility to infectious disease, *Science*, 184, 952, 1974.

Willert, H.-G. and Semlitsch, M., Reactions of the articular capsule to wear products of artificial joint prostheses, *J. Biomed. Mater. Res.*, 11, 157, 1977.

Wood, N.K., Kaminski, E.J. and Oglesby, R.J., The significance of implant shape in experimental testing of biological materials: disc vs. rod, *J. Biomed. Mater. Res.*, 4, 1, 1970.

Younger, A.S. et al., The outcome of two-stage arthroplasty using a custom-made interval spacer to treat the infected hip, *J. Arthoplasty*, 12(6), 615, 1997.

Ziats, N.P., Miller, K.M. and Anderson, J.M., *In vitro* and *in vivo* interactions of cells with biomaterials, *Biomaterials*, 9, 5, 1988.

Bibliography

Aderem, A., How to eat something bigger than your head, *Cell*, 110, 5, 2002.

Bauer, T.W., Particles and peri-implant bone resorption, *Clin. Orthop. Rel. Res.*, 405, 138, 2002.

Berry C.L. (Ed.), *The Pathology of Devices*, Springer–Verlag, Berlin, 1994.

Bisno, A.L. and Waldvogel, F.A., *Infections Associated with Indwelling Medical Devices*, American Society of Microbiologists, Washington, D.C., 1989.

Brandwood, A. et al., Phagocytosis of carbon particles by macrophages *in vitro*, *Biomatials*, 13, 646, 1992.

Cameron, H.U. (Ed.), *Bone Implant Interface*, Mosby-Year Book, St. Louis, 1994.

Chang, C.C. and Merritt, K., Infection at the site of implanted materials with and without preadhered bacteria, *J. Orthop. Res.*, 12, 526, 1994.

Coleman, D.L., King, R.N. and Andrade, J.D., The foreign body reaction: a chronic inflammatory response, *J. Biomed. Mater. Res.*, 8, 199, 1974.

Costerton, J.W. et al., Microbial biofilms, *Annu. Rev. Microbiol.*, 49, 711, 1995.

Craig, M.R. et al., A novel total knee arthroplasty infection model in rabbits, *J. Orthop. Res.*, 23(5), 1100, 2005.

Duffield, J.S., The inflammatory macrophage: a story of Jekyll and Hyde, *Clin. Sci.*, 104, 27, 2003.

Delle Valle, C.J., Zuckerman, J.D. and Di Cesare, P.E., Periprosthetic sepsis, *Clin. Orthop. Rel. Res.*, 420, 26, 2004.

Ellingsen, J.F. and Lyngstadaas, S.P., *Bio-implant Interface: Improving Biomaterials and Tissue Reactions*, CRC Press, Boca Raton, 2003.

Esterhai, J.L., Jr., Gristina, A.G. and Poss, R. (Eds.), *Musculoskeletal Infections*, American Academy of Orthopedic Surgeons, Park Ridge, IL, 1992, 153–300.

Gatti, A.M., Biocompatibility of micro- and nanoparticles in the colon, *Biomaterials*, 25, 385, 2004.

Greco, R.S. (Ed.), *Implantation Biology. The Host Response and Biomedical Devices*, CRC Press, Boca Raton, FL, 1994.

Heggeness, M.H. et al., Late infection of spinal instrumentation by hematogenous seeding, *Spine*, 18, 492, 1993.

Hunt, J.A., Remes, A. and Williams, D.F., Stimulation of neutrophil movement by metal ions, *J. Biomed. Mater. Res.*, 26, 819, 1992.

Ingham, E. and Fisher, J., Biological reactions to wear debris in total joint replacement, *Proc. Inst. Mech. Eng., Part H*, 214, 21, 2000.

Inghram, J.H. et al., The influence of molecular weight, crosslinking, and counterface roughness on TNF-alpha production by macrophages in response to ultra high molecular weight polyethylene particles, *Biomaterials*, 25, 3511, 2004.

Ito, A. et al., *In-vitro* analysis of metallic particles, colloidal nanoparticles, and ions in wear-corosion products of SUS317L stainless steel, *Mater. Sci. Eng.*, C17, 161, 2001.

Kawaguchi, H. et al., Phagocytosis of latex particles by leucocytes. I. Dependence of phagocytosis on the size and surface potential of particles, *Biomaterials*, 7, 61, 1986.

Leibovich, S.J. and Ross, R., The role of the macrophage in wound repair, *Am. J. Pathol.*, 78, 71, 1975.

Maloney, W.J. et al., Isolation and characterization of wear particles generated in patients who have had failure of a hip arthroplasty without cement, *J. Bone Joint Surg.*, 77A, 1301, 1995.

Merritt, K., Role of medical materials, both in implant and surface applications, in immune response and in resistance to infection, *Biomaterials*, 5, 47, 1984.

Nagase, M., Host reactions to particulate biomaterials, in *Encyclopedic Handbook of Biomaterials and Bioengineering, Part A: Materials*, Vol. 1, Wise, D.L. et al. (Eds.), Marcel Dekker, New York, 1995, 269.

Peters, K. et al., Effects of nanoscaled particles on endothelial cell function *in vitro*: studies on viability, proliferation, and inflammation, *J. Mater. Sci.: Mater. Med.*, 15, 321, 2004.

Rae, T., Cell biochemistry in relation to the inflammatory response to foreign materials, in *Fundamental Aspects of Biocompatibility*, Vol. 1, Williams, D.F. (Ed.), CRC Press, Boca Raton, FL, 1981, 159.

Rae, T., Localized tissue infection and the influence of foreign bodies, in *Fundamental Aspects of Biocompatibility*, Vol. 2, Williams, D.F. (Ed.), CRC Press, Boca Raton, FL, 1981, 139.

Revell, P.A., *Pathology of Bone*, Springer–Verlag, Berlin, 1986, 217–223.

Rimondini, L., Fini, M. and Giardino, R., The microbial infection of biomaterials: A challenge for clinicians and researchers, *J. Appl. Biomater. Biomech.*, 3(1), 1, 2005.

Sanzén, L. and Linder, L., Infection adjacent to titanium and bone cement implants: an experimental study in rabbits, *Biomaterials*, 16, 1273, 1995.

Schoen, F.J., *Interventional and Surgical Cardiovascular Pathology: Clinical Correlations and Basic Principles*, W.B. Saunders, Philadelphia, 1989.

Sethi, R.K. et al., Macrophage response to cross-linked and conventional UHMWPE, *Biomaterials*, 24, 2561, 2003.

Spector, W.G. and Wynne, K.M., Proliferation of macrophages in inflammation, *Agents Actions*, 6, 123, 1976.

Sugarman, B. and Young, E.J. (Eds.), *Infections Associated with Prosthetic Devices*, CRC Press, Boca Raton, FL, 1984.

Trowbridge, H.O. and Emling, R.C., *Inflammation: A Review of the Process*, 5th ed., Quintessence Pub., Carol Stream, IL, 1997.

Vogler, E.A., Water and the acute biological response to surfaces, *J. Biomater. Sci. Polymer Edn.*, 10(10), 1015, 1999.

Williams, D.F., Tissue–biomaterial interactions, *J. Mater. Sci.*, 22, 3421, 1987.

Yamamoto, A. et al., Cytoxicity evaluation of ceramic particles of different sizes and shapes, *J. Biomed. Mater. Res.*, 68A, 244, 2004.

9

Coagulation and Hemolysis

9.1 Introduction

In the previous chapter, inflammation was presented as a nonspecific response to tissue damage. This chapter will consider responses to two more specific events involving the circulatory system and its tributaries:

- Damage to blood carrying vessels and/or contact with foreign materials leading to coagulation
- Damage to the tissue of blood, leading most generally to cellular destruction or hemolysis

9.2 The Coagulation Cascade

9.2.1 Intrinsic Pathway

The coagulation cascade may be thought of as a biological amplifier that permits an initiating event to be magnified into a process sufficiently widespread to produce local homeostasis, prevents further loss of blood (if the vascular process has been breached), and permits repair of the damaged tissue. The overall process is referred to as coagulation or thrombosis and the resulting hemostatic plug is termed a thrombus. If damage to the wall of a blood vessel (endothelium) is the initiation factor, then coagulation proceeds by an intrinsic pathway.

In this case, the first two events closely parallel those of inflammation. In fact, they are essentially those of the inflammatory process. Initially, the smooth muscle in the vessel wall dilates and then constricts, probably stimulated by activated factor XII (also called Hageman factor) (see Figure 9.1). Although this is formally the first step in the intrinsic pathway, it is preceded by surface contact (and denaturation) of other molecules, including kininogen and prekallikrein. Endothelial permeation also increases but is masked

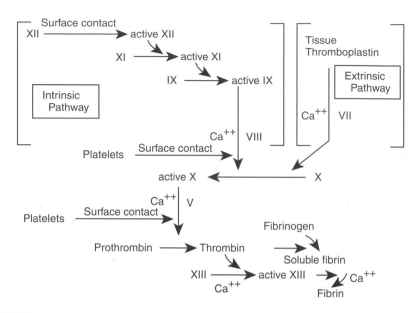

FIGURE 9.1

The coagulation cascade. (Adapted from Salzman, E.W., in *The Chemistry of Biosurfaces*, Vol. II. Hair, M.L., Ed., Marcel Dekker, New York, 1972, 489.)

by the release of serum and blood-borne cells if the vessel wall is ruptured. In addition, the endothelial lining becomes sticky.

The combination of the presence of activated factor XII and the sticky quality of the endothelial lining triggers the first step unique to coagulation, the adhesion and aggregation of platelets. Adhered platelets rapidly lyse (undergo membrane rupture) through mechanical and biochemical paths, releasing adenosine diphosphate (ADP), serotonin, and epinephrine. ADP encourages further platelet adhesion, and the latter two agents cause vasoconstriction. The combination of these agents rapidly produces a platelet "plug" that serves to staunch further blood loss from the area.

Activation of factor XII and platelet adhesion trigger a complex chain of events leading to transformation of inactive fibrinogen into an active molecule, fibrin. This transformation, accompanied by a shrinking or retraction of the platelet plug, produces a mature clot, a mesh of polymerized fibrin strands trapping leukocytes, erythrocytes, and platelet fragments. Within minutes to hours this clot is invaded by the same series of cells seen in pure inflammation and then later is perfused by numerous new capillaries. Eventually, the clot is removed and replaced by fibrous scar and remodeled tissue.

9.2.2   Extrinsic Pathway

The intrinsic pathway to coagulation, as previously described, depends upon interaction of normal blood components (macromolecules, cells, platelets, etc.) after alteration by an initiation event, usually surface contact. An alternate initial coagulation pathway, the extrinsic pathway, involves release of materials from cells external to the vascular processes. The released material is termed tissue thromboplastin. This is a protein–phospholipid complex derived from normal cell contents (otherwise termed factor III) that, with factor VII and Ca^{++}, activates factor X (Figure 9.1). The intrinsic and extrinsic coagulation pathways merge in this common event leading to the terminal event of fibrin production and clot formation.

9.2.3   Implant-Induced Coagulation*

The events of the intrinsic pathway are triggered, as previously stated, by contact between blood elements and a surface. The normal endothelial lining of blood vessels is not able, fortunately, to induce this response. Damage to the endothelium may expose collagen, its major structural molecule. Normally, collagen is rendered nonthrombotic (not able to induce coagulation) by a covering of a family of macromolecules, glycopolysaccharides. This coating is electropositive, which attracts a layer of neutralizing negative ions and thus repels the negatively charged erythrocytes and platelets. Exposed collagen is electronegative, and thus highly thrombotic. This property is utilized in surgery when powdered crystalline collagen may be used as a topical hemostatic agent on highly vascular tissues in which electrocauterization and/or ligation are not possible — for example, the liver.

The intrinsic pathway may also be triggered by contact with a foreign body** (such as an implant) and the resulting events are quite similar. In this case, however, the implant persists after the initial insult. This difference from the case of isolated vessel wall damage has several possible consequences (Figure 9.2):

- Blood-borne proteins retaining native structure may coat the surface and prevent activation of factor XII or adhesion of platelets. Such a surface would have a high degree of hemocompatibility.

- Even if platelet adhesion occurs, it may not be accompanied by sufficiently rapid lysis to promote further progression of the cascade. Such a surface would not actively form a thrombus. However, it would deplete the circulating blood of platelets and thus might reduce the coagulatibility of the host. Such an effect is common in chronic (repeated) hemodialysis, or intraoperatively when an *ex vivo* blood oxygenator is used. Brash (Skarja et al. 1997) has developed

---

* See Banerjee et al. (1997) for a review of the interaction between blood and biomaterials.
** We speak here of contact with the surface of a "foreign body"; however, the surface of an implant so rapidly becomes coated with serum proteins and coagulation factors that it is better to think of the foreign body contact effect as mediated by surface adhered and denatured organic molecules. See Vroman (1971) and Chapter 5, particularly Section 5.5.

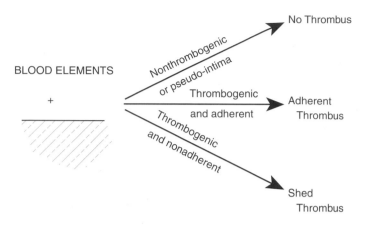

FIGURE 9.2
Interaction of implants with blood elements.

an *in vitro* test for quantification of platelet adhesion under flow conditions (see Section 17.4.3).

- A thrombus may form but be rapidly removed by blood dynamic forces. Such an implant will "shed" emboli and cause damage by infarction at a remote site. This effect is utilized in the Kusserow test for whole blood compatibility of materials (see Section 18.2.3).

- Remodeling will not remove the obstruction but will tend to encapsulate it, as in the case of the fibrous encapsulation found around implants in soft tissue. If the implant surface is structured (such as a felt or velour) to encourage cellular trapping, the surface exposed to the blood may come to function as the endothelial wall of a normal vessel and is termed "pseudointima" (see Section 10.3.2). It differs, of course, from the normal intima because it has no smooth muscle component and thus no ability to dilate or constrict.

These effects have been summarized by Baier (1972) as seen in Figure 9.3. In this figure, Baier also indicates possible points and methods of intervention that may reduce the thrombogenic potential of implant surfaces.

In the ordinary (implant-free) progression of the intrinsic pathway, the fibrin clot gradually isolates flowing blood from the site of possible surface contact insult. However, on a foreign (implant) surface, it is possible for fibrin to initiate coagulation by itself due to its altered configuration after surface binding (Lindon et al. 1986). Implants may also initiate coagulation by binding (and possible activation) of molecules such as complement C3* that are not normally involved in the intrinsic pathway (Hayashi 1990; Herzlinger et al. 1981).

---

* The proteins involved in the complement system are usually associated with blood plasma, where they are present in abundance. However, due to the close association between complement and immune response, this topic is discussed in Section 12.2.2.

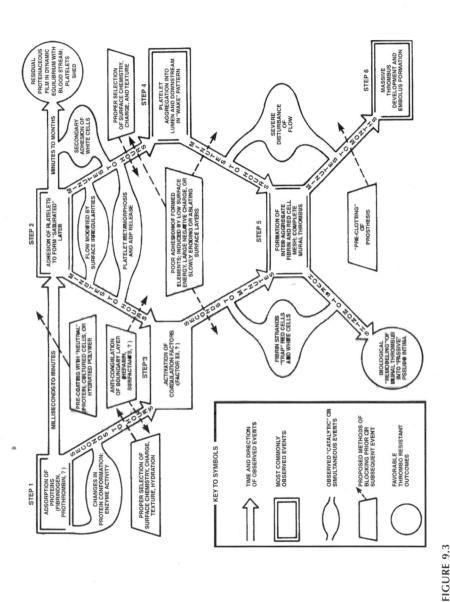

FIGURE 9.3
Coagulation events, timing, and intervention strategies. (From Baier, R.E., *Bull. N.Y. Acad. Med.*, 48, 257, 1972. With permission.)

9.3   Approaches to Thromboresistant Materials Development

9.3.1   General Considerations

In the same article from which Figure 9.3 is drawn (Baier 1972), the various historical approaches taken to design new surfaces or to render surfaces of older materials less thrombogenic were summarized (Figure 9.4). The approaches shown by the solid-line arrows pointing to the left are those that mimic properties that the natural intact endothelium is known to have. Those shown by the dotted lines pointing to the right are other proposals not based so directly upon known natural properties, but rather on theoretical approaches. All have met with mixed success and failure because, with the limited exceptions of knitted polyester grafts; felted polyurethane; poly (tetrafluoro) ethylene and related materials that can sustain "pseudointimal" linings; certain bulk polymers; and graphites, most materials evoke unacceptable host responses for chronic exposure to blood. Even satisfactory materials tend to thrombose in prosthetic devices with blood conduit internal diameter less than 6 mm.

Although Figure 9.4 is now more than 30 years old, it is interesting that no really new approaches to solution of the so-called "blood contact" problem have been developed. The only addition that could be made to this schematic, other than subtopics under each of the eight main headings, would be the addition of viable biomaterials as a fifth mimicking approach

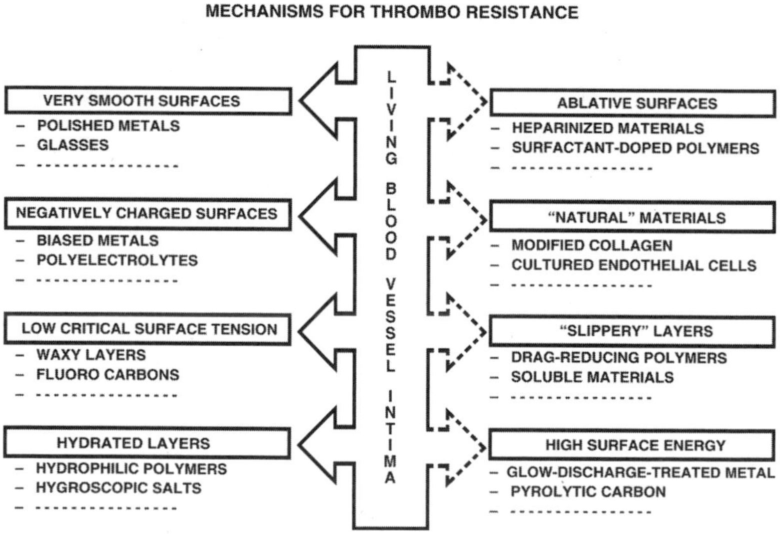

MECHANISMS FOR THROMBO RESISTANCE

FIGURE 9.4
Approaches to producing thromboresistant surfaces. (From Baier, R.E., *Bull. N.Y. Acad. Med.*, 48, 257, 1972. With permission.)

(right side). This is an extension of the "natural" materials approach, which is specifically the modification of permanent implantable materials with natural molecules or a surface-dwelling cell population. In the newer approach, a composite of resorbable materials and living cells (smooth muscle cells, endothelial cells, etc.) is made and implanted with the hope that it will eventually remodel into native (host) tissue (Weinberg and Bell 1986).

The lack of new approaches to producing noncoagulating biomaterial surfaces reflects the complexity of the natural system and the difficulty of performing reproducible blood contact experiments with generality of results, whether *in vitro* or in animal models. This natural complexity has aroused considerable interest in finding simplifying or dominant factors in surface properties that affect thrombogenesis. Several of the directions of biomaterials efforts indicated in Figure 9.4 reflect such a search and are of historical and practical interest. Three of these will be considered: negative surface charge, critical surface tension, and "natural" surfaces. Each has yielded important results and contributed to a better understanding of thrombogenesis, but has failed to produce the final answer in suppressing host response to materials in contact with blood.

9.3.2 Negative Surface Charge

The recognition that erythrocytes and platelets have net negative surface charges has suggested to many investigators that electrostatic repulsion could be utilized to keep them away from implant surfaces, thus suppressing thrombogenesis. Sawyer and Srinivasan (1972) were the most active initiators and proponents of this idea. A series of early experiments suggested that a relative positive potential on a biomaterial surface exposed to blood promotes thrombogenesis and negative potentials tend to suppress thrombogenesis proportionally to the potential depression below local neutral. These conclusions arise from a complex series of experiments. Perhaps the most convincing data are given in Figure 9.5 (Sawyer and Srinivasan 1972), summarizing the results of implantation of Gott rings in the canine vena cava (see Section 18.2.3) and of a related design (Edwards) made from various materials in the canine aorta.

Under biophysiological conditions, metals with a negative electromotive potential form a positive interfacial potential with blood (due to the attraction of counter ions, as previously noted) and vice versa. Here, one can see the rapid and complete occlusion (coagulation sufficient to prevent blood flow) for silver and platinum, which have positive interface potentials *in vivo*, and the increasing patency (proportion of devices permitting flow) at increasing times for metals, such as iron (in stainless steel), aluminum, and magnesium, that have negative interface potentials.

The approach is, however, quite limited. The use of rigid metallic surfaces for vascular prostheses might prove nonthrombogenic by surface interaction but might produce a pseudoextrinsic thrombogenesis through mechanical

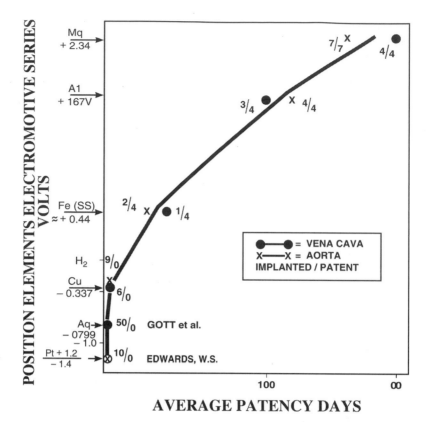

FIGURE 9.5

Relationship between interface potential of vascular implants and patency. (From Sawyer, P.N. and Kaplitt, M.J., Eds., *Vascular Grafts*, Appleton–Crofts, New York, 1978.)

damage to blood-borne cells.* Furthermore, control of interfacial potential might require an active power source, thus making the implant far more complex and less reliable than the knitted prostheses discussed in Section 10.3.2.**

---

* However, such considerations might well play a role in selection of materials for uncoated metallic vascular stents.

** A personal note: as an experimental physicist, I have always been fascinated by Sawyer's results in this area of research. While I was a predoctoral student in the late 1960s, I conceived an experiment, based on Milliken's classic oil drop experiment for determination of the charge of a single electron, to study the approach of platelets to charged surfaces in serum-free saline solution. I had the pleasure of discussing this idea with Phil Sawyer at the First World Biomaterials Congress (Baden, Austria, 1980). Although he thought it was an interesting idea, neither he nor anyone else to his knowledge had ever done this study (to my knowledge it has not subsequently been done).

9.3.3   Critical Surface Tension

The critical surface tension approach was proposed some time ago and has been strongly advanced by Baier (1972) as a significant but not necessarily dominant solution to the problem of surface thrombogenesis. The basic idea is to utilize the Young–Dupree equation (Section 5.4; Equation 5.4):

$$\gamma_{SL} = \gamma_{PS} + \gamma_{PL}\cos\theta \tag{9.1}$$

If surface tensions combine so that $\theta = 180°$, no adhesion of the particle, p, may occur. Then, of necessity, cosine θ must equal -1. This condition can be achieved if:

$$\gamma_{SL} = \gamma_C = \gamma_{PS} - \gamma_{PL} \tag{9.2}$$

(γ_C = critical surface tension).

Because γ_C is determined by the biological system, the trick is to find a surface with a suitable surface tension so that Equation 9.2 is satisfied; then no adhesion would occur for a particular molecular or cellular species and one or more of the surface contact steps in Figure 9.1 could be prevented. This can be done at two points in the coagulation cascade:

- The surface may have the appropriate critical surface tension to prevent adhesion of factor XII.
- The surface may have the appropriate critical surface tension to prevent adhesion of platelets in the intrinsic or the final (common) pathway.

This turns out to be far more difficult in practice than in principle. For instance, a surface might be selected that does not permit adherence of factor XII. However, other molecular species will probably adhere, γ_{SL} may change, and adhesion of factor XII may then become possible. Measurements of surface tension of nonbiological surfaces, such as silicon, exposed *in vitro* or *ex vivo* to sera or whole blood suggest complex time-dependent changes in γ_{SL}.

Notwithstanding these practical problems, a theoretical range of the material–blood interfacial critical surface tension, γ_C, should suppress thrombogenesis (Figure 9.6). Because most blood contact materials are polymeric, a fruitful embodiment of this approach has been chemical surface modification of implants. Studies of a wide variety of as-synthesized and surface-modified materials show relative improved thromboresistance in this range (20 to 30 dyn/cm*) of surface tension. It is interesting to note that 30 dyn/cm is the so-called "Berg limit" (Vogler 1998); the essential balance point between hydrophobic and hydrophobic interfacial forces at which the solid/liquid phase boundary should exert a minimum deforming effect on proteins.

---

* Older units; preserved for historical purposes in Figure 9.6. 1 dyn/cm = 10^{-3} N·m^{-1}.

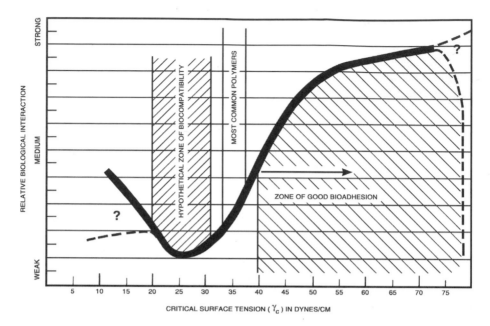

FIGURE 9.6

Proposed relationship of critical surface tension (γ_c) to biological response. (From Baier, R.E., *Bull. N.Y. Acad. Med.*, 48, 257, 1972. With permission.)

9.3.4 "Natural" Surfaces

The thromboresistance of the undamaged internal surfaces of blood vessels has attracted the surgeon and the bioengineer for a long time. Direct transplants (allografts) and implants of animal material (xenografts) are limited in utility by host rejection of the implant through an immune response (see Section 12.1) and by biological degradation of the foreign material. Various methods of processing have been tried to reduce the immune response and to improve resistance to degradation. A number of processes in use involve cleaning the tissue, removing cellular debris, and crosslinking the collagen component ("tanning") by a variety of agents such as glutaraldehyde, formaldehyde, etc. Although human material has been used, the pig is a favorite donor. Kiraly and Nosé (1974) have summarized some of the early applications of such materials.

These materials seem to have considerable degrees of thromboresistance. However, they are not incorporated into the body in the same way that knitted grafts are (Nosé et al. 1977). Thus, a pseudointima does not form and the surfaces exposed to blood are slow to mature. Although cells are found on their surfaces, the same low surface tensions that suppress thrombogenesis seem to retard cellular adhesion. Additionally, these processed materials are relatively impervious to diffusion of fluids and tend to develop late calcification, similar to that which occurs naturally in arteriosclerosis.

However, the approach remains interesting, particularly as how calcification can be inhibited becomes known (Levy et al. 1995), and bears considerable promise for the future, perhaps utilizing cultured (grown *in vitro*) tissue. The "natural" approach is an obvious precursor to the more recent ideas involving viable biomaterials for blood-contacting surfaces (see earlier discussion).

9.3.5 An Overview of Thromboresistant Materials Development

It is difficult to consider in further detail the efforts at bulk and surface modification that have been made to render implant surfaces friendlier to blood. In general, the experiments with bulk materials are straightforward, but their interpretation depends strongly on the validity of the blood exposure test used to evaluate them. Chapter 17 and Chapter 18 will return to this point.

I think that the experiments in surface modification and coating remain open to broad, general criticism. In the first place, there is rarely very good characterization of the bulk materials used. One may ask what the actual (rather than calculated) structural and energetic properties of the surfaces of these materials are and how these properties affect the resulting surface exposed to cells. Furthermore, there is rarely good evidence that the surface treatments or coatings are homogeneous or even cover the surface completely. The "catalytic" nature and inherent amplification of coagulation processes suggest that the presence of occasional high-energy defects may be highly effective as foci for initiation of thrombogenesis and may be far more important than the anti- or nonthrombogenic properties of the balance of the surface.

As pointed out previously, it can be generally assumed that implant surfaces become rapidly protein coated after insertion and that the proteins are denatured in some degree. I have suggested (Section 5.4) that if a normally free protein adheres to a biomaterial surface, by definition it must be denatured. Whether this is mild and reversible (3 or 4°), moderate (2°), or severe and essentially irreversible (1°) depends upon the nature of the protein–surface interaction forces.* Thus, the central issues concerning adhesion of proteins to surfaces are whether they are uniformly distributed or associated with surface defects and whether the type of denaturation that occurs will evoke a specific cellular response — in this case, the initiation of coagulation.

Finally, most studies neglect to measure the important physiochemical properties of the actual material/surface/protein complex during and/or after blood contact and instead rely on secondary determinations, frequently in simplified systems with only one or two proteins present at low concentration or on theoretical considerations. It seems most likely that, in the absence of surface-bound molecules for which target cells (platelets, erythrocytes, etc.) have specific surface receptors, cells involved in coagulation are affected by the following properties of biomaterials:

---

* See Chapter 5 for a more complete discussion.

- Potential gradients and associated ion fluxes near surfaces
- Features of surface geometry with dimensions between 0.1 and 5 μm
- Actual surface/solution interfacial free energy
- Stresses at impact (governed by the preceding three points as well as surface hardness and conditions of the experiment or clinical exposure)
- Presence of specific proteins sufficiently denatured to evoke a biological response

9.4   Hemolysis

9.4.1   General Description

Foreign materials may trigger thrombosis by contact with blood in the absence of motion at the blood–surface interface. However, motion may trigger thrombus formation or may cause damage to blood cells in the absence of thrombosis. Such initially nonthrombotic damage resulting in cell death and release of cell contents is termed hemolysis. Although hemolysis can be detected by a reduction in red cell (erythrocyte) count or by the presence of cell "ghosts" (fragments of empty cell membranes), it is most usually followed by measuring the level of serum hemoglobin.

Presence of hemoglobin in blood serum is a direct result of erythrocyte lysis. The normal concentration of serum hemoglobin (in humans) of <1.1 g/l represents in toto no more than 0.4% of hemoglobin in the blood. Serum hemoglobin is normally bound to a carrier molecule, haptoglobin; however, the maximum capacity of this fraction in normal serum is 1.4 g/l. Hemolysis rates above the release due to cell death in normal turnover may overpower the ability of haptoglobin to bind and thus "detoxify" otherwise free hemoglobin. Modest increases lead to increases in excretion of hemoglobin and may cause anemia if sustained for long periods. Greater elevations (25 g/l and higher) will cause systemic clinical symptoms including cyanosis and hematuria; still higher levels may lead to kidney failure and toxemia.

Hemolysis may occur in freely flowing blood in the absence of foreign surfaces. Turbulent flow and shear stresses above 150 to 300 Pa will cause direct lysis. If stagnation points exist, as in some device designs, this lysis may lead directly to thrombus formation in the apparent absence of surface contact. Of course, in this case, the initiating surface is damaged cell membrane exposed by cell lysis.

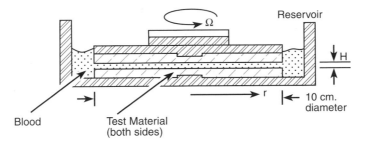

FIGURE 9.7
Schematic of apparatus for study of shear-induced hemolysis. (Adapted from Lampert, R.H. and Williams, M.C., *J. Biomed. Mater. Res.*, 6, 499, 1972.)

9.4.2 Experimental Relation to Flow Velocity

However, flow effects can be seen in the contact between blood and foreign surfaces at much lower ranges of shear stress. A large number of studies have demonstrated this effect. One of the best is still that of Lampert and Williams (1972). These investigators studied hemolysis rates of various materials compared to a standard material, aluminum, at a variety of flow rates. Their apparatus consisted of a fixed disc with an opposed rotating disc at a fixed separation distance, both on a common axis (see Figure 9.7 for a schematic representation). The interdisc separation (H) and the speed of relative rotation (Ω) could be varied.

The Reynolds numbers (R_e) for this apparatus were calculated as shown below. With respect to separation (H) at the edge of the disc (max r):

$$R_e\left(H\right)=\frac{\rho\Omega H^2}{\eta} \tag{9.3}$$

where
  ρ = density of blood
  Ω = angular velocity
  η = viscosity of blood

$R_e(H) \leq 1.5$; laminar flow to $R_e(H) = 10^2$.
  With respect to radius (r) at maximum separation (max H):

$$R_e\left(H\right)=\frac{\rho\Omega r^2}{\eta} \tag{9.4}$$

$R_e(r) \leq 4.4 \times 10^4$, laminar flow to $R_e(r) = 10^5$.
  These conditions yield shear rates, $G \leq 11,200$ sec^{-1}, ($r \leq 5$ cm), and shear stresses that do not exceed 44.8 Pa. In this low shear regime, Lampert and

Williams (1972) defined a relative plasma hemoglobin concentration increase, ΔC, with respect to aluminum:

$$\Delta C = \frac{\left[\Delta C_{hb}\right]\left(m, t\left(\text{secs}\right)\right)}{\left[\Delta C_{hb}\right]\left(A1, 30\right)} \tag{9.5}$$

For a number of materials tested, the following relationship was found:

$$\Delta C = At^{\beta} \tag{9.6}$$

For instance, for heat-cured poly (methyl) methacrylate (Plexiglass™):

$$\Delta C = 0.047t^{0.84} \tag{9.7}$$

In general, A was found to be apparatus dependent for this experiment and is given by the following relationship:

$$A = 0.020\beta^{-5.6} \tag{9.8}$$

On the other hand, β was found to be a constant characteristic of the test material and to have a single unique value for each material composition tested. For a group of five polymers (both test surfaces made from the same material), β correlated to the critical interfacial tension, γ_C, by a linear negative relationship of the form:

$$\beta = D - E\,\gamma_C \tag{9.9}$$

where D and E are experimentally derived constants.

This can be understood by the following argument. A high value of γ_C (with respect to a low value) favors rapid early protein absorption from the plasma. This increases the adhesion of platelets (increases the negative work of adhesion), leading to rapid maturation of a fibrin layer. This mature fibrin layer discourages further platelet and cell adhesion, thus lowering hemolysis rates with respect to those of the surface with lower γ_C. Thus, although high γ_C leads to rapid thrombus formation, it may reduce free cell hemolysis. These experiments suggest that the ideal blood-compatible surface may not be the least reactive one.

These results were obtained with a constant shear stress. Performing experiments at varying values of Ω, Lampert and Williams (1972) formed the ratio, R, to examine shear stress effects:

$$R = \frac{\Delta C(m,\Omega)}{\Delta C(m,640(\text{rpm}))} \qquad t = 100\,\text{sec} \qquad (9.10)$$

The results of this analysis are equivocal due to uncertainties in the true fluid dynamics of the system. They are consistent with a linear rise of R at low stress (below 40 Pa) and a nonlinear increase at higher apparent stresses. These results are interpreted as reflecting a constant boundary layer effect (material effect) and a superimposed bulk shear effect (turbulence effect) at higher rotational speeds. Thus, this experiment neatly shows the merging of the two flow regimes.

Although extremely enlightening, this series of studies may be criticized on three grounds:

- The blood is exposed to an air–liquid interface and to materials other than the test materials. Thus, hemolysis may be associated with increased cell fragility and with contact with nontest surfaces. These effects are contained within the constant A; however, they prevent the derivation of an absolute hemolysis rate for a material.

- The results obtained are specific for the surfaces actually used and not representative to the general material classes from which they are selected. Specimen-specific features, such as type and degree of roughness, clearly affect the outcome (Monroe et al. 1981).

- The experiment is conducted *in vitro* and under conditions in which significant hemolysis rates will occur in brief periods; thus, it is very difficult to relate these results to those that might be obtained *in vivo* at more realistic low hemolysis rates.

9.5 Final Comments

It should be clear from the brief remarks in this chapter that understanding and controlling the host response of materials exposed to blood represents one of the great unsolved problems of biomaterials science. Valve and vascular replacements, left ventricular assist devices, and total artificial heart replacements, as well as dialyzers and oxygenators used for shorter periods, have become very sophisticated in design and control. However, their clinical utility continues to be severely limited by unwanted interactions between their materials of manufacture, the degradation products of those materials, and circulating blood proteins and cells, especially those affected by shear forces and foreign surface contact. Thus, it is difficult to overemphasize the need for progress in developing materials that can function well in the cardiovascular system for long periods of time.

The problem is complicated by several factors:

- The phenomena of coagulation and hemolysis are complex and multifactorial.

- There seems to be a broad range of host response, particularly in temporal variations in response by individuals, unlike the less specific response to inflammation, with only quite modest responses tolerable chronically.

- Partly because of the first two points, as well as the rapidity of development of the coagulation cascade, adequate experimental models and techniques for research in this field are acutely lacking.

Fortunately, the search for improved "blood compatibility" as an attribute of biomaterials continues to be vigorous. Harker et al. (1993) provide an excellent overview of this difficult problem. Part III of this book will return to the specific issue of deficiencies in testing and evaluation.

References

Baier, R.E., The role of surface energy in thrombogenesis, *Bull. N.Y. Acad. Med.*, 48, 257, 1972.

Banerjee, R. et al., Hematological aspects of biocompatibility — review article, *J. Biomater. Appl.*, 12, 57, 1997.

Harker, L.A., Ratner, B.D. and Didisheim, P. (Eds.), *Cardiovascular Biomaterials and Biocompatibility. Cardio. Pathol.*, 2(3) (Suppl), 1993, 1.

Hayashi, K., *In vivo* thrombus formation induced by complement activation on polymer surfaces, *J. Biomed. Mater. Res.*, 24, 1385, 1990.

Herzlinger, G.A. et al., Quantitative measurement of C3 activation at polymer surfaces, *Blood*, 57, 764, 1981.

Kiraly, R.J. and Nosé, Y., Natural tissue as a biomaterial, *Biomat. Med. Dev. Art. Org.*, 2(3), 207, 1974.

Lampert, R.H. and Williams, M.C., Effect of surface materials on shear-induced hemolysis, *J. Biomed. Mater. Res.*, 6, 499, 1972.

Levy, R.J. et al., Calcification of valved aortic allografts in rats: effects of age, crosslinking, and inhibitors, *J. Biomed. Mater. Res.*, 29, 217, 1995.

Lindon, J.N. et al., Does the conformation of adsorbed fibrinogen dictate platelet interactions with artificial surfaces?, *Blood*, 68, 355, 1986.

Monroe, J.M. et al., Surface roughness and edge geometries in hemolysis with rotating disk flow, *J. Biomed. Mater. Res.*, 15, 923, 1981.

Nosé, Y. et al., Surface characteristics of cardiac prostheses *in vivo*, *J. Biomed. Mater. Res. Symp.*, 8, 85, 1977.

Salzman, E.W., Surface effects in hemostasis and thrombosis, in *The Chemistry of Biosurfaces*, Vol. II. Hair, M.L. (Ed.), Marcel Dekker, New York, 1972, 489.

Sawyer, P.N. and Kaplitt, M.J. (Eds.), *Vascular Grafts*, Appleton–Crofts, New York, 1978.

Sawyer, P.N. and Srinivasan, S., The role of electrochemical surface properties in thrombosis at vascular interfaces: cumulative experience of studies in animals and man, *Bull. N.Y. Acad. Med.*, 48, 235, 1972.

Skarja, G.A. et al., A cone-and-plate device for the investigation of platelet biomaterial interactions, *J. Biomed. Mater. Res.*, 34, 427, 1997.

Vogler, E.A., Structure and reactivity of water at biomaterial surfaces, *Adv. Colloid Interface Sci.*, 74, 69, 1998.

Vroman, L., Summation: protein at the interface, *Fed. Proc.*, 30, 1703, 1971.

Weinberg, C.B. and Bell, E., A blood vessel model constructed from collagen and cultured vascular cells, *Science*, 231, 397, 1986.

Bibliography

Department of Health and Human Services, *Guidelines for Blood–Material Interactions*, NIH Publication 85-2185, Public Health Service, National Institutes of Health, U.S. Government Printing Office, Washington, D.C., 1986.

Bamford, C.H. (Ed.), *The Vroman Effect*, Coronet, Philadelphia, 1992.

Barbanel, J.C. et al., *Blood Flow in Artificial Organs and Cardiovascular Prostheses*, Clarendon Press, Oxford, 1989.

Basmadjian, D. et al., Coagulation on biomaterials in flowing blood: some theoretical considerations, *Biomaterials*, 18, 1511, 1972.

Bodnar, E. and Frater, R., *Replacement Cardiac Valves*, McGraw–Hill, New York, 1991.

Bruck, S.D., *Blood Compatible Synthetic Polymers*, Charles C Thomas, Springfield, IL, 1974.

Ellis, J.T. et al., Prosthesis-induced hemolysis: mechanism and quantification of shear stress, *J. Heart Valve Dis.*, 7(4), 376, 1998.

Gott, V.L. and Furuse, A., Antithrombogenic surfaces, classification and *in vivo* evaluation, *Fed. Proc.*, 30, 1679, 1971.

Hanson, S.R., Blood–material interactions, in Black, J. and Hastings, G. (Eds.), *Handbook of Biomaterial Properties*, Chapman & Hall, London, 1998, 545.

Hastings, G., *Cardiovascular Biomaterials*, Springer–Verlag, Berlin, 1991.

Hughes–Jones, N.C., *Lecture Notes on Haematology*, 7th ed., Blackwell Scientific, London, 2003.

Kambic, H.E., Kantrowitz, A. and Sung, P. (Eds.), *Vascular Graft Update, Safety and Performance*. ASTM STP 898. American Society for Testing and Materials, Philadelphia, 1986.

Lefrak, E.A. and Starr, A., *Cardiac Valve Prostheses*. Appleton–Century–Crofts, New York, 1979.

Leonard, E.F., Turitto, V.T. and Vroman, L. (Ed.), *Blood in Contact with Natural and Artificial Surfaces*. Ann. N.Y. Acad. Sci., 516, 1988.

Magnani, A. and Barbucci, R., Hemocompatible materials, surface and interface aspects, in *Encyclopedic Handbook of Biomaterials and Bioengineering, Part B, Applications*, Vol. 2. Wise, D.L. et al. (Eds.), Marcel Dekker, New York, 1995, 1101.

Merrill, E.W., Properties of materials affecting the behavior of blood at their surfaces, *Ann. N.Y. Acad. Sci.*, 283, 6, 1977.

Sawyer, P.N. et al., Physical chemistry of the vascular interface, in *Vascular Grafts*, Sawyer P.N. and Kaplitt M.J. (Eds.), Appleton–Crofts, New York, 1978, 53.

Smith, J.P. and Sawyer, P.N. (Eds.), *Modern Vascular Grafts*, McGraw–Hill, New York, 1986.

Schoen, F.J., *Interventional and Surgical Cardiovascular Pathology*, W.B. Saunders, Philadelphia, 1989.

Thubrikar, M. et al., Study of surface charge of the intima and artificial materials in relation to thrombogenicity, *J. Biomech.*, 13, 663, 1980.

Van Kampen, C.L. et al., Effect of implant surface chemistry upon arterial thrombosis, *J. Biomed. Mater. Res.*, 13, 517, 1979.

Vroman, L., *Blood*, American Museum Science Books, B26, Doubleday, New York, 1968.*

Wagner, W.R. et al., Blood biocompatibility analysis in the setting of ventricular assist devices, *J. Biomater. Sci. Polym. Ed.*, 11(11), 1239, 2000.

---

* *Blood*, by Leo Vroman, is a marvelous, amusing, and witty account of blood biochemistry and surface interactions by one of the leading blood physiologists of the 20th century. Although one will enjoy it as recreational reading, one cannot avoid learning a great deal about blood. In addition to being a researcher, Leo Vroman is an author of poetry and children's books. Unfortunately, most have only been published in Dutch, his native language. *Love, Greatly Enlarged* (1991, Cross-Cultural Communications) is a major poem in English and, given the author, is about many things, not the least of which is blood.

10

Adaptation

10.1 Introduction

So far in Part II, acute host responses to singular events have been considered. The insertion of an implant may evoke inflammation, with an acute course and a longer chronic phase. Interruption of a blood vessel by injury or insertion of an implant may trigger acute coagulation and, perhaps, chronic hemolysis. Chapter 13 will take up the subject of neoplastic transformation: abnormal tissue development and elaboration as a result of chemical or foreign-body challenge.

Between these two types of events — acute response and abnormal development —is another class of tissue response; that is, the presence of an implant, perhaps due to the implant's chemical, physical, or electrical properties, affects the organization and elaboration of tissue elements in the vicinity. These events must be considered because of the well known ability of many of the tissues to remodel adaptively, in response to physical induction factors, to reflect changes in demand and function. From the phrase "adaptively remodel," I shall purloin the term "adaptation" to describe such events, especially as influenced by implants. The recognition and management of adaptation is an important aspect of the design, development, and use of interactive (type 2) biomaterials.

10.2 Tissue Growth Strategies

10.2.1 General Principles

Goss (1978, p. 2) discusses the strategy of growth of tissue in terms of three patterns previously recognized by Bizzozero (1894):

- Expanding tissues grow by mitosis to increase cell number (for instance, the liver).

- Static tissues retain essentially constant cell number but grow by individual hypertrophy (for instance, muscle).
- Renewing tissues retain essentially constant cell number by replacing losses from differentiation of proliferating stem cells (for instance, skin).

In the rapidly developing immature individual, all tissues expand by mitosis. As maturation proceeds, the cells of some tissues lose their mitotic ability and the tissues become static or renewing. It is also possible for tissues to continue to display a combination of two of these patterns, varying their response to the challenge.

The question of control of these processes is still to a certain degree unresolved. Because all of these processes tend towards limits, a variety of negative-feedback control systems have been proposed (see Section 10.3.6 for one example). However, a response is evoked in each cell type by death of a portion of the tissue or by surgical removal. Less significant challenges, such as blunt trauma or change in mechanical functional requirements, may also evoke responses. These observations suggest the existence of a wide variety of control processes regulating the quantity and, to some degree, the type of tissue in any location in a mammalian body. It is altogether reasonable to assume that the response of any such active biological control system facing a challenge may be affected by the presence of an implant.

10.2.2   Fracture Healing

The process of fracture healing — the restoration of the integrity and continuity of mineralized tissue after mechanical injury — includes an interesting example of natural adaptation in the absence of implants. Successful fracture healing can be considered most generally to entail four stages:

1. Hematoma: from injury to formation of a "soft" callus
2. Soft callus: from initiation of soft callus formation until its condensation into a "hard" callus
3. Hard callus: from initiation of hard callus until normal stiffness is restored
4. Remodeling: from restoration of normal stiffness to full restoration of normal structure

Stages 1 and 2 (see Figure 10.1) represent the acute or healing phase leading to the formation of a natural splint or *callus*. This is a weak provisional tissue consisting of fibrocartilage and fibrous bone with little internal organization. However, when 50 to 75% of the normal stiffness is reached, the healing fracture undergoes a very dramatic and fairly rapid transformation. The soft

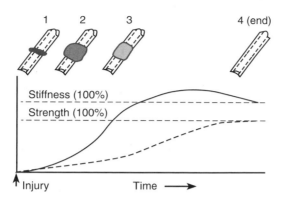

FIGURE 10.1
Stages of fracture healing.

callus rapidly condenses and shrinks to form a more organized hard callus, then is slowly resorbed through a progressive remodeling process leading to full restoration of normal structure (including reopening of the medullary canal in long bones). These latter two stages appear to be mediated by mechanical requirements through Wolff's law (see Section 10.3.4) and lead to an efficient structure with normal properties. Thus, stages 3 and 4 of fracture healing can be thought of as a chronic phase and appear to represent adaptive remodeling of a functionally healed bone (end of stage 2).

Note that normal stiffness is obtained first and, in fact, generally exceeded, due to the combined presence of callus and healing cortical bone in the defect; normal strength is obtained only towards the end of the remodeling phase.

In any particular bone, fracture healing, with a certain degree of injury, can be expected to progress to completion in an average time characteristic of the initial condition and, to some degree, the type of treatment (internal fixation, external splinting, etc.). If there is a significant delay but eventual complete healing and remodeling, the condition is termed delayed union. However, it is possible for the process to be interrupted at any stage. If this occurs in stages 1 and 2, before any degree of structural integrity is obtained, and is permanent, the result is a nonunion, sometimes called a "pseudarthrosis."* Nonunions are frequently sites of active tissue turnover but rarely heal without additional intervention, validating the distinction made here between nonadaptive stages (1 and 2) and the adaptive ones (3 and 4).

---

* Black (1987) includes a more detailed discussion of these diagnostic distinctions.

10.3   Examples of Adaptation in Implant Applications

10.3.1   Introduction

Implant applications offer a wide variety of possible examples of adaptation. Consideration here will be restricted to the following examples:

- Growth of the "neointima" in arterial prostheses
- Attachment of tendon prostheses to soft tissue
- Hard tissue remodeling in the presence of implants
- Bone response to electrified implants

Many other examples of adaptation to the presence of implants can be found. In fact, it may be useful to consider that, when resolution to a stable situation is possible (see Section 8.2.6), accommodation of the local host tissues to implants consists most generally of two phases: an acute or healing phase and a chronic or adaptive phase.

In all of the adaptive processes, the control mechanism invoked is phenomenologically described by a unifying principle. In hard tissue, this principle is termed Wolff's law. Julius Wolff, a 19th century German anatomist, suggested in 1892 that bone (and, by inference, other load-bearing tissues) remodels in an attempt to maintain a constant (optimal) pressure or local stress. Although he did not make such a specific statement, it is usual to say that Wolff's law is: "The form being given, tissue adapts to best fulfill its mechanical function."

Thus, as load increases over a period of time, bone mass would be expected to increase to maintain a constant level of stress. Conversely, a reduction in load should produce a loss of tissue. In a more sophisticated interpretation, realignment of principal stresses should be reflected by a modification of tissue structure. Observations in a variety of static and renewing tissues suggest a considerable pragmatic generality for Wolff's law.

10.3.2   Vascular Adaptation

The growth of a new tissue layer, or neointima, on the internal surfaces of knitted arterial prostheses is an interesting example of adaptation. Here, the prosthesis is introduced to serve as a framework to support host tissue that will serve as a long-term nonthrombogenic blood contact surface. The body of the prosthesis, which is most commonly made of polyester or similar polymeric fiber, provides the mechanical resistance to internal pressures that was once provided by the original vessel.

Upon insertion of the prosthesis, the features of the clotting cascade described in Section 9.2 take place. In fact, the surgeon usually preclots the prosthesis using the patient's blood in an effort to provide a smooth, defect-free surface and to reduce blood loss. The fibrin surface, inside and outside, matures and achieves stable dimensions within 24 hours. At this point, healing is clearly initiated. Within a few weeks, the outside (tissue side) of the prosthesis is covered by granulation tissue, and a capsule of fibrous tissue matures with increasing organization. The resolution or healing response of the internal surface facing flowing blood is a different matter.

Schoen (1989) distinguishes between two forms of vascular resolution: pseudointimal formation, the mere coating of the implant's surface with proteins and cells other than endothelial cells, and neointimal formation, the formation of an endothelial lined surface, usually overlying a layer of smooth muscle cells. The choice of outcome is apparently governed by the nature of the biomaterial surface and, as will be seen, can be considered as an example of adaptation of the natural healing process to the properties of the prosthesis.

During ideal or optimal healing, blood vessels penetrate to the lumen of the prosthesis and "tufts" of tissue spread along the inner surface, merging to form a smooth neointimal surface that functions like the natural arterial lining. Some investigators (e.g., Annis et al. 1978) suggest that this process of "through-growth" is not essential to the formation of the neointima and that longitudinal growth from the ends inward is possible in impermeable vascular prostheses. In a pig, this process is completed within a month, but it takes up to a year in a human patient.

However, this healthy adaptive vascular maturation has been shown (Wesolowski et al. 1968) to be critically dependent upon the prosthesis porosity. Figure 10.2a displays the relationship developed for a variety of porous prosthetic materials tested as arterial grafts in the pig. The porosity is given in units of liters/min/cm^2 of water expressed from the lumen through the wall of an unclotted non-blood-exposed graft with a pressure differential of 120 mmHg. The calcification index is the product of the average calcification (on a subjective scale of 1+ to 4+) of all animals implanted with a given material and the percentage of all specimens of the same material that display calcification. Here, high porosity above a value of 1 favors maturation of the neointima; lower porosity leads to failure of microvascular ingrowth, focal necrosis of the neointima, and possible calcification of the resulting pseudointima, in many respects mirroring the events of arteriosclerosis in natural tissue.

Attempts have been made to moderate this process by "seeding" the lumen wall with autologous cells (Kahn and Burkel 1973), with cultured endothelial cells (Mansfield et al. 1975), and by various pretreatments; however, the relationship found by Wesolowski et al. (1968) appears to be well founded.

The generality of this relationship is suggested by Figure 10.2b. This displays the relationship of a "net acceptability index" and the previously discussed physical water porosity. It represents the results of the evaluation of a variety of knit and velour polyester arterial prostheses (Sawyer et al. 1979). The net acceptability index is a transformation of the "net evaluation index" used by the authors so that the low scores are satisfactory, as in Figure

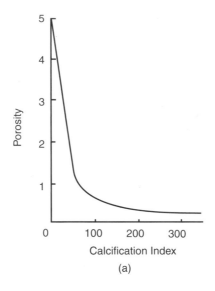

(a)

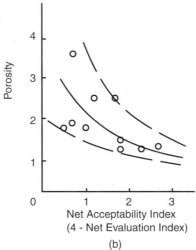

(b)

FIGURE 10.2

(a) Relationship between physical water porosity of arterial (woven) prostheses and calcification in the pig. (b) Relationship between physical water porosity and net acceptability index of arterial grafts (dashed lines indicate range). (Figure 10.2a adapted from Wesolowski, S.A. et al., *Ann. N.Y. Acad. Sci.*, 146(1), 325, 1968; Figure 10.2b adapted from Sawyer, P.N. et al., *J. Biomed. Mater. Res.*, 13, 937, 1979.)

10.2a. The net evaluation index is a combined score based upon *in vivo* performance and postimplantation evaluation. It is clear that the same result is obtained as that found by Wesolowski et al. (1968); high porosity favors good *in vivo* performance. This is clearly an example of a structural attribute of an implant strongly affecting tissue adaptation after surgery. Unlike the case of Wolff's law adaptation in bone, where the amount of tissue is affected by the implant attribute, here the type of tissue is affected by the (nonchemical) implant attribute.

10.3.3 Prosthetic Replacement of Tendons

The second area of adaptation to be considered is in the area of tendon prostheses. Here, the natural system provides a junction between the soft tissue (tendon) and the hard tissue (bone) by a series of collagenous fibers (Sharpey's fibers) that pass into the bone. There has been considerable interest in reproducing such a system by inserting a porous material into the bone or by providing a porous bridge between the end of the natural tendon insertion and a tendon remnant or the muscle. In either case, a situation is desired in which the natural tissue will grow into the prosthesis and provide mechanical strength. The topic of bony ingrowth will be discussed later.

Homsy et al. (1972) performed an interesting study of this subject using a porous graphite-reinforced poly (tetrafluoro) ethylene (Proplast™, Vitek, Inc., Houston, TX).* Blocks of this material were inserted in the rabbit calcaneal tendon, replacing segments of the natural structure, and sutured in place to be load bearing immediately. At periods of up to 26 weeks, the rabbits were sacrificed and the strength of the bond between natural and prosthetic material was tested in tension. The results are shown in Figure 10.3. These results are reported to be the same for tendon/prosthesis and muscle (gluteal)/prosthesis interfaces and to reach a plateau value of rupture strength shortly after 8 weeks — about 5 weeks later than for collagenous

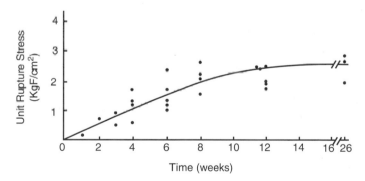

FIGURE 10.3
Prosthesis/tissue anastamosis strength. (From Homsy, C.A. et al., *Clin. Orthop. Rel. Res.*, 89, 220, 1972.)

---

* I discussed this study in the first edition of this work (published in 1981). Since then, the sad story of the misapplication of this material to load-bearing applications in bone, such as in the attempted replacement of the human temperomandibular joint, has become well known. However, in preparing this edition, I elected again to retain this study for two reasons: (1) it is, for its time, a well done piece of work; and (2) it is an object lesson concerning the limits of animal studies and the reality of the need to define biological performance in relationship to specific applications.

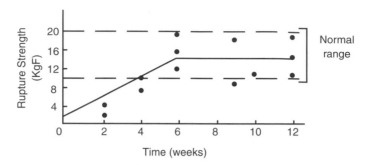

FIGURE 10.4
Breaking strength of pseudotendon. (Adapted from Jenkins, D.H.R. et al., *J. Bone Joint Surg.*, 59B, 53, 1977.)

ingrowth in bony sites. Here the gradual development of strength, as contrasted with the rapid (within 3 weeks) complete penetration of unorganized collagen that the authors would have predicted from earlier studies suggests that an organized structure is forming under control of the axial mechanical load exerted by the muscle.

This picture is substantiated by studies of a different system in this application. Here, the system is a complete tendon prosthesis that gradually disintegrates under use. Studies with a braided carbon ligament in rabbits (Forster et al. 1978) and sheep (Jenkins et al. 1977) showed that, as the prosthesis frayed and fatigued, it served as a scaffold for the growth of fibrous tissue that took over the function of the prosthesis. Figure 10.4 shows the breaking strength of the rabbit calcaneal tendon prostheses from this study. The authors ascribe the rapid development of strength to a stimulation effect of the carbon, but one might equally suggest that the gradual transfer of stress to the ingrowing tissue evoked this adaptive response. The development of maximum strength at 6 weeks (somewhat earlier than in the study of Homsy et al. in 1972) suggests that the disintegration of the prosthesis served to transfer stress more rapidly than was the case with a more durable material.

This experiment has been carried to a natural conclusion by incorporating the carbon fibers in a matrix that is degradable in the internal environment (Alexander et al. 1979). The matrix used here was polylactic acid, and the implant was inserted as a replacement for the canine patellar tendon. A gradual dynamic replacement of prosthesis with organized fibrous tissue was reported as the prosthesis matrix disintegrated, with reasonable maturity and linear tissue arrangement after 2 months of implantation. However, in neither of these experiments did the resulting tissue closely come to resemble normal tendon. Thus, it should be best termed neotendon, in parallel with Schoen's (1989) terms for healing vascular endothelial tissue. In more extreme cases when the new tissue more resembles a fibrous scar or capsule, it is more appropriately termed pseudotendon and its long-term durability under mechanical loads must surely be questioned. Balduini at al. (1986) have summarized further clinical developments that attempted to build on these observations.

10.3.4 Adaptive Remodeling of Bone near Implants

10.3.4.1 Stress Shielding

Wolff's law suggests that the introduction of a load-bearing implant coupled to a previously load-bearing natural structure should result in some atrophy or tissue loss. Because the assumption of a portion of the tensile load or bending moment by the implant must necessarily reduce the local stress in the adjacent tissue, this phenomenon has come to be called "stress shielding" (Huiskes 1988). The most commonly cited example is that of the progressive loss of bone material in the proximal medial femoral cortex (calcar) observed in animals and humans after total replacement of the hip joint. However, observation of the remodeling response is complicated by a simultaneous presence of an osteolytic response mediated by the presence of wear debris released from the articulating interface (Amstutz et al. 1992).

A more easily examined example is an unfortunate concomitant of the use of metallic internal fracture fixation devices. These devices are usually far more rigid than the bone to which they are attached, even if the bone is intact (as in experimental situations). Although they provide excellent support and maintain reduction and fixation during healing, a considerable amount of osteoporosis,* or loss of bone mass without external change of shape, occurs in the bone under the plate or adjacent to the rod. A study of experimental fractures in rabbits (Brown and Mayor 1978) seems to reinforce this point. Fractures were produced in the tibias of rabbits and were internally fixed with rods made of a variety of metals and polymers. The rods were a constant diameter to provide a range of stiffness relative to the intact bone from 10 to 0.03×. The animals were sacrificed and studied at 9 and 16 weeks after fracture and fixation. The results were confused by an anomalous response to one metal alloy (Ti6Al4V); however, at 16 weeks, fractures fixed with rods that were less stiff than the intact bone were significantly stronger and tougher in torsion than those fixed with rods that were stiffer than the intact bone. Additionally, in the weaker, less tough bones (fixed with the stiffer rods), a greater degree of osteoporosis was seen histologically.

This experiment is difficult to interpret solely in terms of an adaptive response to implants because the changes in bone are presumably caused by two factors: a healing response and an adaptive response. Moyen et al. (1978) conducted an experiment in dogs in which no fracture was involved and obtained somewhat similar results. In this experiment, metallic plates of two

---

* The term osteoporosis is more generally applied to metabolic rather than adaptive loss of bone. (See NIH Consensus Statement, Vol. 17 (1)), Osteoporosis Prevention, Diagnosis and Therapy, Washington, D.C., 2000.) However, the structural and mechanical consequences are essentially the same as in adaptive remodeling, so the same term is used here.

different stiffnesses varying by a factor of approximately 5 were attached to the midshaft of the femur in the dog. The bone mass under the plates was compared with the control (unplated) side after 6 and 9 months implantation. Interestingly, a small constant porosity of 1 to 3% was seen. However, after 6 months, the bone mass under the rigid plate had decreased 26.4% vs. only 16.4% under the more flexible plate. The decreases in bone mass continued to develop more slowly up to 9 months and showed modest reversals in another group implanted for 6 months and studied 3 months after plate removal. The authors ascribed the failure to observe the greater porosity seen in other studies (such as the one by Brown and Mayor in 1978) to the absence of the fracture-healing process accompanying the remodeling (adaptive) process.

Perren et al. (1988) further criticized the possible adaptive role in the production of porosity near fracture fixation devices and suggested that the physical presence of the device interferes with revascularization after fracture. He showed an inverse relationship between the area of plate–bone contact and cortical porosity in a sheep tibial model. One may, in turn, criticize this work because reducing the plate–bone contact area probably reduces the coupling between plate and bone, thus rendering the plate effectively less stiff — that is, less able to remove load (and thus reduce local stress) from the bone.

Another study by Bradley et al. (1979) combined some of the aspects of the studies of Brown and Mayor (1978) and Moyen et al. (1978). In this case, a variety of fracture fixation plates, with stiffnesses between 4 and 40% of the bone to be fixed, were used in a 16-week study of the healing of femoral midshaft osteotomies in dogs. A definite relationship was seen between plate rigidity and strength of the bony material and the femoral midshaft as a structure. This is shown in Figure 10.5.

Two comments should be made about this study. In the first place, the parameter examined was *strength* rather than *rigidity*, as in the case of the previous two studies. Although rigidity may parallel strength, the correlation is not exact, even in materials that are simpler in microstructure than bone. Furthermore, restoration of rigidity is probably more important in the early phases of fracture healing because it confers functional ability before adaptation is complete. In the second place, porosity was not studied, as in the work of Moyen et al. (1978). Porosity was suggested by Moyen to be a concomitant of trauma rather than simply adaptation (my term) and by Perren et al. (1988) as secondary to interference with revascularization; it may severely affect material and structural strength due to stress concentration effects, but have a modest volume-fraction effect upon modulus and thus upon material and structural bending rigidity (see Section 6.3.2). It is impossible to isolate this effect in this study.

One should not assume from these studies that large changes in stress are necessary to modify bone growth — that is, to produce adaptive changes in bone. Modest changes in stress, such as those that might be produced by simple, soft polymeric caps of bone shafts after segmental excision, have been shown to produce profound adaptive changes (Lusskin et al. 1972).

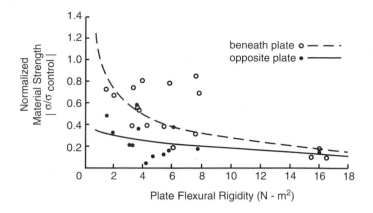

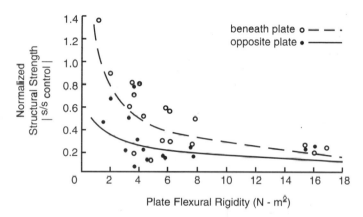

FIGURE 10.5

Changes in bone material and structural strength with fixation plate rigidity. (Adapted from Bradley, G.W. et al., *J. Bone Joint Surg.*, 61A, 866, 1979.)

10.3.4.2 Ingrowth into Porous Biomaterials

It is an easy step from the earlier discussion of the ingrowth associated with the prosthetic replacement of tendons to consideration of the more general problem of ingrowth into porous bodies. One of the responses to implants is the formation of a fibrous capsule, so it is no surprise that tissue will invade the internal spaces of an implant with an open, connected pore structure.

Extensive studies of this phenomenon have been conducted. Ingrowth occurs into porous implants fabricated from a wide variety of metals, polymers, and ceramics. The nature of the ingrowing tissue in the presence of sufficient interfacial mechanical stability* depends upon the size of the

---

* The issue of the role of interfacial shear (producing the so-called "micromotion") on tissue ingrowth remains sufficiently confused that an analytical discussion of this point is not possible. However, see Brunski (1988) and Prendergast et al. (1997) for fuller discussions of this topic.

pore (Friedenberg and Lawrence 1959) or, more properly, on the minimum size of the interconnections between pores (Klawitter and Weinstein 1974). Soft tissue elements will be found in interconnects as small as 1 to 5 μm; at some minimum interconnect diameter between 50 and 100 μm, mineralized tissue will be found and organized osteonal bone will grow into interconnects as small as 250 μm. Maximum interfacial shear strengths develop between 8 and 16 weeks after implantation, depending upon anatomical locations, species of animal, and type of tissue ingrowth. Velocity of ingrowth appears to increase with pore sizes above 50 μm and to reach a peak near pore sizes of 400 and 500 μm, as determined in a single pore model (Howe et al. 1974).

The ability of tissue to mineralize and organize as interconnect size increases is another clear example of adaptation. A study of Proplast™ (Vitek, Inc., Houston, TX) by Spector et al. (1979) confirmed this finding and demonstrated that it is not a false conclusion based upon comparison of studies with different materials and/or test conditions. If implanted directly, this material exhibits a pore size near 76 μm with an interconnect size of 50 μm. In a canine cortical bone site, only fibrous ingrowth was observed for periods of up to 20 weeks. However, if the material was "teased" before implantation to increase the size of interconnects, a variable degree of bony ingrowth occurred.

There appears to be a difference of opinion over the interpretation of the findings in this report (Homsy 1979; Spector 1979). This finding, combined with earlier reports (Klawitter and Hulbert 1971), suggests a practical lower interconnect limit of 100 μm for bone ingrowth. The mechanism of control of ingrowth and the manner in which pore interconnect size controls mineralization are unknown. Although Wolff's law arguments can be invoked to explain tissue remodeling near the bone–implant interface, it is presumed that tissue more than one pore diameter deep within the implant porosity will be essentially load free if the modulus of the implant exceeds that of bone to any significant degree. However, tissue maturation internal to porous implants appears to have little dependence on implant material modulus, but may be related more to electrical, chemical, and morphological effects on the pericellular environment.

10.3.4.3   Adhesion

Tissue is not inherently "sticky." Cells adhere to each other and to their extracellular matrices through the interaction of a variety of specific and nonspecific adhesion molecules and specific cell surface receptors for portions of these molecules (see Section 11.3.3), in addition to more diffuse Van der Waals bonding mechanisms. However, attempts to cause implants purposefully to adhere to tissue have aroused considerable interest.

When such adhesion is produced by the mere close (molecular-scale) approximation of tissue and implant, without an intervening fibrous capsule or other elements of an inflammatory response, it is termed most generally tissue integration; in the case of bone, the more specific term is osseointegration (Albrektsson and Hansson 1986). In the latter case, the apparent adhesion is produced by cellular binding to proteins adsorbed to the implant surface. Originally thought to be a property of pure titanium alone, such tissue integration has now been shown for a variety of metallic implant surfaces (Linder 1989), including tantalum (Black 1994). In fact, Linder (1989) has suggested that, in general, "osseointegration is a response of bone to a tolerable implant material inserted under tolerable conditions" without specifying the meaning of "tolerable" in either case.

When tissue adhesion to an implant is accompanied by a chemical alteration of the implant surface, a true bonding process with a continuous gradation of structure and composition across the tissue–implant interface may occur. Although there is no generally accepted term for this condition, interactive biomaterials that produce it have been termed *surface active* (Hench and Wilson 1984) in recognition of the necessity of chemical reaction with the local host environment prior to bond formation.* A number of ceramic and glassy materials have been produced that develop such bonds to bone and soft tissue (Figure 10.6).

In the case of integration or of bonding, the implant becomes mechanically coupled to the adjacent tissue. In the case of hard tissue, this results in a strain incompatibility due to the differences in moduli between bone and the implant. Several adaptive changes are possible. The most common situations are:

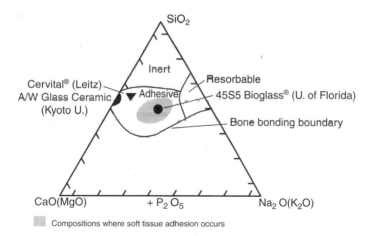

FIGURE 10.6
Ceramic and glassy tissue-bonding materials. (From Hench, L.L. and Wilson, J., *Science*, 226, 630, 1984. With permission: L.L. Hench.)

---

* The term bioactive has also been used for such materials (see Section 1.4). However, this is an apparent misnomer because it appears that the necessary surface modification is a consequence of exposure to the physiological environment, rather than to life processes.

- The implant is placed in cancellous bone and is of very significantly higher modulus than the surrounding tissue. The frequently observed response in this case is the formation of a bony "plate" much resembling a subchondral plate in an articular joint and a relative rarefaction of the cancellous trabeculae behind the plate. This results in introducing a relatively compliant tissue zone adjacent to the implant and "shielding" the bone further away from the mechanical consequences of the stiff implant.

- The implant is placed in cortical bone and is of significantly higher modulus than surrounding tissue. In this case, bone near the implant becomes porous, much as in the stress-shielding examples previously discussed (Section 10.3.4.1). However, this porosity may increase and proceed to a remodeled condition resembling cancellous bone. Thus, this process is termed cancellization.

In either case, the tissue structure changes are a result of the change in mechanical conditions near the newly formed interface and thus are true examples of adaptive remodeling.

10.3.5   Bone Response to Electrified Implants

It has been frequently suggested that the mechanism of Wolff's law in bone is electrically controlled. Bone and other tissues produce potentials when deformed; these potentials are called piezoelectric potentials or, more generally, strain-related potentials. A variety of other potential sources also exists.

Bassett (1971) proposed a generalized, closed-loop control system (as shown in Figure 10.7) to relate these signals to hard tissue remodeling. There is a conceptual error in his scheme because, presumably, the structural response (to adjust stress) results in a change in the osseous transducer (see added dashed line), rather than in a modification of the extrinsic force as proposed. Nevertheless, this general idea, first proposed some years before this early review was published, has been a motivating factor in the investigation of the effects of electrical phenomena on the modification of bony growth and remodeling. Numerous studies have shown a correspondence between endogenous electrical phenomena and growth, repair, and remodeling processes; however, no critical experiments that show that these signals are necessary and sufficient to serve as stimuli for the observed processes have yet been performed.

Although it is not clear that electrical control of bone growth, remodeling, and repair is an example of adaptive response to implants, it is worth noting some general conclusions from research in this area for completeness of this discussion (Black 1987). A physical electrode may be considered as a special case of metallic implantation: one in which the electrode, instead of being allowed to find its appropriate mixed corrosion potential (see Section 4.6), is maintained under a controlled relative potential or current condition. The

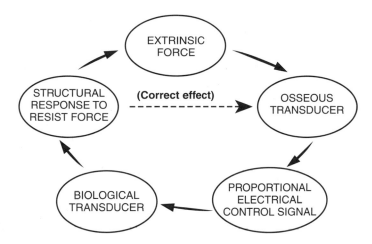

FIGURE 10.7
Negative feedback control system proposed as a basis for Wolff's law. (Adapted from Bassett, C.A.L., in *Biochemistry and Physiology of Bone*, Vol. 2, 2nd ed., Bourne, G.H., Ed., Academic Press, New York, 1971, 1.)

responses to implantation of such a physical electrode in or near hard tissue are summarized as:

- The presence of a metallic cathode, with a negative potential, stimulates the conduct of cells involved in bone formation.
- In particular, bony repair in sites of trauma is accelerated, and cells in medullary sites may be induced to form bone in the absence of bony trauma or to maintain bone formed in response to transient trauma.
- In all cases, apparently a narrow stimulatory "window" is defined by limits on current and electrode potential.
- Finally, monophasic negative pulses of frequencies from 10 to 730 Hz, with duty cycles between 50 and 5%, provide stimulation that approaches but does not exceed that of direct uninterrupted current.

Although the relationship of this line of research to the more general problem of adaptive growth is unclear, it does represent one of the more systematic attempts to elucidate the phenomena involved.

10.4   A Final Comment on Adaptation

It now seems clear that one of the original goals of implantation — that is, to produce minimal tissue (host) response — is an outmoded view that may limit further development of implant materials and devices. It is proper to ask that adverse host response be kept within bounds acceptable to the application. This is the necessary condition of biocompatibility. It is essential to rule out *a priori* certain classes of response, such as neoplastic transformation, as unacceptable. Now it appears equally reasonable to pursue active tissue response in the form of adaptation so that natural tissue can take over the role of the implant as completely as possible.

One of the ways of viewing the research literature on local host response is to note that it has three somewhat unconnected parts:

- The majority of the studies reported emphasize the chemical composition of the implant and its degradation products. The local host response is seen as a physiological response to soluble chemical species.

- A smaller body of work, primarily oriented to orthopaedic surgery, emphasizes the stiffness of the implant in relation to surrounding tissues, strains imposed by function, and, especially recently, the surface texture and configuration of the implant surface. The local host response is seen as a structural embodiment of consequences of Wolff's law.

- A still smaller set of studies report the cellular and tissue response to imposed electrical fields and currents, especially in the context of biomaterials, by implanted electrodes. The local host response is seen, primarily, as mediated by information content of the electrical effects and secondarily by local electrochemically induced pericellular environmental changes.

Figure 10.8 illustrates the general schematic form of the proposition: physical factors induce local host response through various mechanisms.

However, it may well be the case that these effects are not independent, but interdependent and perhaps, in some cases, synergistic. Figure 10.9 summarizes the local host effects discussed in Chapter 8, Chapter 9, Chapter 12, and Chapter 13 and their relationships to the degree or intensity ("dose")

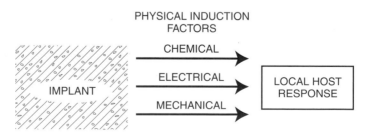

FIGURE 10.8
Physical induction factors in local host response.

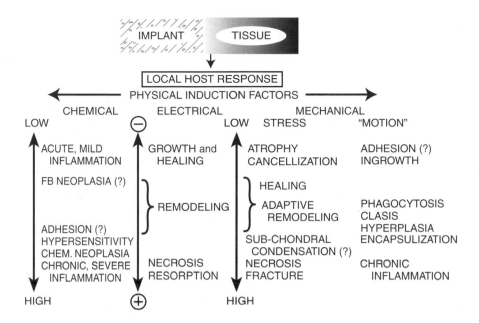

(?): Possible effect

FIGURE 10.9
Adaptive responses to physical induction factors. (Adapted from Black, J., *Orthopaedic Bio-materials in Research and Practice*, Churchill–Livingstone, New York, 1988, 288.)

of physical induction factors. Here I distinguish between interfacial stress and resulting shear displacement (motion): these are, in fact, coupled because the latter depends upon the former and on the surface structure of the implant. A "rough" implant permits far smaller interfacial displacements than a "smooth" nonadhesive one under the same stress. Normal host response, the quiescent state after full, acceptable resolution has occurred (see Section 8.2.6), is most generally characterized by low chemical activity, intermediate (near charge neutral) electrical activity, and intermediate interfacial stress, accompanied by an appropriate physical configuration of the implant surface. Particular cases, such as direct tissue adhesion, require other combinations of levels of these factors.

Much work remains to be done until the principles of adaptation are fully understood and harnessed to the solution of patient problems.

References

Albrektsson, T. and Hansson, H.-A., An ultrastructural characterization of the interface between bone and sputtered titanium or stainless steel surfaces, *Biomaterials*, 7, 201, 1986.

Alexander, H. et al., Ligament and tendon replacement with resorbable polymer-filamentous carbon tissue scaffolds, *Trans. Orthop. Res. Soc.*, 4, 27, 1979.

Amstutz, H.C. et al., Mechanism and clinical significance of wear debris-induced osteolysis. *Clin. Orthop. Rel. Res.*, 276, 7, 1992.

Annis, D. et al., An elastomeric vascular prosthesis, *Trans. Am. Soc. Artif. Intern. Organs*, XXIV, 209, 1978.

Balduini, F.C., Clemow, A.J.T. and Lehman, R.C., *Synthetic Ligaments: Scaffolds, Stents, and Prostheses*, Slack, Thorofare, NJ, 1986.

Bassett, C.A.L. Byophysical principles affecting bone structure, in *Biochemistry and Physiology of Bone*, Vol. 2, 2nd ed., Bourne, G.H. (Ed.), Academic Press, New York, 1971, 1.

Bizzozero, G., *Brit. Med. J.*, 1, 728, 1894 (cited in Goss, 1978).

Black, J., *Electrical Stimulation: Its Role in Growth, Repair, and Remodeling of the Musculoskeletal System*, Praeger, New York, 1987.

Black, J., *Orthopaedic Biomaterials in Research and Practice*, Churchill–Livingstone, New York, 1988, 288.

Black, J., Biological performance of tantalum: a review, *Clin. Mater.*, 16(3), 167, 1994.

Bradley, G.W. et al., Effects of flexural rigidity of plates on bone healing, *J. Bone Joint Surg.*, 61A, 866, 1979.

Brown, S.A. and Mayor, M.B., The biocompatibility of materials for internal fixation of fractures, *J. Biomed. Mater. Res.*, 12, 67, 1978.

Brunski, J.B., The influence of force, motion, and related quantities on the response of bone to implants, in *Non-Cemented Total Hip Arthroplasty*, Fitzgerald, R.H., Jr. (Ed.), Raven, New York, 1988, 7.

Forster, I.W. et al., Biological reaction to carbon fiber implants: the formation and structure of a carbon-induced "neotendon," *Clin. Orthop. Rel. Res.*, 131, 299, 1978.

Friedenberg, Z.B. and Lawrence, R., Bone growth in polyvinyl sponge, *Surg. Gynecol. Obstet.*, 109, 291, 1959.

Goss, R.J., *The Physiology of Growth*, Academic Press, New York, 1978.

Hench, L.L. and Wilson, J., Surface active biomaterials, *Science*, 226, 630, 1984.

Homsy, C.A., Comments on "characteristics of tissue growth into Proplast and porous polyethylene implants in bone," *J. Biomed. Mater. Res.*, 13, 987, 1979.

Homsy, C.A. et al., Porous implant systems for prosthesis stabilization, *Clin. Orthop. Rel. Res.*, 89, 220, 1972.

Howe, D.F., Svare, C.W. and Tock, R.W., Some effects of pore diameter on single-pore bony ingression patterns in Teflon, *J. Biomed. Mater. Res.*, 8, 399, 1974.

Huiskes, R., Stress patterns, failure modes, and bone remodeling, in *Non-Cemented Total Hip Arthroplasty*, Fitzgerald, R.H., Jr. (Ed.), Raven, New York, 1988, 283.

Jenkins, D.H.R. et al., Induction of tendon and ligament formation by carbon implants, *J. Bone Joint Surg.*, 59B, 53, 1977.

Kahn, R.H. and Burkel, W.E., Propagation of pseudointimal linings of vascular prostheses, *In Vitro*, 8, 451, 1973.

Klawitter, J.J. and Hulbert, S.F., Application of porous ceramics for the attachment of load-bearing internal orthopedic applications, *J. Biomed. Mater. Res. Symp.*, 2, 161, 1971.

Klawitter, J.J. and Weinstein, A.M., The status of porous materials to obtain direct skeletal attachment by tissue ingrowth, *Acta Orthop. Belgica*, 40, 755. 1974.

Linder, L., Osseointegration of metallic implants. I. Light microcopy in the rabbit, *Acta Orthop. Scand.*, 60, 129, 1989.

Lusskin, R. et al., Bone contouring under silicone polymer implants, *Clin. Orthop. Rel. Res.*, 83, 300, 1972.

Mansfield, P.B., Wechezak, A.R. and Sauvage, L.R., Preventing thrombus on artificial vascular surfaces: true endothelial cell linings, *Trans. Am. Soc. Artif. Intern. Organs*, XXI, 264, 1975.

Moyen, B.J.-L. et al., Effects on intact femora of dogs of the application and removal of metal plates, *J. Bone Joint Surg.*, 60A, 940, 1978.

Perren, S.M. et al., Early temporary porosis of bone induced by internal fixation implants. A reaction to necrosis, not stress protection? *Clin. Orthop. Rel. Res.*, 232, 139, 1988.

Prendergast, P.J., Husikes, R. and Soballe, K., ESB research award 1996. Biophysical stimuli on cells during tissue differentiation at implant interfaces, *J. Biomech.*, 30, 539, 1997.

Sawyer, P.N. et al., *In vitro* and *in vivo* evaluations of Dacron velour and knit prostheses, *J. Biomed. Mater. Res.*, 13, 937, 1979.

Schoen, F.J., *Interventional and Surgical Cardiovascular Pathology: Clinical Correlations and Basic Principles*, W.B. Saunders, Philadelphia, 1989, 36.

Spector, M., Reply to comments on "characteristics of tissue growth into Proplast and porous polyethylene implants in bone," *J. Biomed. Mater. Res.*, 13, 991, 1979.

Spector, M., Harmon, S.L. and Kreutner, A., Characteristics of tissue growth into proplast and porous polyethylene implants in bone, *J. Biomed. Mater. Res.*, 13, 677, 1979.

Wesolowski, S.A. et al., Arterial prosthetic materials, *Ann. N.Y. Acad. Sci.*, 146(1), 325, 1968.

Wolff, J., *Das Gesetz der Transformation der Knochen*, A. Hirschwald, Berlin, 1892.

Bibliography

Brighton, C.T., Black, J. and Pollack, S.R. (Eds.), *Electrical Properties of Bone and Cartilage: Experimental Effects and Clinical Applications*, Grune & Stratton, New York, 1979.

Burke, J.F. et al., Successful use of a physiologically acceptable artificial skin in the treatment of extensive burn injury, *Ann. Surg.*, 194, 413, 1981.

Chehroudi, B. and Brunette, D.M., in *Encyclopedic Handbook of Biomaterials and Bioengineering*, Part A, Vol. 1, Wise, D.L. et al. (Eds.), Marcel Dekker, New York, 1995, 813.

Dadsetan, M. et al., Surface chemistry mediates adhesive structure, cytoskeletal organization, and fusion of macrophages, *J. Biomed. Mater. Res.*, 71A, 439, 2004.

Draenert, K.D. et al., Strain adaptive remodeling in total joint replacement, *Clin. Orthop. Rel. Res.*, 430, 12, 2005.

Fitzgerald, R.H., Jr. (Ed.), *Non-Cemented Total Hip Arthroplasty*, Raven, New York, 1998.

Giavaresi, G. et al., Mechanical and histomorphometric evaluations of titanium implants with different surface treatments inserted in sheep cortical bone, *Biomaterials*, 24, 1583, 2003.

Homsy, C.A., Implant stabilization. Chemical and biomechanical considerations, *Orthop. Clin. N. Am.*, 4, 295, 1973.

Huiskes, R. et al., A biomechanical regulatory model for periprosthetic fibrous-tissue differentiation, *J. Mater. Sci. Mater. Med.*, 8, 785, 1997.

Lane, J.M. (Ed.), *Fracture Healing*, Churchill Livingstone, New York, 1987.

Lossdörfer, S. et al., Microrough implant surface topographies increase osteogenesis by reducing osteoclast formation and activity, *J. Biomed. Mater. Res.*, 70A, 361, 2004.

Rubin, C.T. and Hausman, M.R., The cellular basis of Wolff's law. Transduction of physical stimuli to skeletal adaptation, *Rhem. Clin. N. Am.*, 14, 503, 1988.

Smith, I.O., Baumann, M.J. and McCabe, L.R., Electrostatic interactions as a predictor for osteoblast attachment to biomaterials, *J. Biomed. Mater. Res.*, 70A, 436, 2004.

Søballe, K. et al., Tissue ingrowth into titanium and hydroxyapatite-coated implants during stable and unstable mechanical conditions, *J. Orthop. Res.*, 10, 285, 1992.

Thompson, D'A.W. *On Growth and Form*, Bonner, J.T. (Ed.), Cambridge University Press, Cambridge, 1977.

Vogel, S., *Life's Devices*, Princeton, NJ, Princeton University Press, 1988.

Wainwright, S.A. et al., *Mechanical Design in Organisms*, John Wiley & Sons, New York, 1976, 348.

Woo, S. L.-Y. et al., Less rigid internal fixation plates: historical perspectives and new concepts, *J. Orthop. Res.*, 1, 431, 1984.

11

In Vitro Tissue Growth and Replantation

11.1 General Considerations

In 1992, I defined the field of biomaterials (Section 1.4) as having four historic phases and, in turn, identified four classes or types of biomaterials:

- Type 1: inert
- Type 2: interactive
- Type 3: viable ([bio]hybrid)
- Type 4: replant

The current increasing interest in tissue engineering (TE) represents a shift in focus from types 1 and 2 to types 3 and 4 biomaterials. The earlier biomaterials, especially type 2, are not passé; on the contrary, they will continue to be represented in devices used in the bulk of conventional clinical applications, will be incorporated in some phase 3 devices, and will serve in devices intended as bridges to replantation* of phase 4 "devices" (organs). In some applications, due to problems of cost, supply, etc., types 1 and 2 will continue to be the biomaterials of choice indefinitely. Research and development of type 2 materials also continues very actively: in fact, the use of such materials to produce adaptive affects in the host tissues (see Chapter 10) can be considered, in many cases, as *in vivo* precursors of tissue engineering. Nevertheless, tissue engineering is a rapidly growing area of biomaterials science and engineering (BSE). This chapter will begin to define the field, explore its early progress, and foresee its near future.

---

* The surgical literature uses the term "replantation" to describe reattachment of severed body parts (fingers, etc.). If the severed part is viable and circulation is restored, such procedures can be highly successful. I retain the term (Section 1.4 and here) because, in each case, the inserted or reattached portion is mature, autologous tissue.

11.2 What Is Tissue Engineering?

The clearest early definition of tissue engineering of which I am aware is: "Tissue engineering is the application of principles and methods of engineering and life sciences toward fundamental understanding of structure-function relationships in normal and pathological mammalian tissues and the development of biological substitutes to restore, maintain, or improve tissue function" (Skalak et al. 1988). After providing this definition, Skalak went on to remark that

> The basic point of the above definition is that tissue engineering involves the use of living cells.... The definition is intended to encompass procedures in which the replacements may consist of cells in suspension, cells implanted on a scaffold such as collagen and in cases in which the replacement consists entirely of cells and their extracellular products.

Skalak was correct and prescient: the use of engineering principles and techniques to elaborate and incorporate living cells into constructs for therapeutic use distinguishes tissue engineering from more conventional biomaterials studies and from the concerns of other fields of physical and biological science and medicine. However, his definition has not been generally accepted and there are many interpretations of the scope and breadth of tissue engineering today.

The best global discussion of this term is provided by Vacanti and colleagues (2000):

> In essence, new functional living tissue is fabricated using living cells which are usually associated in one way or another to a matrix or scaffolding which can be natural, man-made, or a composite of both. The living cells can migrate into the implant after implantation or can be associated with the matrix in cell culture before implantation. Conceptually, the field (tissue engineering) differs from the field of cell transplantation insofar as organized three-dimensional tissue is desired and designed.

However, Vacanti et al. conflate types 2, 3, and 4 biomaterials as they have been previously defined (Section 1.4):

- Type 2 consists of materials engineered *in vitro* to produce a desired host response *in vivo*, such as ingrowth into a porous surfaced medullary stem.

- Type 3 consists of composites of cells and matrix (natural, man-made, or a combination) produced *in vitro* for implantation, such as synthetic vascular grafts incorporating one or several cell types in a resorbable matrix.

- Type 4 consists of cells, but more generally tissue and, eventually, organs, grown and/or modified *in vitro* for replantation. Carticel™ (autologous hyaline cartilage cells cultured and replanted) is a primitive type 4 biomaterial because, although it is fully viable, it lacks the (differentiated) three-dimensional aspect referred to by Vacanti.

I will not attempt a final definition of "tissue engineering" here: as is the case for any emerging field, the definition will mature as the field does. However, any widely adopted, successful definition (one that can clearly delimit TE and distinguish it from other pre-existing efforts) must contain four elements:

- TE must involve engineering — that is, the utilization of fundamental physical, chemical, and electromagnetic laws and principles as well as proven design and development methodology to produce practical solutions to clinical problems. Thus, merely renaming another research field "tissue engineering" will not contribute to progress. A sad example of this is the parallel emerging field of "genetic engineering," which apparently involves neither an engineering design component nor any appeal to basic physical laws or principles.
- TE must involve engineering manipulation of live cells or tissue, not merely the preparation of interactive (type 2) biomaterials. Thus, there may be type 3 and 4 tissue-engineered materials, but type 1 or 2 materials cannot be reasonably said to be tissue engineered because they affect, attract, or incorporate viable cells and tissues only after being placed *in vivo*.
- The organic component of a tissue-engineered product must include viable cells (or, at the very least, functional genes). The use of processed natural products as type 1 and 2 biomaterials in medical devices (such as gluteraldehyde-treated porcine tissue) is very well established and, although it has considerable clinical utility, it cannot be fairly said to constitute TE. Such products are probably better grouped with other "biologics": nonviable agents or materials of essentially natural (rather than synthetic) origin.
- The production of a tissue-engineered product must also involve some *in vitro* manipulation of viable tissue, cells, or organs. If this is not the case, it will be very difficult to distinguish, as Vacanti et al. (2000) try to do, between tissue engineering and transplantation of cells, tissue, and organs; the latter is a purely medical, not engineering, procedure.

Tissue engineering has a considerable overlap with the emerging field of regenerative medicine. It is as yet unclear where one can draw the line between the two; in fact, interdisciplinary academic programs already combine the two. In general, one can distinguish tissue engineering as primarily comprising efforts to replace damaged or absent tissue, using engineering techniques as outlined earlier. Regenerative medicine currently embodies more traditional therapeutic approaches, utilizing stem cells and genetic transfection, to restore inadequate or lost function *in situ*, as in treatment of diabetes, heart disease, spinal cord injury, and Parkinson's disease (National Resource Council 2002).

11.3 The Cell–Receptor Paradigm

11.3.1 Early Ideas

The advent of the "unit cell" concept in materials science had a revolutionary effect on understanding of materials properties and their dependence on structure. Thus, it was natural, as physical scientists and engineers moved into interdisciplinary biological research, for them to seek a similar unifying, simplifying paradigm. In early BSE studies, tissues were regarded as continuous, largely homogenous materials possessing only limited anisotropy of structure and properties. Because most early characterization studies were performed on dead tissue, cells were viewed as imperfections in structure, rather like defects or grain boundaries in polycrystalline materials, and were largely overlooked. It was understood that cellular function defined the living state, but that was not a concern for engineers and the general, usually unspoken, nonvitalist assumption was that living and dead materials had the same physical properties. This has turned out to be untrue in the general case (Black 1984).

As BSE became more sophisticated, the biological cell came to be seen as an equivalent, in tissues, of the unit cell in engineering materials. However, much of the bulk of tissues is made up of water and of various molecules, collectively termed extracellular matrix. This matrix, as well as the small partial volume contributed by the cell walls of dead cells, is, in fact, being characterized when investigations of structure–property relations are performed on tissues. Only in particular hypercellular structures, such as the epiphyseal growth plates of long bones or in the contents of the circulatory system, do the physical structure and properties of biological cells dominate in mechanical property determinations.

The cell wall, more generally termed the plasma membrane, was originally described as a phospholipid bilayer, with a hydrophobic core, possessing general permeability and numerous pores, some passive but others with active ion-pumping mechanisms. The cell content was regarded as an amorphous gel with specialized organelles, such as the nucleus and mitochondria, simply floating in essentially random locations. This simple model has proven inadequate to describe and explain the details of cell morphology and function and, in particular, the association of cells with each other and with their extracellular matrix, in all of the specialized profusion found in mammalian as well as nonmammalian tissues. For instance, such a simple model predicts that, through surface tension arguments, all cells should be spherical in solution and sessile on surfaces. This is clearly not the case.

Fortunately, in parallel with the development of BSE, mammalian cell biology and physiology was making great strides. A new unifying paradigm has emerged: receptor–ligand binding. Tissues are now seen as associations of cells and matrix, connected by specific and nonspecific receptor–ligand binding and receptors crossing the plasma membrane, providing bidirectional linkages capable of transducing information among the interior of the cell, its nearest neighbors, and its environment. Furthermore, most cells are now recognized to have well defined internal structures; active and passive molecular scaffolding links many of the organelles. Thus, the receptor–ligand-binding model in normal tissues provides the key to understanding the elaboration of those tissues and therefore the association between cells and synthetic matrices of types 1 through 3 biomaterials.

Tissues, as always, remain artifacts of the lives of cells. However, through the receptor–ligand paradigm, how cells make tissue matrices and, in turn, how these matrices influence the conduct of their lives can be understood.

11.3.2 The Membrane Receptor

In its most general form, a cellular receptor is a complex of two molecular chains traversing the cell membrane. The receptors are grouped together into types, such as integrins, selectins, cadherins, etc., based upon similarity of structure and of function. Within each type, the individual molecular chains are grouped together into families, depending upon general features of structure — primarily, the possession of a common subunit (see following).

The integrin type is perhaps of primary importance to TE studies because these receptors play key roles in cell–cell and cell–matrix association. Integrins are heterodimers made up of one each from subunits or chains termed "α" and "β" (see Figure 11.1). There are large numbers of α- and β-chains and thus very large numbers of possible different receptor structures and functions. The α- and β-chains are distinguished by the use of numerical subscripts: for example, the $\alpha_6\beta_1$ is a common receptor specialized for binding to the matrix protein laminin (Wei et al. 1997). However, all integrins share the following characteristics:

- The two chains, as combined, reside in the cell membrane so that they have three principal domains, or subsections:
  - An intracellular domain that can link with intracellular molecules and, in particular, can bind to the internal molecular skeleton of the cell
  - An intramembrane domain

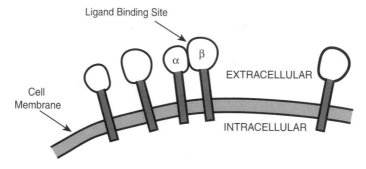

FIGURE 11.1
Schematic arrangement of the integrin receptor.

- An extracellular domain that forms the binding site for extracellular ligands, such as free molecules (cytokines, peptides, etc.) or portions of the extracellular matrix
- The receptors are free to move along the surface of the membrane and, under certain conditions, such as phagocytosis, can be internalized, recycled, and reappear on the cell surface.
- Intracellular and extracellular binding is reversible and, as such, the bound state represents an equilibrium:

$$\text{Receptor + Ligand} \quad \overset{k_b}{\underset{k_d}{}} \quad \text{Receptor-ligand complex}$$

Thus, the action of a receptor depends upon its population concentration on the cell membrane, the concentration of the ligand, and the energetics of binding and dissociation, as represented by k_b and k_d, respectively. Furthermore, divalent ions, such as Ca^{++}, are also frequently involved in forming or stabilizing receptor–ligand complexes. In addition, the population concentration on the cell membrane depends upon equilibrium between the assembled receptor and the intracellular concentrations of the respective α- and β-chains. Thus, receptor activity can be affected in many ways and receptor–ligand association has the potential to exert well differentiated effects on the cell.

11.3.3 Receptor–Matrix Interactions

The primary interest here is in the consequences of binding of receptors to molecules in the extracellular matrix. Again, although this complex material holds many molecules and the appearance and concentration of the spectrum vary from tissue to tissue, certain motifs recur. Ligand binding by receptors depends on recognizing short sequences of three or more amino acids. One such sequence is (-arginine-glycine-aspartamine-) (abbreviated: RGD). The

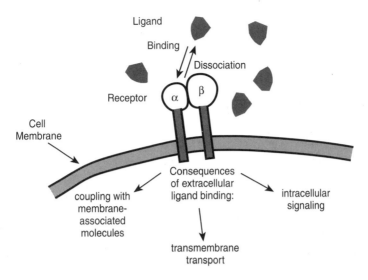

FIGURE 11.2
Possible consequences of extracellular receptor–ligand binding.

$\alpha_5\beta_1$ integrin binds to the RGD sequence, which is found in the very common extracellular matrix molecule fibronectin. Thus, the formation of $\alpha_5\beta_1$RGD complexes plays a strong role in association between cells and the extracellular matrix (MacDonald 1989). This observation has been utilized in the fabrication of interactive substrates that will bind cells through receptor–ligand association rather than through nonspecific chemical affinity (Massia and Hubbell 1990).

Once receptor–ligand binding takes place, several consequences can occur (Lauffenburger and Lindermann 1993) (Figure 11.2):

- The extracellular receptor–ligand complex formation may change the nature and/or affinity of the intracellular domains for intracellular species. Such intracellular binding, in turn, may alter the behavior of the extracellular domain of the receptor.
- The complex may be internalized, as in phagocytosis, thus playing a role in transmembrane transport of the ligand.
- Changes in the extracellular domain may "transduce" information, via the intracellular molecular skeleton (not shown in Figure 11.2 for clarity) to organelles such as the nucleus. In the short term, this may result in modification of cellular behavior (modulation), but in the longer term, it may produce activation of DNA, resulting in expression of new RNA and thus a possibly irreversible change in cell function (differentiation).

The emerging understanding of the consequences of the receptor–ligand paradigm is profound. In regard to BSE in general and TE in particular, the following conclusions can be drawn:

- Cells are in constant communication with their external environment; therefore, maintenance and/or alteration of the pericellular conditions are important considerations in understanding host response to biomaterials.

- In their native habitat, cells depend upon signals received (transduced) from their extracellular matrix in order to develop normally and to maintain their appropriate phenotype. Thus, the design of synthetic matrices for type 3 biomaterials must focus not merely on avoiding cytotoxic or inhibitory responses but also on providing appropriate information so as to encourage cells to maintain their normal habit and function or stimulate specific behavior.

- The appropriate consideration of biomaterial–(local) host interactions must now move from the so-called "tissue–material" interface to the cell–material or, more properly, the receptor–ligand interaction realm.

11.4   Matrices and Cell Sources

11.4.1   Cells*

Whether consisting entirely of cells and their extracellular products, like more traditional tissue grafts and organ transplants, or merely incorporating living cells, tissue replacements come in three types: auto-, allo-, and xeno, reflecting the original cell source (respectively, autobiopsy, allobiopsy, and xenobiopsy). The issue of xenohybrids (type 3) or xenoreplants** (type 4) will not be considered here because they represent special cases of xenografts and, except in the minds of animal rights advocates, do not raise any of the objections that will be discussed later. However, the success in transplanting human immune systems to small rodents such as mice suggests that, in the future, the availability of "pseudo" xenotissue and organ sources may help to resolve some of my present concerns. It has even been proposed to use genetically transformed larger animals such as pigs to grow immunologically matched xeno-organs, which I would term xenoreplants (Fox 1997).

Of the two remaining tissue types, the autoreplant, or true replant, as employed by Peterson (Brittberg et al. 1994) (see Section 11.5) in attempting

---

* Portions of this subsection, as well as Section 11.5, were published previously in different form (Black 1997).

** Strictly speaking, such replants could only be into animals, such as seeing eye dogs, unless transgenic hosts were used.

to repair articular cartilage, appears to raise the lesser concern. The availability of true cultured autografts would certainly definitively dispel some of the generic problems with transplants: each replant would exactly match the donor genetically (especially immunologically), it would introduce no additional infectious agents (if carefully handled *in vitro* and during replantation), and the supply would always match the demand. The downside would be high cost, significant delay (which in the case of culturing a full organ such as the kidney might be several years), and availability of support technology. The commercial and legal issues are fairly straightforward: the cost would reflect the processing (growth and handling) of tissue removed from the ultimate user and then returned, as well as some amortization of research and development costs.

However, the alloreplant seems to pose more problems. On the face of it, the use of cells from a single, possibly fetal or newborn, human donor and the elaboration of very large quantities of tissue appear attractive. This offers the theoretical prospects of lower costs (through economy of scale), better quality control, and a more manageable commercial manufacturing process. Early efforts in this area feature, in some cases, a self-contained cassette or cartridge: a support enclosure in which the cells can be maintained, nourished, and kept sterile until delivered to the sterile field within the operating room for implantation.

However, several areas of concern arise:

- The possible use of tissue from a single source — not for 15 to 25 recipients as is commonly the case for organ transplantation, but for perhaps as many as 25,000 recipients — raises the prospect of real clinical catastrophe if something goes wrong, such as inadvertent transmission of an undetected (possible previously unrecognized) slow virus. Unfortunately, one can only test for those viri and bacteria that have already been detected and even such tests have a significant rate of false negative findings.

- The use of an allobiopsy rather than autobiopsy cell source probably enables the future identification of the replant by karotyping, especially in the case of long lived tissue such as articular cartilage or cultured functional organs. This has potential implications for legal proceedings related to mal-outcome of the clinical procedure.

- In the U.S., the Uniform Anatomical Gift Act (1968) and the National Organ Transplant Act (1984) essentially forbid the sale or other commercial use of dead or live human body parts. The motivation for these laws is very clear and straightforward: they were intended to make human material available for teaching, research, and therapeutic purposes without creating a market in such materials. The concern about market forces stems from three bases:

- A recognition that the human body is special; emboding the moral sense that human beings are ends in themselves and should not be used as means to achieve other purposes

- A desire to prevent the poor and powerless from selling parts of their body, perhaps under duress

- A more general need to prevent the creation of an analog of the autobody chop shop that converts stolen cars into far more valuable subassemblies and parts

In the case of postmortuum organ donation, the organ is donated by the next of kin, frequently carrying out the desires of the donor, and the charges to the recipient cover only "harvesting," testing, transport, and implantation (although donor funeral expenses are also sometimes provided for). However, what about the donation of cells or portions of organs, perhaps by surviving donors, that could benefit thousands of recipients and are incorporated into "products" with significant value added by manufacturers? What would be sold then? Who should benefit financially? Can it be done legally and ethically?

- The need to obtain allogenic cells with pluripotentiality has turned interest first to human adult and then to fetal and embryonic stem cells. The former can be obtained with little or no injury to the donor, but harvesting the latter invariably results in death of the fetus or embryo. This latter situation has produced a wide range of national responses related, in large part, to local attitudes towards early-life issues such as abortion. In some countries, such cell sources may not be used and, in others, there is wide latitude, under ethical supervision. In the U.S., a hybrid approach is followed, permitting fetal stem cells to be used but limiting their sources narrowly to previously* established cell lines when public funding is involved.

Thus, one of the barriers to successful TE appears to be a need to understand and reach agreement concerning implications of choosing among various cell sources. As I have suggested previously, some of these objections may be overcome, potentially, by the use of transgenic xeno- (animal) sources. In the near term, however, the issues raised by current practices must be addressed and workable answers provided. Similar issues, particularly of ownership and its transfer, have already arisen in the commercial preparation of biological products from human cell sources. The litigation record, although instructive, does not resolve these questions definitively. Furthermore, even if it did, one would still be constrained to consider the ethical aspects of the questions. I will return to these points again in Section 11.5.

---

* Before August 9, 2001 (speech, 11/11/01, President G.W. Bush).

11.4.2   Matrices

There are also less ethically challenging but more pragmatic problems with the choice of matrix material, in the case of design and fabrication of a type 3 biomaterial.

Matrices may be natural in origin, such as collagen, keratin, or chitosan. Natural matrices are, to a lesser or greater degree, inherently "biodegradable," depending upon the amount of molecular structure change during processing, because mammalian systems possess a wide repertoire of degradative enzymes for self- and foreign organic molecules. A further attraction of natural sources is that a matrix familiar to the selected cells can be chosen; thus, type II collagen can be combined with chondrocytes in an attempt to fabricate a tissue-engineered hyaline cartilage. Collagen is perhaps the most widely used of such natural materials (Silver and Pins 1992; Bell 1995), although concerns still remain about immune response to some types (Lynn et al. 2004).

Matrices may also be prepared by deliberately modifying natural materials through physical, chemical, and enzymatic treatment. This is a practice of great antiquity, used in attempts to process natural structures, such as demineralized bone or tendon segments, to reduce their antigenic properties and improve their physical handling and postimplantation behavior. Many such materials derived from allo- and xeno- sources are in clinical use as type 2 biomaterials.

However, both of these approaches, although still popular, seem too crude today. A far more promising approach is the direct synthesis of polymers with specific structures and properties, such as including receptor recognition sequences, as the previously noted (-RGD-). Capello (1992) and his coworkers have been pioneers in this approach, using recombinant techniques to select DNA sequences that code for specific molecular arrangements and then transfecting these pseudogenes into bacteria such as *Escherichia coli*. They then induce them to synthesize large quantities of the desired material, which can then be spun into fibers, coated onto surfaces, etc. Such materials can be designed to be nonresorbable, partially resorbable, or fully resorbable, depending upon the demands of the application. One of the first achievements of this technique was the synthesis of spider silk modified to include receptor recognition domains (Anderson et al. 1994).

11.4.3   Combining Cells and Matrices

The issue of combining cells with matrices will not, in the long run, be a problem as the technology of TE moves increasingly towards type 4 or replant materials. In the meantime, considerable concern and argument will involve which combinations of cell and matrix sources are the most appropriate. Although it is hard to generalize, I suggest that, at this moment, the possible combinations can be grouped into three classes, in order of decreasing preference (Figure 11.3):

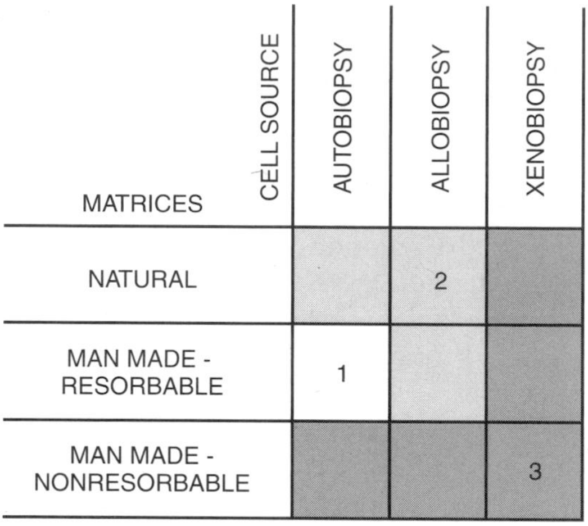

MATRICES	CELL SOURCE	AUTOBIOPSY	ALLOBIOPSY	XENOBIOPSY
NATURAL			2	
MAN MADE - RESORBABLE		1		
MAN MADE - NONRESORBABLE				3

FIGURE 11.3
Possible combinations of matrices and cell sources (numbers identify classes; see text).

- Class 1: the most desirable from pragmatic and ethical points of view appears to be the use of autobiopsy cells with partially or fully resorbable, synthetic matrices.

- Class 2: this can be extended, with care and consideration, to include natural matrices such as collagen and chitosan, perhaps with some chemical modification, and allobiopsy cell sources, particularly primitive stem cells. This class is the one now enjoying the most attention from industrial developers.

- Class 3: finally, and likely to be least satisfactory in the long run, is the use of xenobiopsy cell sources and the permanent incorporation of nonresorbable matrix elements. In some cases, such as in early studies using encapsulated xenobiotic cells for experimental human therapy, these approaches are unavoidable. It may continue to prove economically desirable in certain external applications, such as burn treatment. However, I hope that this approach will fall into disuse, due to permanent concerns about the possibility of unsought gene transfer and presence of undetected infectious agents.

11.5 Thinking Twice about Tissue Engineering

The dividing line between traditional biomaterials (in particular, the search for the Philosopher's Stone), the truly inert (type 1) biomaterial, and the field of tissue engineering was crossed on October 2, 1967 when Dr. Christiaan Barnard transplanted a live human heart into a patient with heart failure

(Barnard 1967). Although his first patient succumbed to a variety of clinical complications 18 days later, the possibility of routine transplantation of major functioning organs drew worldwide attention. An immediate impact felt in the U.S. was a radical curtailment of funds for the multicontractor federal program directed towards the development of an implantable (permanent) artificial heart. It is worth noting that this research and development program never recovered from this setback; today, successor devices such as active left ventricular assist devices (LVADs) are seen only as "bridges" to transplantation: as devices to sustain a patient's life until a suitable donor organ becomes available. In the same way, blood and peritoneal dialysis, which were originally viewed as miraculous but last-stage interventions in kidney disease and failure, are now widely employed for prolonged periods for patients awaiting definitive treatment by allotransplantation.

The success of organ transplantation from cadavers or, in the case of kidneys, from related or unrelated live donors cannot be denied. Perhaps as many as 340,000* U.S. patients have received transplants of living organs, including kidneys (the most commonly transplanted), heart, lung, liver, pancreas, and intestinal segments. Many patients receive multiple organ transplants, such as ex-governor of Pennsylvania Robert Casey, who received a combined heart and liver transplant in 1993 (Alexander and Baker 1993). Casey's situation illustrates some popular concerns about organ donation and transplantation:

- Organs for transplantation are rare in comparison to need and waiting times may be long. In 1995, it was estimated that 38,000 U.S. patients were on waiting lists as possible organ recipients; a new name was added very 30 minutes and at least 8 patients per day died while awaiting transplants. Nevertheless, a match was fortuitously found for Casey within 1 day of the decision to perform his transplant. Today, some 88,500 people await transplants.
- The donor involved was young and relatively disenfranchised: a 34 year old murder victim. This had been the situation in Dr. Barnard's initial heart transplantation; the donor was a young man killed in a vehicular accident (Barnard 1967).
- The recipient was older and, to a considerable degree, privileged. This issue was also highlighted by Barnard's first transplant: in a country still in the coils of apartheid, the donor was black and the recipient was a retired white civil servant. This issue of status privilege was also raised when the legendary baseball star Mickey Mantle received an unsuccessful liver transplant (Meyerson 1995).

Without question, organ transplantation is difficult and expensive. It is extremely difficult to screen donors for transmissible disease and accurately match donor organs to recipients so that the best possible blood and tissue

---

* http://www.optn.org/latestData/rptData.asp.

compatibility, as well as appropriate size, can be obtained. It must be done in a very short time span because organs generally become available on short notice and deteriorate rapidly with time, even when the donor is maintained on life support. Thus, statewide and regional networks and a national network, the United Network for Organ Sharing (UNOS),* have sprung up in the U.S. in response to the National Organ Transplant Act (1986) to facilitate optimal usage of organs. As a result, it is now possible for organs and tissues from a single donor to be given to many geographically widely separated recipients. Extensive publicity drives have been conducted to encourage individuals, especially people obtaining driver's licenses, to register as prospective organ donors. However, the fundamental problems remain: demand far exceeds supply and costs of the procedures involved tend pragmatically to reduce access by less well off and disenfranchised patients; as a result, nagging questions of social justice remain.

It is fair to state that these moral, ethical, and pragmatic considerations have also played strong roles in the development of TE so far. Early efforts in TE, although surrounded by high enthusiasm and attracting large quantities of venture capital, were relatively noncontroversial. These included, primarily in animal experimental studies and, in some cases, early human clinical trials, the encapsulation of Langerhans' islet cells for the treatment of diabetes (Scharp et al. 1994); the separation, culturing, and reinfusion of specific lymphocyte subpopulations for cancer therapy (Chen 2000); and the fabrication of a variety of hybrid skin replacements for use in burn treatment (Yannas and Burke 1980; Yannas 1997). In each case, the goal was transient therapy rather than definitive replacement, the conditions addressed were severe and life threatening, and an easy distinction could be maintained between "implant" and recipient.

However, in 1994, another phase began. Dr. Peterson and coworkers from the University of Göteborg, Sweden (Brittberg et al. 1994), reported early clinical trials of growth and replantation of articular chondrocytes in a procedure to replace full thickness focal defects in the tibial plateau. Autologous cells were removed from non-load-bearing areas of articular cartilage, separated from their matrix, cultured *in vitro* for 14 to 21 days, and then replanted in articular cartilage defects in the tibial plateaus of each donor; autologous periosteal membrane was used to retain the replant. In this application, the therapy is expected to be definitive (in the same way that implanting a metal and plastic total joint "replacement" is), the disease treated is not life threatening, and the replant is expected to become fully integrated with the patient's tissues.

This technique was introduced into the U.S. on an experimental basis and received FDA approval for some medical indications in August 1997. The "product," as commercialized by Genzyme Tissue Repair (GTR) (a division of Genzyme Inc.) and now distributed by U.S. Biosciences, is called Carticel™ (autologous replant chrondocytes). The technique of Brittberg et al. (1994)

---

* http://www.unos.org.

is generally followed, with a 3- to 6-week interval between autobiopsy and replantation. The culture process currently costs (nominally) $19,750 of an estimated average total treatment cost, including surgeon's fees, of $40,000.* The general technique, now termed articular cartilage implantation or ACI, has been essentially duplicated by several other companies and is in use in a number of countries.

This development requires taking a second look at the entire concept of TE. Before going too far down this path, it is worthwhile to think twice — to consider the implications and ask whether some things should not be done even when they appear to be possible. Section 11.4 discussed some of the trade-offs necessary between benefit and risk in the selection of matrices and cell sources for type 3 and 4 biomaterials. It is still too early to do more than muse about which of the risks will emerge as true clinical and legal problems and, as a result, which of the conflicting viewpoints among TE researchers and developers will come to dominate clinical practice in replantation.

I would like to note a more fundamental concern about TE. This concern was raised a half a century ago by Jack Vance (1956) in a novel entitled *To Live Forever*. Vance imagined a city society, Clarges, on a remote world in the last stages of societal decay. On one hand, its citizens possess an obsession about immortality, but, on the other, they submit to an agreement for State limitation of life span through the use of public assassins, with postponement of "termination" based upon a continual measurement of one's individual contribution to the public good. However, as one would suspect, in Clarges some people are more equal than others and society, in Vance's account, has evolved into five social classes: Brood, Wedge, Third, Verge, and Amaranth. It is the privileged Amaranth, the social and economic elite, who have solved the problem of immortality. Those few judged to have achieved the most and contributed the most to Clarges' society are admitted into the Amaranth class and undergo the following procedure:

> ...Five cells were extracted from [the] body. After such modification of genes as might be desired, they were immersed in a solution of nutrients, hormones and various special stimulants, where they rapidly evolved through the stages of embryo, infant, child and adolescent.... When invested with the prototype's memory-bank, they became the identity of the original: full-fledged surrogates (Vance 1965).

Amaranths zealously keep their memory-bank recordings up to date and their surrogates are carefully guarded against the day that the original (the prototype) might have a fatal accident, develop an incurable disease, or be irrecoverably injured or killed by violence.

Vance's novel centers on a problematic situation: one of the surrogates escapes and tries to lead a life independently of its prototype. Issues concerning the meaning of self, the value of life, involuntary servitude, and

---

* http://www.firstdatabank.com; Dr. T. Minas (personal communication).

manipulation of the fundamental elements of human existence are raised. In this prescient novel, the logical, although perhaps impossible, consequence of the promise of Dolly, the first successful report of cloning a sheep by nuclear transfer (Campbell et al. 1996), can be recognized. A dark reflection of the "baby factories" of an earlier visionary novel, *Brave New World* (Huxley 1932), in which all fetal development occurs *in vitro* (rather than *in utero*) and chemical manipulation is employed to fit each individual to his or her predestined place in society can also be seen. Rather than rejecting such disturbing visions out of hand as incredible, one should be aware of the widespread current efforts in therapeutic gene implantation and of anecdotal rumors of conception of babies to serve as marrow donors for older siblings.

The question that ought to be raised by Vance, Huxley, and visionaries is essentially, "When is enough, enough?" That is to say, where is the line between legitimate therapeutic intervention and a morbid preoccupation with life enhancement at all costs, and who shall judge its location? This is not a problem unique to the fields of BSE and TE. It can be recognized in the use of life support for the terminally ill, in radical interventional surgery, including multiple organ transplants in the elderly, in fetal (*in utero*) surgery, and so forth.

In his work, *Enough: Staying Human in an Engineered Age* (2003), McKibben wrote:

> ...[T]hese new technologies show us that human meaning dangles by a far thinner thread than we thought. What if the ending to our story has already been written, our compass set? What if we have been programmed, or at least must suspect each time we choose a path that we have been nudged in that direction by our engineered cells. Who then *are we*?

One can properly object that my suggesting connections between TE and, on one hand, the fictional visions of Huxley and Vance and, on the other, biotechnological research into gene transplantation and mammalian cloning is extreme and far fetched. In principle, I agree. However, this is a situation in which one can only see the extreme ends of a spectrum: at one end are research and medical procedures, which are simple and raise no ethical issues; at the other are dark dreams of clearly morally objectionable acts. The reason for creating this spectrum, or linkage, is to raise the questions: how will the boundary between the acceptable and the unacceptable be recognized? What are the moral mileposts that should warn one to slow down and, perhaps, to stop when, in McKibben's view, enough has been achieved?

Consider an illustrative example of such a spectrum, one relating to kidney transplantation. The implantation of cadaveric kidneys can be placed at one end; at the other, assume Vance's hypothesis but suggest only that the cloned human surrogate be maintained as an "organ bank" for the prototype.

Clearly, the former situation is found to be acceptable and the latter rejected as unthinkable.*

Now consider some possible intermediate points on this spectrum of possible organ sources, in no particular order:

- Live organ transplantation:
  - From a parent
  - From a child
  - From a sibling
  - From a sibling expressly conceived for the purpose
  - From a late term aborted fetus
  - From a transgenic anima
  - From a paid donor
  - From an executed criminal
  - From a condemned criminal
  - From a criminal seeking reduction or remission of sentence
- Implantation of artificial constructs (hybrid artificial organs) with cells from one or more of such sources or from a cloned surrogate

The potential use of each of these organ or cell sources raises interesting, different, and, in some cases, morally complex problems. Their rank order of moral acceptability is not obvious and a marker or threshold of unacceptability is not clear.

Traditionally, such questions have been referred to philosophers, ethicists, and religious leaders while scientists, engineers, and physicians have gone on with their studies and clinical treatment. I have no simple answers to the questions raised here. However, I am sufficiently disturbed by long-term implications of TE to suggest that engineers and scientists need to open a broad and deep dialogue with a cross-section of interested parties rather than simply going ahead with a narrow focus on possible technological solutions to human problems. The road to hell is, as Ambrose Bierce commented, paved with good intentions (1906).

Finally, I want to suggest a simple functional test for engineers and scientists in these (or, for that matter, other related) fields of investigation. Even if one can personally resolve the issues raised, as one must, it is worthwhile considering this question: will this work ultimately benefit refugees in Rwanda** or in the other parts of the world mired in desperate, apparently chronic, poverty and deprivation?

---

* If one has any doubt of this statement, simply replace "kidney" with "heart" or "pancreas" in the first sentence of this paragraph.
** As this is written (in 2005), more than three-fourths of a million refugees still are unable or afraid to return home, despite the best efforts of international organizations, more than a decade after the massive intertribal massacres that occurred in Rwanda.

I have come to call this question the "Rwanda test." I offer it to readers, experienced professionals, and students alike — not with the suggestion that a negative response is a necessary "show stopper," but rather with the hope that, among all the good and promising questions that can be asked, increasingly often those that have the potential to bring the greatest good to the most with the least risk of catastrophe will be selected. To fail to apply such a test to future investigations runs the risk of losing oneself and one's society.

11.6   Some Final Comments

Tissue engineering, with its hints of Frankenstein's monster and the seduction of dealing with the very substance of life — living tissue — is enormously alluring to beginning and long-time investigators in BSE, as well as in many other more traditional fields. Beyond the ethical concerns raised in the previous section, I want to close this discussion with a few practical concerns.

Without question, TE will continue to grow and flourish, although many of the early extravagant visions of the pioneers may be long delayed or prove unattainable. In the meantime, it is important not to lose sight of these points:

- Like the larger field of BSE, TE has three primary aspects: it is a materials science, a biological science, and a clinical science. Thus, TE cannot be expected to be successful unless it is moved forward by integrated multidisciplinary teams of physical and biological scientists, engineers, and clinicians and physicians. It would be easy for newer TE workers (such as materials specialists beginning to work in TE) to become second-rate biochemists, biophysicists, cell biologists, etc. This is a bad idea; it is far better to leave these more fundamental fields to their traditional practitioners, harvest their intellectual product, and focus on being broad integrators and innovators, as workers in BSE have always been.

- Interdisciplinary or innovative studies are no excuse for mediocrity. TE should not be allowed to become a refuge for workers who cannot compete successfully elsewhere in BSE or in its foundation fields of biological and physical sciences and engineering. On the contrary, difficult interdisciplinary fields such as TE have little room for the otherwise blameless but merely average investigator.

- Nothing is really new: many challenging problems faced in TE have been investigated in other contexts and, in many cases, practical solutions already exist. The emergence of online publications, new journals, and fledgling scientific societies are welcome as signs of intellectual vigor; however, abandoning the traditional literature and forums of biological and physical science and engineering and, particularly, of BSE will only handicap students and advanced workers alike in TE.

- TE products will continue to need a supporting superstructure of types 1 and 2 biomaterials for their fabrication, evaluation, preservation, handling, implantation, and clinical monitoring. Care must be taken that older, successful biomaterials technologies are not neglected in the haste to move ahead. Otherwise, future workers will repeat old mistakes and be faced with continually "reinventing the wheel."

- Clinical success of TE products will require a much more sophisticated understanding of the physical property differences between normal and diseased tissues than is currently available. I have long argued this point in the broader field of BSE, saying that, in particular, tissue mechanics is an essential prerequisite to and should be a component of any research effort directed towards support or replacement of natural tissues or organs with structural attributes. With the emergence of TE, I hope for an accompanying revival of tissue mechanics and morphometrics, with an increased focus on changes associated with medical and surgical procedures, disease, age, and interaction with implants.

- In any newer aspect of research such as TE, traditional methods and procedures continue to have a place. Vision is no excuse for abandonment of rigorous process; good science will always require the sequence of conception of new ideas; hypothesis formulation; careful observation; replication of experiments; critical, skeptical statistical analysis of outcomes; and testing and retesting of earlier hypotheses. Good engineering practice requires clear statements of problems; examination, development, and perfection of alternate approaches; and exhaustive testing* and verification of numerical, process, and hardware solutions. With regard to outcomes in science or engineering, if something seems too good to be true, it probably is, whether it is a laboratory result or a vacation travel offer.

Nevertheless, I have significant enthusiasm for TE; I only hope that the field and its workers are able to fulfill its great promise in responsible and ethical ways.

---

* Many years ago, to my amusement and dismay, I heard a podium presentation about an implant study in which two dogs had been used to examine local host response to a wide variety of candidate biomaterials. When I questioned the presenter, I suffered a *lapsus lingua* and asked why two dogs were used (rather than why *only* two were used!). The answer, after much reflection, was, "Well, I suppose I could have used just one." Since then, at each meeting I have attended, I have mentally bestowed the "one dog" award to the presentation containing the greatest amount of data gained from the smallest number of test subjects, animal or human. Regretfully, there has been a continuing need to make this award at TE as well as BSE meetings. (See also Chapter 18, Appendix 1.)

References

Alexander, K.L. and Baker, S., Governor Casey's timely transplant, *Bus. Week*, June 28, 1993.

Anderson, J.P. et al., Structural evolution of genetically engineered silk like protein polymers, in *Silk Polymers: Materials Science and Biotechnology* (ACS Symposium Series #544). Kaplan, D., Adams, W.W., Farmer, B. and Viney, C. (Eds.), American Chemical Society, Washington, D.C., 1994, p. 137.

Barnard, C.N., The operation. A human cardiac transplant: an interim report of a successful operation performed at Groote Schuur Hospital, Cape Town, *S. Afr. Med. J.*, 41(48), 1271, 1967.

Bell, E., Strategy for the selection of scaffolds for tissue engineering, *Tissue Eng.*, 1(2), 163, 1995.

Black, J., Tissue properties: relationship of *in vitro* studies to *in vivo* behavior, in *Natural and Living Biomaterials*, Hastings, G.W. and Ducheyne, P. (Eds.), CRC Press, Boca Raton, FL, 1984, 5.

Black, J., Thinking twice about tissue engineering, *IEEE Eng. Biol. Med.*, 16(4), 102, 1997.

Brittberg, M. et al., Treatment of deep cartilage defects in the knee with autologous chondrocyte transplantation, *New Engl. J. Med.*, 331(14), 889, 1994.

Campbell, K.H. et al., Implications of cloning, *Nature*, 6573, 383, 1996.

Capello, J., Genetic production of synthetic protein polymers, *Mater. Res. Soc. Bull.*, 17, 48, 1992.

Chen, U., Lymphoid cells, in Lanza, R.P., Langer, R. and Chick, W.L. (Eds.), *Principles of Tissue Engineering*, 2nd ed., Elsevier Science, New York, 2000, 611.

Fox, M., Sheep-cloners PPL to breed for transplants, *Reuters News Service*, 3/24/97, 1997.

Huxley, A.L., *Brave New World*, Doubleday, Doran & Co., Garden City, NJ, 1932.

Lauffenburger, D.A. and Linderman, J.J., *Receptors: Models for Binding, Trafficking, and Signaling*, Oxford University Press, New York, 1993.

Lynn, A.K. et al., Antigenicity and immunogenicity of collagen, *J. Biomed. Mater. Res., Part B: Appl. Biomater.*, 71B, 343, 2004.

MacDonald, J.A., Receptors for extracellular matrix components, *J. Physiol.*, 257, L331, 1989.

Massia, S.P. and Hubbell, J.A., Covalent surface immobilization of Arg-Gly-Asp- and Tyr-Ile-Gly-Ser-Arg-containing peptides to obtain well-defined cell-adhesive substrates, *Anal. Biochem.*, 187(2), 292, 1990.

McKibben, B., *Enough: Staying Human in an Engineered Age*, Henry Holt, New York, 2003, 65.

Meyerson, A.R., Final stats: Mantle's last medical bills, *NY Times*, 8/20/95.

National Organ Transplant Act, Public Law No: 98-507, 1984.

National Research Council, *Stem Cells and the Future of Regenerative Medicine*, National Academy Press: Washington, D.C., 2002, 4.

Scharp, D.W. et al., Protection of encapsulated human islets implanted without immunosuppression in patients with type I or type II diabetes and in nondiabetic control subjects, *Diabetes*, 43, 1167, 1994.

Silver, F.H. and Pins, G., Cell growth on collagen: a review of tissue engineering using scaffolds containing extracellular matrix, *J. Long-Term Eff. Med. Impl.*, 2(1), 67, 1992.

Skalak, R. et al., Preface, in Skalak, R. and Fox, C.F. (Eds), *Tissue Engineering*, Alan R. Liss, Inc., New York, 1988, 1.

Uniform Anatomical Gift Act (1968, as amended 1987), National Conference of Commissioners on Uniform State Laws, C. 1:12A-8 (subsequently adopted by individual states (U.S.)).

Vacanti, J.P. and Vacanti, C.A., History and scope of tissue engineering, in Lanza, R.P., Langer, R. and Chick, W.L. (Eds.), *Principles of Tissue Engineering*, 2nd ed., Elsevier Science, New York, 2000, 3.

Vance, J., *To Live Forever*, Ballantine Books, New York, 1965.

Wei, J. et al., Integrin signaling in leukocytes: lessons from the $\alpha_6\beta_1$ integrin, *J. Leukocyte Biol.*, 61, 397, 1997.

Yannas, I.V. and Burke, J.F., Design of an artificial skin. I. Basic design principles, *J. Biomed. Mater. Res.*, 14, 65, 1980.

Yannas, I.V., *In vivo* synthesis of tissues and organs, in Lanza, R.P., Langer, R. and Chick, W.L. (Eds.), *Principles of Tissue Engineering*, 1st ed., Elsevier Science, New York, 1997, 167.

Bibliography

Atala, A. and Lanza, R.P., *Methods of Tissue Engineering*, Academic Press, New York, 2001.

Beauchamp, T.L. and Childress, J.F., *Principles of Biomedical Ethics*, 5th ed., Oxford University Press, New York, 2001.

Bierce, A., *The Cynic's Word Book*, 1906. (Reprinted as: *The Devil's Dictionary*, Castle Books; New York, 1967).

Brodt, P. (Ed.), *Cell Adhesion and Invasion in Cancer Metastasis*, Chapman & Hall, London, 1996.

Germain, L. et al., Engineering human tissues for *in vivo* applications, *Ann. N.Y. Acad. Sci.*, 961, 268, 2002.

Gold, E.R., *Body Parts: Property Rights and the Ownership of Human Biological Materials*, Georgetown University Press, Washington, D.C., 1996.

Fox, R.C. and Swazey, J.P., *Spare Parts. Organ Replacement in American Society*, Oxford University Press (Acadia Institute), New York, 1992.

Hardie, D.G., *Biochemical Messengers: Hormones, Neurotransmitters, and Growth Factors*, Chapman & Hall, London, 1991.

Katz, B.Z. and Yamada, K.M., Integrins in morphogenesis and signaling, *Biochimie*, 79(8), 467, 1997.

Langer, R. and Vacanti, J.P., Tissue engineering, *Science*, 260, 920, 1993.

Lanza, R.P., Langer, R. and Chick, W.L. (Eds.), *Principles of Tissue Engineering*, 2nd ed., Elsevier Science, New York, 2000.

Lysaght, M.J. and Hazelhurst, A.L., Tissue engineering: The end of the beginning, *Tissue Eng.*, 10(1/2), 309, 2004.

Palsson, B., Hubbell, J.A., Plonsey, R. and Bronzino, J.D. (Eds.), *Tissue Engineering*, CRC Press, Boca Raton, 2003.

Ratner, B.D. and Bryant, S.J., Biomaterials: Where we have been and where we are going, *Annu. Rev. Biomed. Eng.*, 6, 41, 2004.

Schwartz, M.A. et al., Integrins: emerging paradigms of signal transduction, *Annu. Rev. Cell Dev. Biol.*, 11, 549, 1995.

Shelly, M., *Frankenstein*, 1818 (reprinted by J.M. Dent, Everyman's Library, London, 1994.)

Skalak, R. and Fox, C.F. (Eds.), *Tissue Engineering*, proceedings for a workshop held at Granlibakken, Lake Tahoe, California, February 26–29, 1988, Alan R. Liss, Inc., New York, 1988.

Younger, S.J. et al., (Eds.), *Organ Transplantation*, University of Wisconsin Press, Madison, 1996.

12

Allergic Foreign Body Response

12.1 Specific vs. Nonspecific Response

In earlier consideration of the inflammatory response (Chapter 8), the actions of neutrophils and macrophages in response to a foreign material are described as a nonspecific defense mechanism. That is, their response is universal in nature and only slightly affected by the structure and chemical composition of the foreign material. This chapter will discuss a second type of response to foreign materials, the specific or immune response.

The aspects of specific response to foreign or nonself materials are grouped together and collectively ascribed to a system of cells and mediating agents, collectively termed the immune system. Immunity is usually understood as the property of being secure or nonsusceptible to the adverse effects of a particular bacterium or foreign material. Conversely, allergy is the property of being especially sensitive (or hypersensitive) to such agents. Figure 12.1 shows the overall system and its general features in mammals.

The immune system is configured or adapts to distinguish between self (things that are part of the natural, intact physiological system) and nonself (all other things). It normally ignores all aspects of self; however, if it mistakes self for nonself, adverse reactions, collectively termed autoimmunity, may occur. Introduction of foreign tissue, also recognized as nonself, produces an inflammatory response termed rejection. Resistance may be conferred by genetic inheritance of a "memory" for certain nonself materials such as proteins in bacterial cell walls, thus producing a natural resistance to certain infections. Perhaps the most important aspect of the system is its ability to adapt by developing a specific memory for particular foreign materials. This may be produced by deliberate exposure to a partial or attenuated organism or material under nonpathogenic conditions (vaccination) or by prior exposure under sensitizing conditions (high dosage, physical stress, presence of an adjuvant material, etc.). The result of this specific memory may be desirable, as in affording acquired (vs. natural) resistance to infection, or undesirable, as in producing a form of adverse reaction to antigens or implants, termed hypersensitivity.

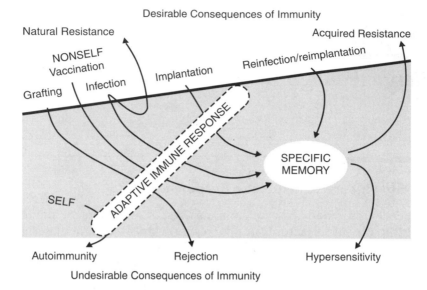

FIGURE 12.1
The immune system. (Adapted from Playfair, J.H., *Immunology at a Glance*, 3rd ed., Blackwell Scientific Publications, Oxford, 1979.)

12.2 Mechanisms of Immune Response

12.2.1 Antigen–Antibody Complex Formation

Specific or immune responses depend upon the exact details of the chemical composition and conformation or structure (see Section 5.2) of the foreign material. This class of response is directed primarily towards recognition of foreign proteins such as toxins, viri, and bacterial cell wall components. The response to these foreign materials takes place through two mechanisms: humoral and cellular (also termed cell-mediated) response. In each case, the foreign body is referred to as an antigen and the body responds by producing an antibody. Antibody is a generic name for a macromolecular complex formed by the association of large immunoglobulins present in serum into a Y-shaped molecule with a molecular weight exceeding 1×10^6. The stem of the Y is essentially the same for all antibodies, permitting it to bind to cell surfaces; regions in the arms are variable in structure, producing the specificity, or ability to bind with a particular antigen, characteristic of an antibody.

The humoral mechanism is based upon the production of freely circulating antibodies. These antibodies are designed to unite with the foreign material and "denature" or neutralize it. That is, the antibody–antigen complex lacks the undesirable or destructive activity of the free antigen. The complex may accumulate locally in tissue, be carried to lymph nodes by phagocytes, or be more easily catabolized than the free antigen. Circulating antibody production is mediated by a class of lymphocytes called B-cells that arise from primitive mesenchymal cells in the bone marrow. Antibody production is initiated by introduction of an antigen consisting in part or whole of a foreign (nonself) material. Whether biological, organic, or inorganic in constitution, such material may be able to act as an antigen; it may combine with native proteins, especially complement fragments of C3 and C5 (see Section 12.2.2), to form an antigen; or it may undergo metabolic processing by a phagocytic cell, usually a macrophage, to become an antigen.

Once antibodies are produced and released into the blood stream, they may persist for long periods of time. This is the principle of immunization to bacterial and viral infection: administering a small provocative dose of a specific antigen or one that produces antibodies specific to the infectious organism of interest. Then, when a later challenge is encountered, immediate antibody–antigen complexing occurs without the delay necessary for new antibody production. The antibody production response is quite variable, depending upon the initiating agent, its concentration, the general state of health of the immune system, and the presence of sensitizing agents such as corticosteroids. Finally, a subpopulation of B-lymphocytes, memory B-cells, are then capable of rapidly synthesizing additional amounts of the specific antibody (which it "remembers") upon stimulus by a later exposure to the same foreign body.

Cell-mediated response depends upon the action of another class of lymphocytes, the T-cells. These cells also arise in bone marrow, but pass through the thymus gland where they undergo a conversion that improves their ability to differentiate. They then collect in lymph nodes and associated tissue. Their activity continues to be affected by a hormone secreted by epithelial cells in the thymus gland. The T-cells cannot be distinguished from B-cells morphologically until challenged by an antigen. As in the case of humoral response, a foreign material or one of its degradation products may be able to act as an antigen; it may combine with native proteins, especially complement molecule C5 (which may be activated to C5a [see Shepard et al. 1984]), to form an antigen or it may undergo metabolic processing by a phagocytic cell, usually a macrophage, to become an antigen.

T-cells may then be distinguished by morphological changes that include the appearance of many polyribosomes and scant rough endoplasmic reticulum. They produce and store a different class of antibodies, primarily bound to the cell membrane surface. These antibodies are highly specific and cannot survive with appreciable activity outside or separate from the T-cell. T-cell antibodies act against intracellular infections, cancer, and foreign materials of nonbiological origin. However, T-cells must be present and aggregate in the region of antigen concentration to be effective because they must externalize and directly present the antibody to the antigen.

In addition to direct neutralization of undesired effects of foreign materials, the formation of antibody–antigen complexes acts to enhance inflammatory response. This can happen directly through a nonspecific phagocytic response because the complexes can grow to microscopic size by accretion of additional antibody and antigen molecules, or it can occur indirectly through complement activation (Chenoweth 1986; Tang et al. 1998).

Because particulate foreign materials such as wear debris from a joint replacement (Urban et al. 1994, 2004) may be distributed widely in the host and lymphocytes and circulating antibodies are also widespread, local response to antibody–antigen complexing may occur anywhere. This results in the wide variety of physiological effects popularly termed "allergic": swelling of the membranes in the respiratory system (hay fever, asthma, etc.), rash or reddening (arthus, etc.), hives (swelling related to local kinin activation), and so forth.

12.2.2 Complement System Activation

The formation of antigen–antibody complexes will interfere with the chemical function of the antigen. However, if the antigen is a surface feature, perhaps a receptor, on the surface of an invading bacteria, then the mere formation of such a complex may not be enough to prevent the bacteria from multiplying, producing toxins, etc. Thus, a humoral system of immune defense exists that has been termed the complement system because it supports and extends the immune system. The complement system consists of approximately 40 proteins of various molecular weights found in serum and interstitial fluid. When activated, its main function is to produce a product (the membrane attack complex [MAC]) that renders bacterial cell wall membranes porous, leading to cell death. Thus, the MAC is directly bactericidal.

The principal molecular elements of the complement system are labeled C1 though C9 and, in a motif similar to the coagulation cascade (see Figure 9.1), they participate in a cleavage and amplification process leading to the formation of MACs. There are two primary pathways: the classical pathway is initiated by the formation of antigen–antibody complexes and thus can become active as a concomitant of humoral or cellular immune responses; an alternate pathway can be triggered in the absence of a specific immune response by certain foreign molecules, such as repeating sugars or proteins (Figure 12.2).

The role of complement activation in immune response to implants is controversial, but has been recognized by some researchers (Chenoweth 1987; Tegnander et al. 1994). It is clearly implicated in the case of T- or B-cell activation. However, the types of materials that may be able to activate the alternate pathway are still not well recognized. Complement activation has several consequences:

- The MAC can attack native cells and foreign cells (as in transplants), as well as bacteria, causing undesirable cellular necrosis.

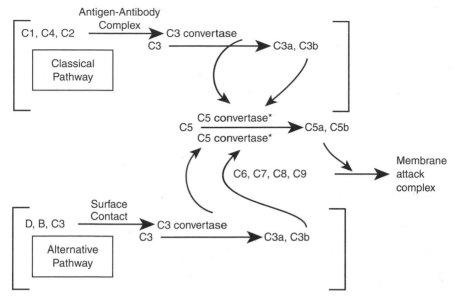

*different structures; same enzymatic activity

FIGURE 12.2
Classical and alternative pathways for complement activation. (Adapted from Elgert, K.D., *Immunology. Understanding the Immune System*, Wiley–Liss, New York, 1996.)

- In sufficient concentration, several of the activated intermediates, such as C5a, are capable of producing an inflammatory process (see Section 8.2).
- Some intermediates, such as C3b, inhibit the growth of antigen–antibody complexes.
- Some intermediates, such as C3b and C5a, serve as opsonins (see Section 8.2.3) and encourage phagocytosis.

The consequences of complement activation are not necessarily adverse. Although cellular necrosis and inflammation are unwanted effects, reduction in antigen–antibody complex size and improvement of phagocytosis through more efficient opsonization may be beneficial in certain settings. The role of complement activation in local (and systemic) host response to implants is still largely unexplored and further investigations may yield new insights in the future.

12.3 Classes of Hypersensitivity Reactions

Allergic responses are more properly categorized collectively as hypersensitivity reactions (Merritt 1998). These may be separated into immediate hypersensitivity, which is mediated by direct antibody–antigen combination, and delayed hypersensitivity, which is cell mediated. Immediate hypersensitivity is further subdivided into three types:

- Anaphylactic or immediate shock response
- Cytolytic/cytotoxic reactions
- Toxic complex syndrome

Delayed hypersensitivity responses are usually called type 4 reactions. If a challenge evokes an immediate reaction (type 1, 2, or 3) and then a further, delayed reaction, the net reaction is termed "mixed" and referred to as type 5. (Note: these responses are frequently designated by Roman numerals.)

The nature of supposed responses to implants (to be discussed later) suggests that they are, collectively, examples of delayed hypersensitivity, or type 4 reactions. The type 4 reaction is clinically similar to a chronic inflammatory response, except that lymphocytes as well as neutrophils are seen in foci of antigen–antibody complex accumulation and additional concomitant symptoms, as discussed in Section 12.4, may occur.

12.4 Hypersensitivity Reactions Associated with Implants

12.4.1 Polymers

Although humoral and cell-mediated immune responses are usually directed toward materials of natural origin, it is of interest to inquire concerning the response to implants. As of now, few responses to polymers used as biomaterials are recognized, except for the special case of implants made from processed natural tissue. The use of such materials, including processed allografts (tissue from human donors) and xenografts (tissue from other species, such as porcine heart valves, etc.) is finally limited by the ability to denature or chemically mask the foreign materials so as to suppress their antigenic activity (Bajpai 1983). Some natural materials used in medicine, but fortunately not as implants (such as latex rubber), are widely recognized to evoke responses (Emans 1992).

Attempts to produce immune responses to bulk polymers (Maurin 1995; Stern et al. 1972) have produced very mild effects. They are most suggestive of immune response to native proteins denatured by adsorption (see Section

5.5) sufficiently so that they are no longer recognized as self and are able to serve as antigens, rather than direct antibody production or T-cell activation by polymer molecules. Clinically, cell-mediated responses have been reported to poly methyl methacrylate "bone cement" (Haddad et al. 1995; Clementi et al. 1980) and to silicone elastomers (Kossovsky et al. 1987).

This latter topic has attracted a wide interest in recent years. Silica (SiO_2) has long been recognized as an antigenic adjuvant; that is, when administered in conjunction with an antigen, in animal models, it produces a heightened immune response. Some animal studies suggest that silicone gel may be an adjuvant (Nicholson et al. 1996; Naim et al. 1995). Thus, scattered reports of apparent autoimmune diseases in patients with silicone elastomer breast augmentation devices raised the question of whether a causal connection might be possible. Kossovsky has been the primary proponent of this view (Kossovsky and Freiman 1994). However, despite continued animal studies and extended human epidemiological studies, no association has been demonstrated between the use of silicone implants and a wide range of connective tissue disorders, many of which are known or suspected to be autoimmunity diseases (Gabriel et al. 1994).*

Despite these isolated reports implicating polymers, concerns about immune or allergic responses to biomaterials have centered primarily on metallic materials on the skin and as implants.**

12.4.2 Metals

12.4.2.1 General

The action of metals on the immune system is a bit of a puzzle. It is generally recognized that they must be dissolved to be active but the low molecular weight and simplicity of structure of the resulting ions argue against their being capable of directly inducing humoral or cell-mediated response. It is thought that they combine with organic molecules such as albumin to form complexes termed haptens, which possess antigenic qualities. It has also been suggested that increases in concentrations of naturally occurring metal–carrier protein complexes, such as Fe–transferrin or thioneins, can render them effective haptens. Details of metal–protein complexing affecting molecular shape changes are complex (Friedberg 1974).

However, Yang and Merritt (1994, 1996) have been able to demonstrate the presence of antibodies to albumin–metal complexes in patients with well functioning cobalt-base alloy joint replacement components and to produce specific monoclonal antibodies to these complexes in a rabbit model. In the presence of excessive wear, these findings may possibly be clinically significant. Nakamura et al. (1997) reported a case of autoimmune hemolytic

---

* The reader may wish to consult Angel (1997) for an account of the practical consequences of this controversy.
** Note: immune responses to ceramic biomaterials have apparently not been reported.

TABLE 12.1

Incidence of Metal Sensitivity

Allergen	Patients Presenting with Skin Problems (%)			Normals (%)		
	Male	Female	Total	Male	Female	Total
Nickel	3.1	12.9	9.6	1.5	8.9	4.2
Chromium	12.7	7.1	9.3	2.0	1.5	1.7
Cobalt	4.7	5.3	6.0	nr	nr	nr

Note: nr: not reported.

Source: Adapted from Hildebrand, H.F. et al., in *Biocompatibility of Co–Cr–Ni Alloys*, Hildebrand, H.F. and Champy, M. (Eds.), Plenum Press, New York, 1988, 201.

anemia associated with abnormal wear of a cobalt-base femoral head by screw impingement.

Metal sensitivity among the general population is not rare; sensitivity to nickel is the most common, followed by cobalt and chromium. The incidence of sensitivity is estimated to be between 1 and 5%, with as much as 10% of the population sensitive to at least one of these metals (Table 12.1). Incidence rates are different for men and women, reflecting differences in home and workplace exposure, and are higher for individuals involved in certain industries, including mining, metal refining, electroplating, printing, etc.

In addition to acting as antigens through hapten formation, some metals of interest for use in implants have been shown to affect directly the response of the host immune system to other antigens. Chromium (Shrivastava et al. 2002) and nickel have been shown to suppress antibody production; the roles of cobalt and manganese are anomalous. Iron, chromium, and nickel also have been shown *in vitro* to bind with T-cell surface antigens (Bravo et al. 1990); this binding may change the specificity of the previously formed antigens.

12.4.2.2   Dermatitis

Only two aspects of immune response to metals will be discussed. The first of these is dermatitis as a direct response to metallic contact. This is important for a number of reasons. It may be a direct and unacceptable side effect of the use of external metallic support devices such as braces or dentures. It has come to be recognized as a general indicator of systemic challenge in the mechanism of hypersensitivity of metals.

A classic account of metallic dermatitis is that of Fisher (1986), who recognizes sensitization by nickel, chromium, cobalt, gold, and platinum among the metals of implant interest (the last two have extensive dental applications). With the exception of nickel, these do not provoke an initial sensitivity in the solid state due to their low solubility. However, in a previously sensitized individual, all can evoke skin inflammations (that is, dermatitis) of various types and degrees of severity. Fisher suggests that little

TABLE 12.2

Sensitivity Thresholds for Metals

Clinical Sensitivity	Challenge Compound	Threshold Conc. (mean, wt%)
Co	$CoCl_2$	0.27
Co, Ni	$CoCl_2$	0.25
Co, Ni, Cr	$CoCl_2$	0.51
Co, Cr	$CoCl_2$	0.30
Cr	K_2CrO_4	0.21
Cr, Co	K_2CrO_4	0.08
Cr, Co, Ni	K_2CrO_4	0.14
Cr	$K_2Cr_2O_7$	0.22
Cr, Co	$K_2Cr_2O_7$	0.22

Source: Adapted from Wahlberg, J.E., *Berufsder-matosen*, 21, 22, 1973.

cross-sensitivity occurs — that is, metal "A" causing a response in a patient sensitized to metal "B" — although nickel sensitivity is often accompanied by cobalt sensitivity.* Chromium appears to cause a response primarily when present as a chromate [Cr^{+6}]; the other metals are active in divalent and trivalent ionic forms. Fisher's chapter is especially valuable for its catalogs of metal-bearing articles and environmental (exposure) settings. It also provides excellent clinical descriptions of the various dermatitides and of techniques for skin testing for sensitivity.

Wahlberg (1973) tested a number of patients with identified clinical sensitivity to metals and determined threshold concentrations for topical application of metal salts. Of interest is his finding that the carrier used in the patch test affects the threshold in many cases. That is, if the carrier aids penetration of the metallic ions, a lower threshold is found. Table 12.2 presents these data for water-based solutions only. At variance with Fisher's conclusion, a subtle pattern of cross-sensitivity, at least with respect to the minimum dose required for response, can be seen. These data should be regarded with some care because individual patients showed a response to concentrations one to two orders of magnitude below mean threshold values for these experimental groups.

Wahlberg also looked for relationships between clinical severity of responses and threshold values for particular patients and found poor correlations except in the case of cobalt, where the correlation coefficient $r = 0.61$. He concluded that "...renewed contact with cobalt plays a greater role in recurrence [of allergenic response] than [with] allergens such as chromium and nickel, where other factors, such as infections, heat, moisture, cold, stress, etc....contribute to the recurrence."

At a more subtle level, Hallab et al. (2004) found a positive correlation between chromium and cobalt serum concentrations in nonsymptomatic

---

* Note that this latter finding may be due simply to the close association of these two metals in alloys, etc. and not to a true cross-sensitivity.

patients with high release rate (metal-on-metal) hip replacements and the responses of their lymphocytes to dissolved cobalt or nickel challenge *in vitro*.

It should be noted here that clinical practice is to use 1 to 5 wt% solutions for skin patch testing (McGillis et al. 1989) for metallic allergenic response. Comparing these concentrations with the threshold data in Table 12.1 lends real weight to the concern that patch testing in the presence of a sensitizing agent or condition may contribute to a later immune response in a previously insensitive individual.

Many clinical reports detail local as well as remote skin response to metallic devices. One that is reported completely (Brendlinger and Tarsitano 1970) will suffice as an example. The patient, a 25-year-old woman, appeared with generalized eruptions on her trunk, arms, and legs. Treatment with topical corticosteroids provided some relief. She sought treatment for dermatitis on her ring finger 8 months later. Despite treatment, she continued to experience a spread and increase in intensity of symptoms. A rash appeared on her feet. She began to experience pain and soreness in her mouth 2 months later — that is, 11 months after her first symptoms appeared. On examination, she was found to have a cobalt-chromium partial denture that she had acquired several months before her initial skin problems and had worn intermittently thereafter. Replacement of the metal denture with an acrylic one resulted in prompt remission of symptoms. Reinsertion of the metal denture resulted in a return of symptoms within 24 hours. At that time, skin testing showed that she was sensitive to chromium as well as nickel in pure solid metallic form.

Sensitivity to chromium, cobalt, and nickel is now well recognized in dental applications in which contact between the device and the oral mucosa occurs. Hildebrand et al. (1988) report a compilation of 149 cases that fulfill three strict criteria:

- Presence of one or more clinical features suggestive of immune response, such as eczema, redness, ulceration, etc.
- Healing (resolution of the clinical features) after removal of the device
- Positive skin (epicutaneous) response to a metallic component of the device

Of particular interest in this report is the observation that only 28 patients (~20%) reported a prior history of symptoms referable to an established metal sensitivity. Thus, it is probable that the use of stainless-steel and cobalt-base alloys in dental applications can result in sensitizing previously non-sensitive patients.

It should not be concluded that skin or mucosal contact by the implant is necessary to produce dermatitis. A report (Cramers and Lucht 1977) documents the cases of three patients with 316L stainless steel and screw implants who developed dermatitis 3 to 3.5 months after surgery. Two patients were found to be sensitive to chromium and cobalt by patch test and one was sensitive to nickel. On surgical exploration, no infection could be cultured in any case, and all immune response symptoms resolved promptly after the devices were removed.

12.4.2.3 Implant Site Inflammation

The second aspect of immune response to metals to be considered is the direct implant site inflammation. Hicks (1958) was probably the first to report this effect. Initially, it was thought to be a simple inflammatory response associated with the relatively high corrosion rates of alloys in use in the 1940s and 1950s. In the 1970s, interest in the problems of loosening of total joint replacements, especially of the hip, reawakened interest in this problem, especially in relation to possible immune response to metals.

An initial study of the possible relationship between sensitivity to metal and problems with total joint replacement conducted by Evans et al. (1974) aroused considerable interest. These researchers reported the results shown in Table 12.3. They also found an apparently greater effect associated with metal-on-metal devices. Several of their conclusions are:

1. Evidence is presented which suggests that after replacement, bone necrosis and consequent loosening of the prosthesis may be due to the development of sensitivity to the metals used.

4. Examination of this material [tissue of joints from sensitive patients] showed necrosis of bone and soft tissue following obliterative changes in the vascular supply.

7. We conclude that prostheses in which metal articulates with polyethylene should be preferred; that any patient in whom loosening or fragmentation occurs should be patch tested and that if sensitivity is found the implant should be removed.

This study suggests a linkage between loosening, perhaps secondary to inflammation, and sensitivity, especially for metal-on-metal devices. Although they have overall lower wear rates, such devices would be

TABLE 12.3

Relationship between THR Loosening and Metal Sensitivity[a]

Patients	Total (#)	Sensitive (#, %)	Insensitive (#, %)
Loose	14	9[b](64)	5 (36)
Not loose	24	—	24 (100)

[a] By skin test.
[b] 11 loose prostheses.

Source: Adapted from Evans, E.M. et al., *J. Bone Joint Surg.*, 56B, 626, 1974.

expected to shed larger amounts of metallic products than metal-on-polymer ones and appear to be involved more often in the supposed linkage than do metal-on-polymer devices. The study was poorly controlled, as was a smaller one later by Elves et al. (1975), who reported the following results:

> Sensitivity to chromium, cobalt, nickel, molybdenum, vanadium and titanium was studied by patch tests in 50 patients who had received total joint replacements. Nineteen (38%) were sensitive to one or more metals, primarily cobalt and nickel. In 23 patients, nontraumatic failure of the prosthesis had occurred and 15 of these failures were sensitive to metal. Out of 27 patients with no evidence of prosthesis loosening, four were sensitive to nickel and cobalt or nickel alone. Dermatological reactions occurred in 13 patients after surgery; however, only eight of these showed evidence of metal sensitivity.

However, several questions remain unanswered. One of particular interest is whether sensitization occurs from an implant or if it is a pre-existing condition. No accurate incidence rates for metal sensitivity in the general population are available. Large-scale studies, yielding the rates quoted in the previous section, have been done only on populations that appear at dermatological clinics — that is, patients with active skin problems — with small control groups. A report published with that of Elves et al. (Benson et al. 1975) favored the presensitization position. Groups of patients awaiting total hip joint replacement were compared with those who had received the devices already and were, in some cases, already symptomatic (device loosening). Although "high" rates were found in both groups, no differential was seen.

A subsequent study of 212 patients awaiting total hip replacement (Deutman et al. 1977) produced more definite data. These patients could be divided into four groups, as shown in Table 12.4. This study showed a modest

TABLE 12.4

Metal Sensitivity[a] and Associated Complications

Patient Classification	Total Number	Sensitive[a]	
		Preoperative	Postoperative
I: no previous bone operation	173	10	14[b]
II: previous metal implant	17	2	2
III: loose THR (to be revised)	16	2	2
IV: normal THR (contralateral)	6	—	—

Note: THR = total hip replacement.

[a] Sensitive to at least one: Co^{+2}, Ni^{+2}, CrO_4^{-2} (by skin test).

[b] From retest, 6 months postoperatively of 66/168 patients with no preoperative sensitivity.

Source: Adapted from Deutman, R. et al., *J. Bone Joint Surg.*, 59A, 862, 1977.

possibility of association between sensitivity and device loosening and a small possibility of sensitization or activation of previous sensitization by metallic implantation.

Another clinical report (Brown et al. 1977) casts further doubt on an easy interpretation. This study reported a group of 20 American patients with 23 hip implants of the metal-on-metal type. At least one implant was loose in each patient. No patients were found to be sensitive to cobalt, nickel, or chromium. This difference in incidence rates of metal sensitivity has been ascribed to different environmental exposure between Brown's American patients and Elves' and Benson's British patients.

The questions of the relationship between immune sensitivity and device loosening and of possible sensitization by implanted device components have remained of interest to the clinical and research communities. Carlsson et al. (1980) examined a group of 112 patients before and 134 patients after metal-on-polymer hip replacement and concluded that little or no relationship existed between previous sensitivity and loosening. They also felt that it was doubtful that devices could induce sensitivity. Waterman and Schrik (1985) studied 85 patients before and after metal-on-polymer hip replacement and, although finding definite evidence of postoperative sensitization to Cr^{+6}, Co^{+2}, Ni^{+2}, and methyl methacrylate, also concluded that no relationship was present between these findings and device loosening.

These latter studies suggest that probably more than one mechanism is involved in device loosening. The results of Brown et al. (1977) would be explained by some, such as Willert and Semlitsch (1977), as being secondary to accumulations of wear debris and response to that accumulation. In small amounts, wear particles are encapsulated or removed to regional lymph nodes. When this system is overwhelmed, a foreign body response with accumulation of giant cells may invade the tissues surrounding the joint, causing resorption of soft and hard tissue. In such cases, device loosening might be secondary to cellular attack of the interface between implant and tissue (Harris 1995) or, as it were, it might be a biological analog of crevice corrosion. However, multiple processes may occur in the same implant site (Santavirta et al. 1990).

There has been continuing interest in the question of a possible relationship between immune sensitivity to metal implants and bone damage in the absence of infection (aseptic loosening) or wear debris. Leynadier and Langlais (1988) reviewed the studies cited here, as well as others, and summarized the outcome of 300 patients. In these studies, they found an overall 7.4% incidence of sensitivity (to Ni, Cr, and/or Co in some valence state) in patients with a good clinical outcome ($N = 163$) vs. a 46% incidence of sensitivity in patients with aseptic loosening ($N = 137$). They further noted an unexpectedly high rate of sensitivity to cobalt (30%) that was more than ten times that expected from their control population. On the basis of this review, they concluded that, except in exceptional cases, loosening was more likely to promote development of sensitivity rather than vice versa.

TABLE 12.5

Relationship of Metal Sensitivity[a] to Loosening in Internal Fixation of Fractures

Postoperative Complications	Number	Sensitive			Sensitive to (#)[b]		
		M (#)	F (#)	Total (%)	Ni	Cr	Co
None	208	—	8	8 (3.9)	7	3	—
Delayed union	230	10	14	24 (10.4)	21	4	3
Infected	267	14	13	27 (10.1)	26	2	4

[a] By skin test.
[b] Some sensitive to more than one metal; no cobalt in alloy used.

Source: Hierholzer, personal communication, 1990.

This view is contradicted by Hierholzer (1990) in a study of patients with nickel-bearing (steel) fracture fixation implants. He found that, although tissue nickel concentrations around fracture fixation hardware were as much as 100 times greater in infected than noninfected sites (Hierholzer et al. 1984), a positive correlation could be found between incidence of all prosthetic loosening (whether associated with delayed union or infection) and metal sensitivity. His results are summarized in Table 12.5.

A major criticism of this entire line of clinical investigation of possible immune responses to implants is the relative crudity of the skin test. Merritt and Brown (1980) have adapted a test termed the leukocyte migration inhibition factor (MIF) test to determine sensitivity to metallic ions more accurately. This test is an *in vitro* measure of the ability of metal ions (incorporated into haptens) to inhibit migration of human leucocytes towards a chemotactic attractant. Inhibition of migration is taken as a measure of production of a leukocyte migration inhibition factor by T-lymphocytes presumably activated by the specific metal-bearing hapten involved. In a later report, Merritt and Brown (1985) reviewed a study of 283 patients who underwent routine or cause-related device removal. Their data (summarized in Table 12.6) suggest a far higher incidence of metal sensitivity in patients with metallic devices than in any other study previously cited. In a parallel test of 629 patients coming to surgery (without prior history of metal implantation), they found, again by the MIF test, that 25% were sensitive to at least one metal among nickel, cobalt, and chromium.

Using a somewhat different approach, Wooley et al. (1997) demonstrated an association between sensitivity to poly (methyl) methacrylate or cobalt-base alloy particles and clinical diagnosis in patients receiving primary total joint replacement or presenting for revision for component loosening and pain, suggesting as expected a role for other health factors in determining immune response to foreign materials.

More recently, using MIF testing, Merritt and Rodrigo (1996) screened a carefully selected group of 22 patients, without metallic implants, who were coming to primary total joint replacement surgery. All were insensitive to

TABLE 12.6

Metal Sensitivity[a] at Device Removal

Alloy	Number	Insensitive (%)	Sensitive (%)	Reacting (%)[b]
Stainless steel	187	43	37	20
Cobalt base	55	26	36	38

[a] Sensitive to one or more of Ni^{+2}, Co^{+2}, Cr^{+6} (by MIF test).
[b] "Nonmigrators" (all chemotaxis suppressed); reverted to sensitive on retest 30 to 60 days after implant removal.

Source: Adapted from Merritt, K. and Brown, S.A., in *Corrosion and Degradation of Implant Materials: Second Symposium. ASTM STP 859,* Fraker, A.C. and Griffin, C.D. (Eds.), American Society of Testing and Materials, Philadelphia, 1985, 195.

TABLE 12.7

Metal Sensitivity Associated with Primary Total Joint Replacement

Element	Postimplantation[a]		
	Insensitive (%)	Sensitive (%)[b]	Reacting (%)[c]
Titanium	17 (77.3)	4 (18.2)	1 (4.5)
Cobalt	19 (86.4)	2 (9.1)	1 (4.5)
Chromium	17 (77.3)	4 (18.2)	1 (4.5)
Nickel	20 (91.0)	1 (4.5)	1 (4.5)

[a] 3 to 12 months postoperative.
[b] Seven patients showed sensitivity to one or more element.
[c] One patient.

Source: Adapted from Merritt, K. and Rodrigo, J.J., *Clin. Orthop. Rel. Res.*, 326, 71, 1996.

the metals for which they were screened (see Table 12.7) but 3 to 12 months later, seven (31.8%) had developed sensitivities to one or more metals and one developed a total nonmigration response characterized as a "severe response." See Hallab et al. (2001) for a full review of this complex topic.

12.4.2.4 Summary

It appears possible to draw the following conclusions concerning specific immune sensitivity to metallic biomaterials:

- A significant level of immune sensitivity to metals is present in the general population.
- Groups of patients who have had nickel-, chromium-, and cobalt-bearing implants display higher than expected incidences of sensitivity.

- Specific instances of symptoms consistent with a type 4 delayed hypersensitivity reaction being specifically related to the presence of a metallic implant have been documented.*
- Sensitivity to metal and sensitivity to other clinical symptoms, especially device loosening, are generally correlated; however, which is cause and which is effect is unclear at this time.

12.5 Final Comment

The lack of basic knowledge and reliable statistics on clinical outcomes associated with hypersensitivity responses to biomaterials has had severe consequences, most notably in the debate over possible immune or autoimmune responses associated with the use of silicone gel-filled breast implant prostheses. Although immune responses associated with implants may well have a low incidence, the consequences for individual patients remain severe. In the present medical treatment environment, in which the possibility of such effects is usually ignored, some patients no doubt experience a high level of frustration and prolonged periods of inappropriate therapy. These possibly include patients with suspected infections that prove impossible to culture from clinical specimens and who receive the working diagnosis of "sterile abscess" without appropriate subsequent testing for delayed hypersensitivity to implanted materials (Hallab et al. 2000).

The entire issue of the role of specific (i.e., immune) vs. general response to implants should remain an exciting one, particularly as biomaterials technology advances. For example, newer total joint replacements with hard-on-hard (metal/metal or ceramic/ceramic) bearings are known to yield very large numbers of submicron (1 to 100 nm)-sized metal oxide particles during locomotion. Recent concerns have been raised (Gatti et al. 2004; Lomer et al. 2002) as to whether such particles may be antigens or adjuvants. Basic and clinical research results can be expected to continue to shed more light on these as well as more traditional concerns in the future. However, it would be fair to say that study of effects of biomaterials on the human immune system is one of the most neglected areas of host response research.

---

* This story may still have additional chapters: current interest in the use of metal/metal articulations in total hip replacements is producing a number of clinical failures of fixation of components to bone with adjacent soft tissues characterized as showing "…necrosis, lymphocyte infiltration, elevated mast cell counts and tissue fibrosis" (Lintner et al. 2005.) This is interpreted as a type 3 toxic or arthus response to cobalt-bearing particles (Lintner, personal communication).

References

Angel, M., *Science on Trial*, W.W. Norton and Co., New York, 1997.

Bajpai, P.K., Antigenicity of glutaraldehyde-stabilized biological materials, in *Biomaterials in Reconstructive Surgery*, Rubin, L.R. (Ed.), C.V. Mosby, St. Louis, 1983, 243.

Benson, M.K.D. et al., Metal sensitivity in patients with joint replacement arthroplasties, *Br. Med. J.*, 4, 374, 1975.

Bravo, I. et al., Differential effects of eight metal ions on lymphocyte differentiation antigens *in vitro*, *J. Biomed. Mater. Res.*, 24, 1059, 1990.

Brendlinger, D.L. and Tarsitano, J.J., Generalized dermatitis due to sensitivity to a chrome cobalt removable partial denture, *J. Am. Dent. Assoc.*, 81, 392, 1970.

Brown, G.C. et al., Sensitivity to metal as a possible cause of sterile loosening after cobalt–chromium total hip-replacement arthroplasty, *J. Bone Joint Surg.*, 59A, 164, 1977.

Carlsson, Å.S. et al., Metal sensitivity in patients with metal-to-plastic total hip arthroplasties, *Acta Orthop. Scand.*, 51, 57, 1980.

Chenoweth, D.E., Complement activation produced by biomaterials, *Trans. Am. Soc. Artif. Intern. Organs*, 32, 226, 1986.

Chenoweth, D.E., Complement activation in extracorporeal circuits, *Ann. N.Y. Acad. Sci.*, 516, 306, 1987.

Clementi, D. et al., Clinical investigations of tolerance to materials and acrylic cement in patients with hip prostheses, *Ital. J. Orthop. Traumatol.*, 6, 97, 1980.

Cramers, M. and Lucht, U., Metal sensitivity in patients treated for tibial fractures with plates of stainless steel, *Acta Orthop. Scand.*, 48, 245, 1977.

Deutman, R. et al., Metal sensitivity before and after total hip arthroplasty, *J. Bone Joint Surg.*, 59A, 862, 1977.

Elgert, K.D., *Immunology. Understanding the Immune System*, Wiley–Liss, New York, 1996.

Elves, M.W. et al., Incidence of metal sensitivity in patients with total joint replacements, *Brit. Med. J.*, 4(Nov. 15), 376, 1975.

Emans, J.B., Current concepts review: allergy to latex in patients with myelodysplasia, *J. Bone Joint Surg.*, 74A, 1103, 1992.

Evans, E.M. et al., Metal sensitivity as a cause of bone necrosis and loosening of the prosthesis in total joint replacement, *J. Bone Joint Surg.*, 56B, 626, 1974.

Fisher, A.A., Dermatitis and discolorations from metals, in, *Contact Dermatitis*, 3rd ed., Fisher, A.A. (Ed.), Lea & Febiger, Philadelphia, 1986, 710.

Friedberg, F., Effects of metal binding on protein structure, *Q. Rev. Biophys.*, 7(1), 1, 1974.

Gabriel, S.E. et al., Risk of connective-tissue diseases and other disorders after breast implantation, *N. Engl. J. Med.*, 330(24), 1697, 1994.

Gatti, A.M., Biocompatibility of micro- and nanoparticles in the colon. Part II., *Biomaterials*, 25, 2004.

Haddad, F.S. et al., Cement hypersensitivity: a cause of aseptic loosening? *J. Bone Joint Surg.*, 77B, 329, 1995.

Hallab, N.J. et al., Immune responses correlate with serum-metal in metal-on-metal hip arthroplasty, *J. Arthrop.* (Suppl 3), 19, 88, 2004.

Hallab, N. et al., Metal sensitivity in patients with orthopaedic implants, *J. Bone Joint Surg.*, 83A, 428, 2001.

Hallab, N. et al., Hypersensitivity to metallic biomaterials: a review of leukocyte migration inhibition assays, *Biomaterials*, 21, 1301, 2000.

Harris, W.H., The problem is osteolysis, *Clin. Orthop. Rel. Res.*, 311, 46, 1995.

Hicks, J.H., Pathological effects from surgical metal, in *Modern Trends in Surgical Materials*, Gillis, L. (Ed.), Butterworth, London, 1958, 29.

Hierholzer, S., Local tissue reactions and sensibilitization in the presence of stainless steel implants, personal communication, 1990.

Hierholzer, S. et al., Increased corrosion of stainless steel implants in infected plated fractures, *Arch. Orthop. Trauma Surg.*, 102, 198, 1984.

Hildebrand, H.F. et al., Nickel, chromium, cobalt dental alloys, and allergic reactions: an overview, in *Biocompatibility of Co-Cr-Ni Alloys*, Hildebrand, H.F. and Champy, M. (Eds.), Plenum Press, New York, 1988, 201.

Kossovsky, N. and Freiman, C.J., Silicone breast implant pathology. Clinical data and immunologic consequences, *Arch. Pathol. Lab. Med.*, 118, 686, 1994.

Kossovsky, N. et al., The bioreactivity of silicone, *CRC Crit. Rev. Biocompat.*, 3, 53, 1987.

Leynadier, F. and Langlais, F., Total hip arthroplasties and allergy to metals, in *Biocompatibility of Co–Cr–Ni Alloys*, Hildebrand, H.F. and Champy, M. (Eds.), Plenum Press, New York, 1988, 193.

Lintner, F. et al., Are multinucleated giant cells indicative of cobalt-related tissue damage after metal-on-metal THR? (Ger.; author's trans), *Osteologie*, 14, 117, 2005.

Lomer, M.C.E. et al., Fine and ultrafine particles of the diet: influence on the muscosal immune response and association with Crohn's disease, *Proc. Nutr. Soc.*, 61, 123, 2002.

Maurin, N., Delayed *in vitro* immune response to long-term intraperitoneal polymer implant in mice, *J. Biomed. Mater. Res.*, 29, 1493, 1995.

McGillis, S.T. et al., Patch testing, *Clin. Rev. Allergy*, 7, 441, 1989.

Merritt, K., Immune response, in *Handbook of Biomaterial Properties*, Black, J. and Hastings, G. (Eds.), Chapman & Hall, London, 1998, 513.

Merritt, K. and Brown. S.A., Tissue reaction and metal sensitivity. An animal study, *Acta Orthop. Scand.*, 51, 403, 1980.

Merritt, K. and Brown, S.A., Biological effects of corrosion products from metals, in *Corrosion and Degradation of Implant Materials: Second Symposium. ASTM STP 859*, Fraker, A.C. and Griffin, C.D. (Eds.), American Society of Testing and Materials, Philadelphia, 1985, 195.

Merritt, K. and Rodrigo, J.J., Immune response to synthetic materials, *Clin. Orthop. Rel. Res.*, 326, 71, 1996.

Naim, J.O. et al., The effect of molecular weight and gel preparation on humoral adjuvancy of silicone oils and silicone gels, *Immunol. Invest.*, 24(3), 537, 1995.

Nakamura, S. et al., Autoantibodies to red cells associated with metallosis — a case report, *Acta Orthop. Scand.*, 68, 495, 1997.

Nicholson, J.J., III et al., Silicone gel and octamethylcyclotetrasiloxane (D4) enhances antibody production to bovine serum albumin in mice, *J. Biomed. Mater. Res.*, 31, 345, 1996.

Playfair, J.H., *Immunology at a Glance*, 3rd ed., Blackwell Scientific Publications, Oxford, 1979.

Santavirta, S. et al., Aggressive granulomatous lesions associated with hip arthroplasty, *J. Bone Joint Surg.*, 72A, 252, 1990.

Shepard, A.D. et al., Complement activation by synthetic vascular prostheses, *J. Vasc. Surg.*, 1(6), 829, 1984.

Shrivastava, R. et al., Mini review: effects of chromium on the immune system, *FEMS Immunol. Med. Microbiol.*, 34, 1, 2002.

Stern, I.J. et al., Immunogenic effects of foreign materials on plasma proteins, *Nature*, 238, 151, 1972.

Tang, L. et al., Complement activation and inflammation triggered by model biomaterial surfaces, *J. Biomed. Mater. Res.*, 41, 333, 1998.

Tegnander, A. et al., Activation of the complement system and adverse effects of biodegradable pins of polylactic acid (Biofix®)) in osteochondritis dissecans, *Acta Orthop. Scand.*, 65, 472, 1994.

Urban, R.M. et al., Accumulation in liver and spleen of metal particles generated at nonbearing surfaces in hip arthroplasty, *J. Arthrop.*, 19(8 Suppl 3), 94, 2004.

Urban, R.M. et al., Migration of corrosion products from modular hip prostheses. Particle microanalysis and histopathological findings, *J. Bone Joint Surg.*, 76A, 1345, 1994.

Wahlberg, J.E., Thresholds of sensitivity in metal contact allergy. 1. Isolated and simultaneous allergy to chromium, cobalt, mercury, and/or nickel, *Berufsdermatosen*, 21, 22, 1973.

Waterman, A.H. and Schrik, J.J., Allergy in hip arthroplasty, *Contact Derm.*, 13, 294, 1985.

Willert, H.-G. and Semlitsch, M., Reactions of the articular capsule to wear products of artificial joint prostheses, *J. Biomed. Mater. Res.*, 11, 157, 1977.

Wooley, P.H. et al., Cellular immune responses to orthopedic implant materials following cemented total joint replacement, *J. Orthop. Res.*, 15, 874, 1997.

Yang, J. and Merritt, K., Detection of antibodies against corrosion products in patients after Co–Cr total joint replacements, *J. Biomed. Mater. Res.*, 28, 1249, 1994.

Yang, J. and Merritt, K., Production of monoclonal antibodies to study corrosion products of Co–Cr biomaterials, *J. Biomed. Mater. Res.*, 31, 71, 1996.

Bibliography

Abbas, A.K. et al., *Cellular and Molecular Immunology*, 5th ed., W.B. Saunders, Philadelphia, 2003.

DeLustro, F. et al., Immune responses to allogenic and xenogenic implants of collagen and collagen derivatives, *Clin. Orthop. Rel. Res.*, 260, 263, 1990.

Ellingsen, J.E., A study on the mechanism of protein adsorption to TiO_2, *Biomaterials*, 12, 593, 1991.

Gabriel, S.E., Soft tissue responses to silicones, in *Handbook of Biomaterial Properties*, Black, J. and Hastings, G. (Eds.), Chapman & Hall, London, 1998, 556.

Guyton, A.C., Resistance of the body to infection: II. Immunity and allergy, in *Textbook of Medical Physiology*, 6th ed., W.B. Saunders, Philadelphia, 1991.

Hennekens, C.H. et al., Self-reported breast implants and connective-tissue diseases in female health professionals, *JAMA*, 275(8), 616, 1996.

Hildebrand, H.F., Veron, C. and Martin, P., Nickel, chromium, cobalt dental alloys, and allergic reactions: an overview, *Biomaterials*, 10, 545, 1989.

Klippel, J.H. (Ed.), *Primer on the Rheumatic Diseases*, 12th ed., Arthritis Foundation, Atlanta, 2001.

Kossovsky, N. and Freiman, C.J., Immunology of silicone breast implants, *J. Appl. Biomater.*, 8(3), 237, 1994.

Kossovsky, N. et al., Self-reported signs and symptoms in breast implant patients with novel antibodies to silicone surface associated antigens [anti-SSAA(x)], *J. Appl. Biomater.*, 6, 153, 1995.

Kumar, P. et al., Metal hypersensitivity in total joint replacement, *Orthopedics*, 6, 1455, 1983.

Merritt, K. and Brown, S.A., Hypersensitivity to metallic biomaterials, in *Systemic Aspects of Biocompatibility*, Vol. II, Williams, D.F. Ed., CRC Press, Boca Raton, FL, 1981, 33.

Merritt, K., Role of medical materials, both in implant and surface applications, in immune response and in resistance to infection, *Biomaterials*, 5, 47, 1984.

Niki, Y. et al., Screening or symptomatic metal sensitivity: a prospective study of 92 patients undergoing total knee arthroplasty, *Biomaterials*, 26, 1019, 2005.

Playfair, J.H.L. and Chain, B.M., *Immunology at a Glance*, 7th ed., Blackwell Scientific Publications, Oxford, 2000.

Rostocker, G. et al., Dermatitis due to orthopedic implants, *J. Bone Joint Surg.*, 69A, 1408, 1987.

Wang, J.Y. et al., Prosthetic metals impair immune response and cytokine release *in vivo* and *in vitro*, *J. Orthop. Res.*, 15, 688, 1997.

Weir, D.M. and Stewart, J., *Immunology*, 8th ed. Churchill–Livingstone, Edinburgh, 1997.

Wooley, P.H. et al., The immune response to implant materials in humans, *Clin. Orthop. Rel. Res.*, 326, 63, 1996.

13

Chemical and Foreign-Body Carcinogenesis

13.1 Definitions

This chapter will consider the role of implants in carcinogenesis. Some definitions are needed to make the arguments clear and unambiguous:

Benign Possessing controlled self-limiting growth without invasiveness or ability to metastasize.

Cancer Perhaps the best definition is that of Roe (1966): "Cancer is a disease of multicellular organisms which is characterized by the seemingly uncontrolled multiplication and spread within the organism of apparently abnormal forms of the organism's own cells." Roe further states that the three key characteristics of cancer are cellular multiplication, autonomy, and invasiveness.

Carcinogen An agent capable of causing cancer.

Carcinogenesis The production of cancer (more properly but less commonly termed cancerogenesis).

Carcinogenic/tumorigenic Used interchangeably to connote agents capable of causing cancer.

Carcinoma A malignant neoplasm arising from cells of epithelial origin.

Leukemia or lymphoma A malignant neoplastic transformation of cells of the circulatory system.

Malignant Possessing uncontrolled growth, invasiveness, and ability to metastasize.

Metastasis A neoplasm arising by "seeding" from a primary malignant neoplasm to a remote site. Also called a secondary neoplasm.

Mutagenesis The production of inheritable (genotypic) changes in cells.

Neoplasm A tissue mass arising from an abnormal, uncoordinated proliferation of cells.

Primary neoplasm A locally arising neoplasm.

Sarcoma   A malignant neoplasm arising from cells of connective tissue.

Tumor   Literally, a swelling; used to refer to neoplasms.

With these terms in mind, first, chemically induced and promoted carcinogenesis as it relates to implants will be examined. Initially, all neoplasms associated with implants in experimental animals and in patients were thought to be chemical in origin. It is now recognized that these tumors can arise, at least in animals, from chemical and nonchemical origins. The nonchemical or so-called "solid-state" mechanism will be taken up in the later parts of this chapter.

13.2   Chemical Carcinogenesis

13.2.1   Introduction

Chemical carcinogens have many different forms, affect a variety of cell types, and produce a variety of neoplasms. The nature of their action leads to neoplastic transformation being possible near implants by direct solution or diffusion; at a distance by transport and concentration; or in the absence of implants by contact, ingestion, or inhalation. It is not within the scope of this book to discuss the details of these processes. However, it should be recognized that there is more than one transformation effect. Neoplastic growth may be initiated by alteration of metabolic processes, by alteration of replication processes (by growth stimulation or by reduction of contact inhibition), or by mutagenesis. Although all carcinogens are now thought to be mutagens, not all mutagenic agents are carcinogenic. A mutation may be lethal (to a cell), prevent cellular replication, or simply not affect metabolic or growth processes sufficiently to produce malignant behavior.

13.2.2   What "Everybody Knows" about Cancer

Before proceeding to a discussion of classes and types of chemical carcinogens, it would be a good idea to discuss some popular misunderstandings about carcinogenesis in general and chemical carcinogenesis in particular. "Everybody knows" at least three things about cancer that probably are not so:

- "Cancer is increasing." Figure 13.1 presents a summary of cancer death rates in the U.S. for the period of 1930 to 2000, adjusted for age (American Cancer Society, 2004). The adjustment for age is necessary because, as life expectancy and thus age at death increase, a fixed annual incidence rate of mortality from one source will produce an increase in actual deaths from that source. Today, most death

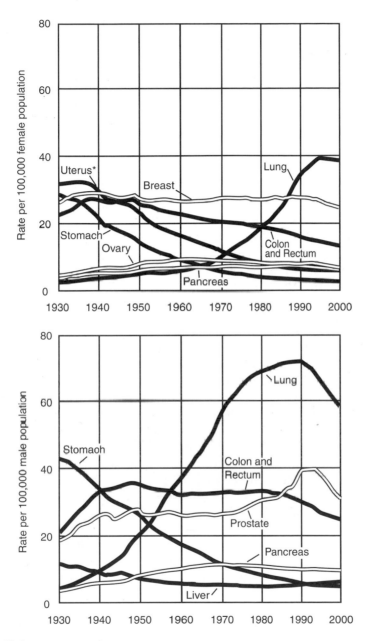

FIGURE 13.1
Cancer death rates, by site, U.S., 1930–2000. Rates adjusted to 1970 standard U.S. population; *cervix and endometrium combined. (Adapted from American Cancer Society, *2004 Cancer Facts and Figures*, American Cancer Society, Atlanta, 2004.)

rates due to particular types of cancer are decreasing. Furthermore, excluding lung cancer, which is related primarily to tobacco smoking and secondarily to environmental effects, death rates due to cancer have been constant or have decreased since 1945 for men and since 1930 for women. Note that, although the rate of death due to prostate cancer appeared to be increasing in the 1980s, this was likely due to better, earlier diagnosis rather than to an actual increase in incidence. Today, although nearly 30% of Americans alive will develop cancer and 25% will die from cancer, the overall 5-year survival rate, despite an aging population, has increased to 63% compared with 33% in the 1960s and 25% in the 1930s. This increased survival rate is due in part to earlier detection, permitting a longer normal course until death and earlier medical intervention, and to improved therapies, especially for some specific cancers.

- "Everything causes cancer." In fact, the contrary seems to be true. Chemical carcinogenesis seems to be the exception rather than the rule. The statistical estimates are as follow. Approximately 1.5 to 2 million compounds and substances are now individually chemically identifiable. An exhaustive literature search concerning the 6000 most likely candidates uncovered evidence that only 17%, or approximately 1000, were possible carcinogens. A survey by the National Institute of Occupational Safety and Health (Christensen 1972) of 2415 suspected carcinogens produced evidence of 1905 reported as carcinogenic effects but only 1000 thought to be carcinogenic in animals. In the most recent compilation available, only 58 substances or groups of related substances or occupational exposures are listed as known to cause cancer in humans; 188 additional ones can reasonably be anticipated to be carcinogenic in humans (U.S. Department of Health and Human Services 2004).

- "Toxic materials cause cancer." The classic study is that of Innes et al. (1969) in which 120 pesticides and toxic industrial chemicals were selected for evaluation. These materials were fed to two strains of mice in the maximum tolerable doses. The animals were sacrificed after a standard period and evaluated for tumor incidence. The results were that 11 compounds (including five insecticides) were significantly carcinogenic; 20 compounds were equivocal — that is, did not show significant elevation of cancer incidence rates in this study; and 89 compounds produced no elevation of cancer incidence rates.

Thus, in this study of compounds specifically selected for their toxicity and given in maximum possible doses, fewer than 10% proved to be carcinogenic. Furthermore, these findings have come under increasing criticism as being too pessimistic. It has been suggested that testing toxic potential carcinogens at high dosages may artificially accentuate their activity by inducing increased rates of cell division (Ames and Gold 1990).

13.2.3 Types of Carcinogens

In the classification of materials that are carcinogens, three types of agents are recognized:

- The complete carcinogen that produces neoplastic transformation by itself
- The procarcinogen, or carcinogen precursor, that is not a carcinogen but is converted to one by metabolic processes in the body of the test animal or man
- The cocarcinogen, which is a weak carcinogen or has no inherent carcinogenic activity but increases the activity of complete carcinogens or procarcinogens when it appears in their company

The exact roles and functions of pro- and cocarcinogens remain unclear. It was suggested early that neoplastic transformation is a two-step process (Friedewald and Rous 1944):

1. *Initiation* produces the primary cellular transformation. The cells enter a latent period and do not ordinarily develop into a tumor.
2. *Promotion* is characterized by the development of previously transformed cells into an active visible tumor.

However, this process is now viewed as having at least three steps, with specific conditions necessary during the latent period if subsequent expression (development of a tumor) is to occur.

Thus, a complete carcinogen is one that is an initiator as well as a promoter, and a cocarcinogen may be promoter or initiator but probably not both. Similarly, a procarcinogen may not be a complete carcinogen after metabolic conversion but its action may depend upon the presence of other initiators and promoters (Berenblum 1969). It is clear that potential chemical carcinogens must be considered in their roles as complete or incomplete agents as well as possible promoters of previously initiated processes of neoplastic transformation.

13.2.4 Chemical Carcinogens

An excellent and still useful review of these three types of agents among organic compounds is that of Weisburger and Williams (1975). Figure 13.2 and Figure 13.3 and Table 13.1 are drawn from this study. Figure 13.2 lists

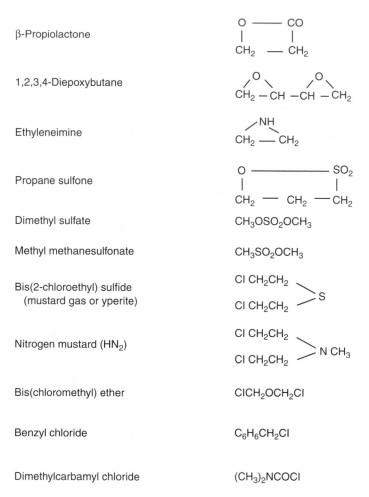

FIGURE 13.2

Typical direct-acting chemical carcinogens. (From Weisburger, J.H. and Williams, G.M., in *Cancer: A Comprehensive Treatise*, Vol. 1, Becker, F.F. (Ed.), Plenum Press, New York, 1975, 185. With permission.)

some of the typical stronger, pure organic carcinogens with their chemical structures. Table 13.1 lists some of the better known procarcinogens. The details of metabolic conversion are still unclear for many of these agents. Table 13.1 suggests the form of the converted carcinogen and Figure 13.3 provides examples of possible intermediates and structures. Of particular interest is the inclusion of vinyl halide or acetate in the procarcinogen list and a variety of epoxides in the activated list in Table 13.1. Polyvinyl chloride (PVC) and polyvinyl acetate (PVA) have some popularity in medical applications and epoxide conversion is possible for many polymeric implant materials.

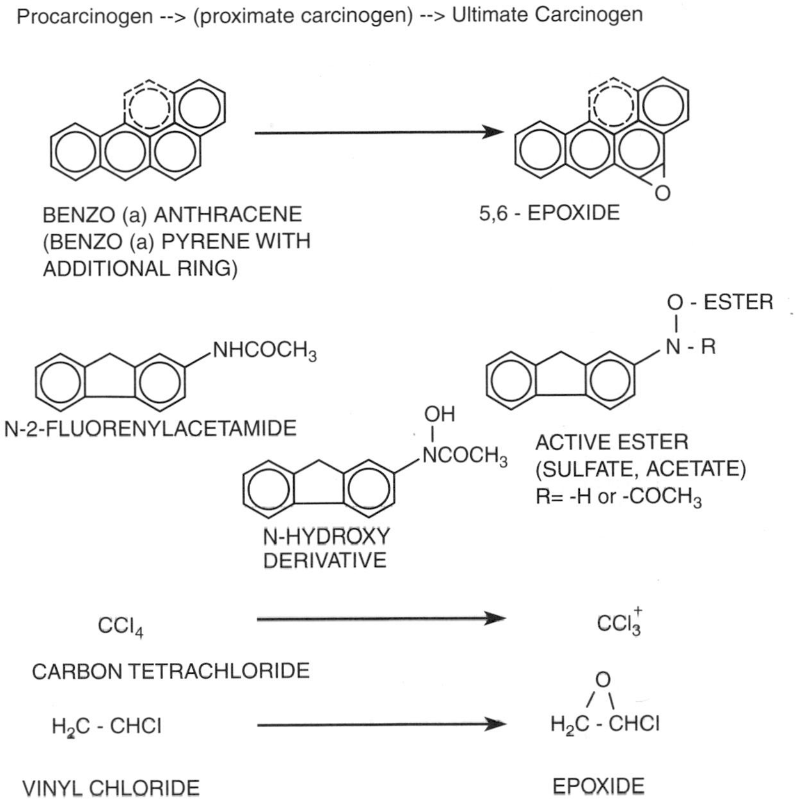

Procarcinogen --> (proximate carcinogen) --> Ultimate Carcinogen

BENZO (a) ANTHRACENE
(BENZO (a) PYRENE WITH
ADDITIONAL RING)

5,6 - EPOXIDE

N-2-FLUORENYLACETAMIDE

NHCOCH$_3$

OH
|
NCOCH$_3$

N-HYDROXY
DERIVATIVE

O - ESTER
|
N - R

ACTIVE ESTER
(SULFATE, ACETATE)
R= -H or -COCH$_3$

CCl$_4$ $\longrightarrow$ CCl$_3^+$

CARBON TETRACHLORIDE

H$_2$C - CHCl $\longrightarrow$ H$_2$C - CHCl (epoxide)

VINYL CHLORIDE

EPOXIDE

FIGURE 13.3

Typical procarcinogen activation reactions. (From Weisburger, J.H. and Williams, G.M., in *Cancer: A Comprehensive Treatise*, Vol. 1, Becker, F.F. (Ed.), Plenum Press, New York, 1975, 185. With permission.)

Testing for possible agents, especially of the pro- or co- type, is quite difficult due to the necessity of following the products through the various steps of the metabolic chain. Also, many of the small animals used for these tests have significant and not inconsiderable rates of spontaneous neoplastic transformation. Although many agents that produce neoplastic transformation in test animals have not been definitely shown to be carcinogenic in man, it is essentially correct to assume that all human carcinogens also produce neoplastic transformation in animals. All known (specifically identified or associated with occupational exposure) chemical carcinogens in humans have been shown to have carcinogenic activity in at least one test animal species. However, the neoplasms may vary widely in location, dose dependency, malignancy, etc. between species.

The vast majority of recognized chemical carcinogens are organic compounds. Ceramic-body induction of carcinogenesis through a chemical route

TABLE 13.1

Principal Procarcinogens and Key Derived Active Metabolites

Procarcinogen Proximate or Ultimate	Actual or Proposed Carcinogen
Polycyclic aromatic hydrocarbons	Epoxide; radical ion?
Aflatoxin	Epoxide
Arylamine or amide; azo dyes	N-Hydroxylamino-O-esters; radical ion (?); epoxide (special case: cutaneous cancers)
Nitro aryl or heterocyclic compounds	N-Hydroxylamino-O-esters
3-Hydroxyxanthine, related purines	O-Esters
Safrole	1'-Hydroxy-O-Esters
Urethane, alkylcarbamates	Active esters
Pyrrolizidine alkaloids	Pyrrolic esters
Alkynitrosamines or -amides, alkyhydrazines or -triazenes	Alkyl carbonium ion
Halogenated hydrocarbons	Haloalkyl carbonium ions
Vinyl halide or acetate	Epoxide?

Source: Adapted from Weisburger, J.H. and Williams, G.M., in *Cancer: A Comprehensive Treatise*, Vol. 1., Becker, F.F. (Ed.), Plenum Press, New York, 1975, 185.

has not been reliably identified in animals at this time. This is probably due to the low solubility of ceramics used in implants and the paucity of testing. The role of metals as possible chemical carcinogens will be examined in the next section.

13.2.5   Metals as Chemical Carcinogens

The status of metals as carcinogens is less clear. One of the difficulties in determining this is the problem of distinguishing between chemical and foreign-body (FB) action (see Section 13.3). Mechanical implantation or inhalation of metal dust may proceed to neoplastic transformation by a chemical route after corrosion, by an FB route by the presence of the residual metal, or perhaps due to aggregation of corrosion products at the implant or at a remote site. Furthermore, unlike most organic molecules, metals can display a wide range of electronic valences.

Metals may be placed in a classification system as given in the earlier discussion. They may be directly (or completely) carcinogenic (pure action) or they may potentiate other agents and their compounds. Reaction products or organometallic complexes may be carcinogenic, thus classing the original form as a procarcinogen. Potentiation (classing metals as cocarcinogens) is a very broad, nonspecific activity because many forms of neoplasms tend to concentrate metallic ions and complexes. It is difficult to distinguish cause and effect here: the concentration of metals may be causal or merely the consequence of the higher level of metabolic activity of the neoplastic cells.

Summarizing a broad range of early animal studies, Sunderman (1971) has made a strong case for carcinogenic roles for chromium, cobalt, iron, nickel, titanium, and for some metals not found in implant alloys. Environmental and industrial workplace studies support the presumed carcinogenicity of chromium, cobalt, nickel, and, perhaps, iron.

Furst (1978) has extensively reviewed the status of metals as carcinogenic agents. This review is noteworthy because the author had previously (Furst and Haro 1969) proposed strict criteria that a material should meet before it could be considered carcinogenic:

> Tumors must appear both at the site and at a distance from the point of application; more than one route [of application] must be effective; more than one species must respond; the growth should be transplantable; and, if malignant, invasion and/or metastasis must be noted. Most important, all histological slides must be evaluated by a pathologist knowledgeable in animal tumors.

These criteria, although more than 35 years old, are still applicable and very relevant today. Of importance are Furst's conclusions drawn from then available *in vitro* and animal studies subject to the preceding criteria:

- Metals for which pure metal and compounds are carcinogenic: Ni
- Metals for which pure metal is carcinogenic but no carcinogenic compound is known: Co
- Metals for which pure metal is not a carcinogen but that have carcinogenic compounds (given in parentheses): Cr (CrO_4^{-2}), Fe (dextran, dextrin), Ti (titanocene?), Mn ($MnCl_2$?) ("?" = there is some doubt)

Only metals of interest in implant applications are included here. Furst (1978) lists several others, including cadmium, lead, and beryllium, that fall into one of these categories. However, it is fair to state that Furst regards metallic carcinogenesis as a well-established, real effect.

The complexity of the problem presented by potentially carcinogenic metallic implants is shown in a study by Gaechter et al. (1977). These investigators implanted polished rods of seven common implant alloys, including common stainless steel and cobalt- and titanium-base implant alloys, in rats and followed them for 2 years. Each of these alloys contained at least one element recognized by Furst as carcinogenic. Neoplasms of a wide variety of types were found, but no statistical elevation above the control (nonimplanted) group incidence rates was seen. This study was possibly suggested by an earlier one by Heath et al. (1971) in which wear-produced particles from a Co–Cr metal-on-metal total joint replacement were shown to be carcinogenic in rat muscle 4 to 15 months after implantation.

There are two possible arguments to explain these conflicting findings. In the first place, the rods used by Gaechter et al. (1977) may have released metal at a slower rate than seen in the works referenced by Sunderman (1971) or in the study of Heath et al. (1971). Thus, dilution may have prevented direct chemical carcinogenesis or indirect (pro-) carcinogenesis by maintaining pool concentrations below critical levels. This possibility is supported by a later, much larger and somewhat longer rat implant study using rods and powder (Memoli et al. 1986), which demonstrated a small but significant increase in incidence of sarcomas and lymphomas in animals with implants containing cobalt, chromium, or nickel.

The possibility that dilution may reduce the risk of neoplastic transformation leads directly to the question of whether a "threshold" of effect exists. That is, is there a concentration of a carcinogenic agent below which it looses its effectiveness? This is a matter of considerable importance in the implant field because corrosion rates of successful alloys are relatively quite low. A high-corrosion-rate alloy would probably be rejected for implant applications because of an acute tissue response. These low corrosion rates result in modest serum and tissue concentration increases, except in instances of local concentration, as will be discussed in Chapter 15.

A great deal of attention has been paid to this possibility of threshold levels by legislators and administrators concerned with food purity and workplace safety. The common view is that no threshold exists; that is, the transforming effect is like a molecular "trigger" and reduced concentration simply reduces the likelihood that the critical event will take place. Therefore, given random chance enhanced by continued exposure, any concentration of a carcinogen can eventually evoke a neoplastic response. This view was the precipitating factor in the adoption in 1958 of the now famous Delaney Amendment to the Pure Food, Drug, and Cosmetic Act. This amendment imposed a zero (!) permissible level of carcinogenic agents as deliberate food additives, stating that "...no additive shall be deemed to be safe if it is found to induce cancer when ingested by man or animal, or if it is found, after tests which are appropriate for the evaluation of the safety of food additives, to induce cancer in man or animals...".* Contrast this with the discussion in Chapter 1 on value judgments inherent in definitions and the carefully enunciated position of Furst (1978) on the carcinogenic status of metals and their compounds.

It is clear that, if one were to apply the Delaney criteria to medical devices, none of the metals listed by Furst (1978) could be judged satisfactory, even for short-term implantation. However, the wide utility of probably carcinogenic food substances, such as certain dyes and saccharin, has resulted in a case-by-case relaxation of the Delaney criteria for deliberate food additives. These decisions have been made by balancing risk against benefit with, admittedly, a portion of political judgment added in some cases. In 1996, the issue of residual materials, such as pesticides, was dealt with by the enactment of the Food Quality Protection Act.** Administered by the U.S.

---

* Cited in *Federal Register* 42(192), Tuesday Oct. 4, 1977, Part VI, page 54166.
** PL 104-170.

Environmental Protection Agency, this law establishes a system of scientific review to establish (and review on a 10-year cycle) tolerable limits for the presence of such materials in food stuffs.

The same careful judgments will probably need to be made concerning metallic implants. To do so, it is necessary to know the dose–response relationship for carcinogenesis accurately in the various animal models, how to project this to low-dose–long-response-time conditions (in which animal experiments become prohibitively expensive), and, most importantly, how to translate the animal projections to rate predictions in humans. Very little of the required information is now available.

The difficulty of doing such studies was illustrated by Bouchard et al. (1996) in a large-scale, essentially lifetime study also performed in rats. In this study, nearly cylindrical metal implants were fabricated from Ti6Al4V (F138) or CoCrMo (F-75) in solid form and the latter in a fully porous form with approximately 20 times the total surface area of the nonporous implants. Groups of approximately 100 rats, with equal numbers of males and females, had an implant placed on the lateral surface of one femur; an additional group received a quantity of 50- to 80-µm F-75 microspheres implanted subcutaneously. Animals were autopsied as they died of apparently natural causes during the experiment and all remaining animals were sacrificed 24 months after implantation. No overall differences in tumor incidence or death rates were found among the groups; however, 55 implant site tumors of various types were observed (Table 13.2).

The data in Table 13.2 show a very significant association between implant fixation ($p < 0.001$) with no apparent association between local dose (presumed to be proportional to implant surface area) of potential carcinogens released by CoCrMo alloys, with the possible expectation of a higher incidence in the highest exposure group (IV) in which the implants might be considered to be fixed due to individual encapsulation. Here, only one complication (implant fixation) was studied closely; others known to affect cancer incidence and prevalence include environmental, dietary, and hereditary factors.

TABLE 13.2

Implant-Associated Tumors

Group	No. Tumors	Implant Fixation Status[a]			
		I	II	III	IV
Solid Ti6Al4V	23	22	0	0	1
Solid CoCrMo	14	12	0	0	2
Porous CoCrMo	3	0	0	3	0
CoCrMo microspheres	15	n/a			

[a] Key: I — loose in soft tissue; II — loose, but in contact with bone; III — fixed to bone (ingrown); IV — unclassified; n/a — not applicable (all microspheres encapsulated in soft fibrous tissue).

Source: Adapted from Bouchard, P.R. et al., *J. Biomed. Mater. Res.*, 32, 37, 1996.

Moreover, one disappointing factor is emerging. It appears that linear projections of response rates to low dose rates, even when the dose–response curve is linear, provide underestimates of the effect. One reason for this is discussed briefly in the following section.

13.2.6   The Latent Period

A second argument that may shed light on the results of Gaechter et al. (1977) is based on the issue of *latency*. It is common in animal and human neoplastic transformation for a period of time to pass between exposure (initiation) and manifestation of neoplastic transformation. This waiting or latent period differs from species to species and is different for each agent. In humans, latency periods are typically 15 to 20 years and may be as long as 40 years (Schottenfeld and Haas 1979). Furthermore, no simple way to "scale" the effect — that is, to predict the latent period for an agent in one species from that observed in another species — is known. Thus, one may argue that the latent period in Gaechter's experiment exceeded the test period, despite the fact that 2 years is more than half the life span of most laboratory rats.

The latency argument is particularly important in the generalization of conclusions such as those of Sunderman (1971) to expectations of implant site tumor incidences in patients. The vast majority of implants have been in patients for only 15 or fewer years because of the advanced age of the average implant patient and the relatively recent advances in total joint replacement. For instance, Table 13.3 suggests that patients 65 years or older at time of surgery have less than a 50% chance of outliving a 20-year latency period, although some 2.5% will live to age 100 or more (Arias 2004). Thus, the appearance of metal carcinogenesis in humans may be awaiting the passage of an unelapsed latency period in the younger patients who have received implants in large numbers in the last decade (however, see Section 13.4). The differences in life expectancy at any age between men and women depend upon a number of factors, including occupational exposure, recreational pursuits, etc., and may not be related merely to gender difference.

Excellent reviews of metal-associated chemical neoplastic transformation have been provided by Sky–Peck (1986), Vahey et al. (1995), Rock (1998), and Adams et al. (2003); the latter three reviews are directed primarily towards human clinical experience.

TABLE 13.3

Life Expectancy[a] by Age in the U.S.

Age (years)	Male	Female
At birth	74.5	79.9
5	70.2	75.4
10	65.3	70.5
15	60.3	65.5
20	55.6	60.7
30	46.3	51.0
40	37.0	41.4
50	28.3	32.2
60	20.2	23.5
65	16.6	19.5
70	13.2	15.8
75	10.3	12.2
80	7.8	9.4
85	5.7	6.9
90	4.2	5.0
95	3.2	3.7
100	2.5	2.8

[a] Mean; all races; alive in 2002.

Source: Arias, E., United States Life Tables, 2002, National Vital Statistic Reports, 53(6), National Center for Health Statistics, U.S. Government Printing Office, Washington, D.C., November 10, 2004.

13.3 Foreign Body Carcinogenesis

13.3.1 Early Observations of Foreign Body Carcinogenesis

So far the various classes of chemical carcinogens have been considered and the available information concerning their metabolism and ability to produce neoplastic transformation has been summarized. Across all the classes of pro-, co-, and complete chemical cocarcinogens, it may be stated that the risk of neoplastic transformation increases at least linearly with the concentration and period of exposure.

Studies of chemical carcinogenesis show interesting differences in action depending upon the manner and form of administration of the agent. Such differences led early investigators to study the influence of the physical form of the carcinogenic agent on its ability to induce transformation. A startling finding was that many agents not previously thought to be carcinogens produced dramatic neoplasm incidence rates in rodents when implanted in a solid form rather than injected or fed in soluble or dispersed form. This effect was called foreign body (FB) carcinogenesis and is known more recently as solid state* carcinogenesis.

Among the early investigators of FB carcinogenesis were E. and B.S. Oppenheimer who, in conjunction with a number of co-investigators, published a long series of papers in the 1940s and 1950s (see Oppenheimer et al. 1955). Their studies and those of other investigators of the period established the following points:

- Solid materials without chemical carcinogenic activity can induce a variety of neoplasms in several small rodent species.
- Induction activity generally increases with the size of the implant.
- Induction activity varies inversely as the inflammatory response; that is, in the long run, well-tolerated materials are more effective FB carcinogens.
- Porosity with an average diameter above 0.22 μm (the smallest size studied) reduces the risk of transformation.

13.3.2   Mechanisms of Foreign Body Carcinogenesis

An excellent contemporary summary of these early investigations, primarily using plastic films as challenge agents, is that of Alexander and Horning (1959), who proposed that "the most likely process [of neoplasm induction] would appear to be that the film alters the normal environment of the neighboring cells in such a way as to favor the induction (or selection) of discontinuous variations leading to malignancy." That is, the survival of viable products of normally occurring cell damage or mutation are somehow favored by the presence of the solid body and protected from physiological processes until they are ready to enter the rapid growth phase characteristic of malignancy.

Two considerations appear to favor this argument. The first is geometric and was discussed briefly in Chapter 8 when the role of implants in infection was examined. A cell is normally surrounded by a volume of tissue subtending a 4π solid angle. As an implant is approached, the solid angle decreases to 2π. Furthermore, if the implant is invaginated with a surface roughness that has a characteristic dimension on the order of cell sizes (2 to 20 μm), the solid angle might even be less than 2π for some selected cells. The results would be less access to microvasculature, poorer diffusional supply, and reduced cell contact inhibition. The flaw in this general line of argument is, of course, the observation that materials with distributed porosity of cellular dimensions are less carcinogenic in rodents than smooth nonporous materials. Perhaps one of these geometric factors is dominant or

---

* I dislike this phrase due to its confusion with semiconducting materials and thus the implication of electronic causality.

perhaps the improved diffusion and cellular activity associated with microporous surfaces offsets the other aspects of the near-surface geometry.

The second consideration that favors the argument proposed by Alexander and Horning (1959) is that chemical and electrical conditions near an implant–tissue interface are different from those at a distance; this has been discussed extensively in previous chapters. The question remains, however, of which field and concentration effects might favor protection of deviant cells. Russian investigators (cited by Bischoff and Bryson 1964) felt that piezoelectric materials with sharp points and asperities were more tumorigenic than the same materials in smooth or colloidal form. This suggested a role for very high gradient electric fields in FB carcinogenesis. A study by Andrews et al. (1979) attempted to investigate this question by subcutaneous implantation of plates of polystyrene resin in mice. The resin was implanted in neutral condition or as poled (polarized) electrets of various strengths. Tumors associated with the control plates were evenly distributed on both sides, and those associated with the electrets were found predominantly on the electronegative side.* The investigators felt that the trend was to higher incidence rates and shorter latency periods for electrets with higher fields.

A more complete review (Bischoff and Bryson 1964) expanded this critique. The authors posed and answered three questions:

- Question 1: "Is the concept of nonspecific (rather than by a specific chemical agent) solid state carcinogenesis justified?"

  Answer: After considerable criticism of experimental method and test subject, Bischoff and Bryson conclude that "on the basis of the responses to rather stable, unrelated substances, there is a type of nonspecific carcinogenesis in rodents that is dependent upon a minimum surface requirement."

- Question 2: "Does solid state carcinogenesis occur in humans?"

  Answer: For humans, the authors note the low reported incidence of neoplasms associated with implants, natural deposits (cholesterol plaques, gall stones, etc.), and chronic low-level inflammatory processes (leading to acellular fibrotic tissue, which has FB attributes). They admit an exception to this basic pattern in the observation of carcinoma associated with silicosis and asbestosis. (Note, however, that in 1964 the very high correlation between a specific type of asbestos [chrysotile] and mesothelioma was not yet known.) They also recognize the problem of the latency period and of the relatively smaller implants (with respect to body weight) used clinically as compared with those in the experiments of Oppenheimer and others. Thus, they concluded that "the incidence of sarcoma [in humans] arising from subcutaneous FB granuloma is minimal."

---

* However, this difference, as well as all other conclusions reported for this study, was not statistically significant.

- Question 3: "Is the subcutaneous site in rodents valid for testing for carcinogenic hazards?"

    Answer: This question reflects their observation of a "widespread disenchantment" with subcutaneous studies in rodents. Their arguments are rather vague, but essentially arrive at the point of view that, through nonspecific irritation, FB carcinogenesis and chemical carcinogenesis may occur together and, without adequate controls, cannot be easily distinguished in the subcutaneous site. They suggest, however, that the determining factor is the difference between response to irritation in the chemical case and transformation after noninflammatory isolation of the foreign body in the FB case. In this latter comment, they presage the more modern studies of FB carcinogenesis.

13.3.3 Additional Studies of Foreign Body Carcinogenesis

Further studies by Ott and by Brand and their students have focused upon the mechanisms of neoplastic transformation in rodents in order to distinguish FB from chemical carcinogenesis. Brand (1975) has more fully summarized his research and theoretical ideas. He made extensive use of related species of mice that will accept tissue transplants without immune response, but in which cells and their daughters can be identified, by species, through an examination of chromosomes (karyotyping). I will paraphrase two sections of his paper dealing with the mechanism of the tumorigenic process and hypotheses concerning initiation and promulgation of the process.

Brand reached the following conclusions, which were documented by thorough and ingenious research:

- The most probable target cell in FB carcinogenesis is the pericyte, a small cell type associated with microvasculature.
- After implantation, the transformation needed to produce a preneoplastic parent cell, with all the genetic information for later expression in the active neoplasm, occurs quite rapidly. In Brand's mice populations, this occurs within 4 to 8 weeks after implantation.
- Although the transformation occurs "near" the FB–tissue interface, actual close contact with the FB is not required.
- Transformation is quite uncommon; thus, neoplasms appear to develop from single parent cells representing one in the several million affected by the presence of the implant.
- Although neoplasm production will occur in a capsule after FB removal, a significant period of implantation after the initial transformation event is required.
- A latent period always occurs between transformation and neoplastic expression. However, this period is characterized more by

inactivity of microphages than of the transformed parent cell that may be cloning (undergoing mitosis without inheritable change) at a slow rate. In the presence of active macrophages, as in moderate to severe chronic inflammation, later neoplastic expression is suppressed.

- When the latent period is over and rapid malignant growth begins, all daughter cells, even if transplanted, appear to act in synchrony.

Boone and coworkers' (1979) set of *in vitro* tissue culture experiments have partially verified Brand's *in vivo* studies. These researchers studied the effects of attachment of mouse fibroblasts to polycarbonate plates in an *in vitro* tissue culture system. Cells implanted after *in vitro* exposure produced transplantable, undifferentiated sarcomas. Notwithstanding a decrease in latent period with increased time in tissue culture, the authors concluded, as had Brand, that the smooth surfaces of the plates acted as an FB carcinogen, for at least initiation, independently of chemical composition.

Brand (1975) cited six proposed mechanistic origins of FB carcinogenesis (with accompanying criticisms):

- Chemical activity of components of the FB. Brand suggested a moderating or modifying role for chemical agents; however, he felt that the nonchemical mechanism for FB carcinogenesis was well established.

- Physiochemical surface properties of the FB. Again, Brand recognized a possible role for interface physical effects but suggested that they are overpowered in importance by other physical factors, such as porosity.

- Interruption of cellular contact or communication. Brand felt that this is an open question, but indicates that it would be expected to play a more important role in neoplasm expression and maturation than in induction.

- Tissue anoxia and insufficient exchange of metabolites. Brand rejected this hypothesis based upon comparison of cell distances from vascular processes in normal and neoplastic tissue and upon induction studies with vascularized microporous surfaces.

- Virus (as an unseen contaminant of FBs). Although some viri are now recognized as mammalian carcinogens, the evidence is still weak for viri playing a role in FB transformation; Brand evidently did not favor it.

- Disturbance of cellular growth regulation. Brand clearly favored this mechanism, based on the heritability of neoplastic behavior in the growing cell population. He suggested a wide variety of possible aberrations in growth control and communication processes in cells.

Thus, his view is that the nonspecific surface effect, whatever its origins, acts in a mutagenic fashion on cell populations.

This discussion of FB carcinogenesis has focused on nonchemical neoplastic transformation effects produced by materials external to cells. However, solid materials in a form that can penetrate cells can also produce FB transformation. The best known example is crysotile asbestos, which was recognized as a human carcinogen only because it produced a relatively rare lung tumor (mesothelioma) (U.S. Department of Health and Human Services, 2004). Studies of asbestos and other fibers in animal models has led to the Stanton hypothesis: mesothelioma can be induced by fibers less than 0.5 to 1 μm in diameter and more than 8 μm in length,* regardless of fiber composition (Lipkin 1980). Lipkin has also shown that *in vitro* fiber cytotoxicity correlates well with these dimensions rather than with fiber composition. Thus, slender stiff fibers, such as mineral whiskers, that are apparently able to penetrate cells and produce direct mechanical damage, presumably to the nucleus, appear to be undesirable components of biomaterials.

Perhaps the best place to end this discussion is with a quotation from Brand (1975, p. 487):

> Despite the rarity of FB tumors in man, it would be irresponsible to look at the situation with complacency. Several measures are at our disposal which would minimize the probability of FB tumors in man.... These include (1) a more restrictive approach to artificial implantations, especially the exclusion of medically unnecessary cosmetic procedures, unless they are indicated for psychiatric reasons; (2) smallest possible size of implants; (3) reexamination of implant carriers at frequent intervals; (4) a centralized registry for gathering information on general complications as well as instances of neoplasia; (5) continued research (a) on implant materials regarding their suitability for specific surgical purposes and (b) on etiological questions concerning this type of neoplasia.

This passage certainly contains food for thought for the bioengineer.

13.4   Nonspecific Carcinogenesis

A final form of neoplastic stimulation is also recognized. Neoplasms can arise in response to chronic irritation (leading to chronic inflammation). Chemicals (as well as foreign bodies), infection, and mechanical trauma have all been recognized as leading to this type of neoplastic transformation. This was possibly a feature in the large, lifetime rodent implantation study

---

* That is, with an aspect ratio $(L/D) > 8$ to 16. However, other factors, such as fiber stiffness, may play a role.

discussed previously (Section 13.2.5; Bouchard et al. 1996). It is characterized by an infidelity of replication (producing a daughter cell not identical to its parent). The formation of keloids (hyperplastic, expansive scars) is a non-malignant example of this effect. The occasional, apparently spontaneous, malignant transformation of benign lesions such as fibrous histiocytomas is a somewhat more ominous example (Heselson et al. 1983).

13.5 Evidence for Implant Carcinogenesis in Humans

In light of the long use of metallic implants in clinical orthopaedics and other surgical specialties, it is fair to ask whether any evidence indicates chemical or FB carcinogenesis associated with implants. The number of reports of tumors at implant sites in animals is mounting. Sinibaldi et al. (1976) reported sarcomas in animals (seven dogs and one cat) occurring 6 months to 4 years after implantation of stainless steel devices. Of interest is the fact that five of the eight cases accompanied the use of the Jonas telescoping splint. With its integral deep "crevice" between parts, this device would be expected to display an abnormally high rate of corrosion (see Chapter 4). Harrison et al. (1976) had earlier reported two cases in dogs, one 6 years and one 12 years after stainless steel implantation during clinical treatment of fractures. An additional case of sarcoma occurring 12 years after Jonas splint implantation in a dog has been reported recently (Madewell et al. 1977). A survey by Stevenson et al. (1982), including these cases, reported 35 fracture-associated sarcomas in animals with an average of 5.8 years between injury (and internal fixation) and diagnosis.

Finally, these tumors in animals are apparently associated with implant site infection. Such infection may be expected to produce elevated rates of corrosion and thus elevated concentrations of metal-bearing species near implants, due to the resulting local acidosis. However, a large-scale case-control study of possible association between tumors and the use of metallic fracture fixation devices in 222 dogs with tumors (Li et al. 1993) failed to show a significant relationship between the incidence of bone and soft-tissue sarcomas and the use of implants predominantly fabricated from stainless steel.

The early human orthopaedic literature reports only three cases of fracture-related implant site tumors: Delgado (1958), sarcoma after fracture of tibia, internally fixed; Dube and Fisher (1972), hemangioendothelioma after fracture of tibia, internally fixed; and McDougall (1956), sarcoma (Ewing's type) in fractured humerus, after internal fixation. The last case is the best known and occurred more than 30 years after the initial injury and metallic implantation. Additional cases continue to be reported, typically occurring more than 5 years after implantation. Although fracture fixation hardware should be removed routinely within 2 years after implantation, if the patient's health permits, less than half is currently removed. Therefore, although such cases are expected to continue to be rare, some concern remains, especially for younger individuals.

More than two dozen cases of tumors associated with partial or total joint replacements in humans have now been published;* the average postoperative period before diagnosis is 7 years. The early reports have been discussed previously (Black 1988); more recent reports are reviewed by Rock (1998) and Adams et al. (2003). These tumors fall into two general groups:

- Tumors of various etiologies occurring in fairly short periods after implantation
- Primarily malignant fibrous histiocytomas occurring 10 to 15 years after implantation

To date, all of these tumors have been associated with stainless-steel or cobalt-base alloy devices. The origin of the former group is somewhat obscure; however, the latter group may reflect direct chemical carcinogenesis (associated with elevated tissue concentrations of metals near the implant; see Chapter 15) or possibly malignant transformation of the previously benign implant capsule.

Orthopaedic devices are placed in soft and hard connective tissues, which are not especially sensitive to primary neoplastic transformation in humans (Black 1984, 1985). Until recently, no evidence had suggested remote site tumors possibly resulting from concentrations of suspected carcinogens, such as chromates, because no large epidemiological study had been done to detect their presence or absence. However, due in part to my suggestions (Black 1984), at least three epidemiological studies have now been completed, the first by Gillespie et al. (1988).

Gillespie and colleagues identified 1358 patients who had received total hip replacements in New Zealand between 1967 and 1978. They investigated the health status of over 1000 of these patients who could be followed for more than 10 years postimplantation and found a highly significant 70% elevated incidence of tumors of lymphatic and hemopoietic origin (Table 13.4). In addition, they observed a significant suppression of soft tissue (colon, bowel, and breast) tumor incidence up to 10 years postimplantation followed by an apparent but nonsignificant increase in incidence. Even 10-year follow-up may be insufficient for expression of primary (chemical) tumors at the low doses encountered at remote sites in implant-bearing human patients. These results may simply reflect an effect of corrosion products producing a chronic immune system stress — that is, playing the part of indirect promoters of soft tissue neoplasias produced by other causes.

---

* The word "published" is operative here: during a career of more than three decades of lecturing on this topic to clinical audiences, almost without fail, after the formal program, I would be approached by a surgeon who knew of someone who had such a case — but as yet unpublished!

TABLE 13.4

Risks of Cancer in Patients with Total Hip Replacement

Feature	Study		
	Gillespie et al. (1988)[a]	Visuri et al. (1991)	Nyrén et al. (1995)[b]
Total patients	1358	433	39,154
Site	New Zealand	Finland	Sweden
Total THRs	unk. (>1358)	511	46,547
Total patient years	14,286	5729	327,922
Average duration, years	10.5	9.6	8.4
Type of THR	Many; mostly McKee–Farrar	McKee–Farrar	Many; no McKee–Farrar
Increased cancer risk[c]	Lymphoma/leukemia (1.38) (total period: 1.68[d])	Lymphoma/ leukemia (3.01[d]); intra-abdominal (2.78)	Bone (2.08); melanoma (1.44[d]); connective tissue (1.42); kidney (1.33[d]); prostate (1.18[d])
Decreased cancer risk[c]	Colon/rectum (0.52[d]); bronchus/lung (0.54); breast (0,30[d])	Respiratory (0.86); female reproductive system (0.56)	Gastric (0.74); lymphoma (0.89)
Overall risk[c]	Decreased (0.77[d])	Unchanged (1.02)	Increased (1.05[d])
Comment	Patients followed > 10 years; SIR = 1.60[e]		

Note: McKee–Farrar is a metal/metal articulating THR device.

[a] SIRs for 5- to 10-year follow-up.
[b] SIRs for 5- to 9-year follow-up.
[c] Standard incidence ratio (SIR).
[d] Significant change in SIR($p < 0.05$).
[e] Significant change in SIR($p < 0.01$).

Source: Adapted from Black, J., *Clin. Orthop. Rel. Res.*, 329S, S244, 1996.

Longer term follow-ups and larger, better defined study groups will be required to explore these preliminary results.

Since this study, two additional ones have been done to explore the same question (Table 13.4). The work by Visuri et al. (1991) appears to support the earlier study, but that of Nyrén et al. (1995) appears to contradict it. However, when viewed in light of the apparent prevalence of metal-on-metal devices, which have been shown to produce perhaps as much as a 10- to 15-fold elevation in circulating serum chromium concentration (Jacobs et al. 1996), one might well conclude that a positive relationship exists between metal release and the incidence of lymphoma and leukemia in patients. This conclusion should be viewed with some caution because it has been known for some time that patients with rheumatoid arthritis are at greater risk than the overall population for developing lymphoma and leukemia (Isomäki et al. 1978). Studies such as those reported in Table 13.5 are based upon comparisons to overall population statistics; in total hip replacement recipient populations, individuals with rheumatoid arthritis are probably over-represented in comparison to the overall population in the country of the study.

In reviewing this growing body of conflicting information, Rock (1998) concludes that "[although] the incidence of primary tumors in close proximity to implants appears consistent with that expected in the general population...the frequency of occurrence and associated individual and group risks of systemic and remote site malignancy remains unresolved."

The question of the occurrence of FB tumors in patients also remains a mystery. Brand (1983) reviewed 43 tumors occurring in humans at implant sites, at up to 53 years after implantation; 25% occurred within 15 years and 50% within 25 years of implantation. In light of the large upsurge in medical and cosmetic implant use in the 1950s and 1960s, he would have expected to find orders of magnitude for more cases if causation in humans was the same as for mice. Thus, although continuing to express concern about the possibilities for FB carcinogenesis in humans, Brand concluded that little clinical evidence for its occurrence existed.

Similarly, Berkel and colleagues (1992) studied a group of 11,676 women with silicone elastomer breast implants, at an average of 10.2 years after implantation, and concluded that they experienced 52% fewer primary breast tumors than expected. Thus, although longer term data still are required, it is beginning to appear likely that the Oppenheimer effect is a consequence of the relatively primitive immune system of rodents in comparison to that in humans.

Perhaps the best overview is provided by a study published by the International Agency for Research on Cancer (IARC 1999). The IARC has classified agents suspected of being carcinogens in a well-defined system based upon balancing animal- and clinically-derived evidence. This system establishes five groups of agents and exposures as carcinogenic, probably or

TABLE 13.5

IARC Classification of Evidence for Human Carcinogenicity Risk

Group Classification in Humans	Degree of Evidence for Carcinogenicity	
	In Humans	In Animals
1: Carcinogenic	< Sufficient *but*	Sufficient
2a: Probably carcinogenic	Limited *and*	Sufficient
	Or inadequate *and*	Sufficient
2b: Possibly carcinogenic	Limited *and*	< Sufficient
	Or inadequate *and*	Sufficient
3: Not classifiable	Inadequate *and*	Limited *or* inadequate
	Or inadequate *and*	Sufficient[a]
4: Not carcinogenic	Suggested lack	??
	Inadequate *but*	Suggested lack

[a] However, mechanism of causation inoperative in humans.

Source: IARC, *Evaluation Carcinogenic Risks Hum.*, Vol. 74, WHO, IARC, Lyon, France, 1999.

possibly carcinogenic, not classifiable, or not carcinogenic (Table 13.5). Based upon an exhaustive study of animal data and human clinical results, the IARC concluded that the following overall evaluation could be made concerning the carcinogenic risk of clinical implants:

- Group 1(carcinogenic): none
- Group 2A (probably carcinogenic): none
- Group 2B (possibly carcinogenic): smooth metallic and polymeric films, solid bodies of metallic cobalt, nickel, and a nickel alloy (66 to 67% Ni, 13 to 16% Cr, 7% Fe)
- Group 3 (not classifiable): orthopaedic implants of complex composition, cardiac pacemakers, silicone breast implants, metallic chromium, titanium, Co-, Cr-, and Ti-based alloys, stainless steels and depleted uranium, as well as dental materials and solid ceramic bodies
- Group 4 (noncarcinogenic): none

It is of interest that, despite the extensive clinical use of biomaterials as human implants, the IARC could not conclude that any are actually carcinogenic (group 1) or totally lacking in risk (group 4).

Two additional ways of approaching this issue parallel Furst's (1978) analysis of metal carcinogenesis in animals. The U.S. Department of Health and Human Services is required by statute* to publish a list of agents (A) known to be human carcinogens or (B) reasonably anticipated to be human carcinogens. These correspond to the IARC groups 1 and 2A, and 2B and 3, respectively (see Table 13.5). The most recent of these lists (U.S. Department of Health and Human Services 2004) contains the following agents, which could be elements of metallic implants or be released by implant degradation:

- Known (A): chromium hexavalent compounds, nickel compounds and metallic nickel
- Reasonably anticipated (B): cobalt sulfate

Additionally, the state of California adopted Proposition 65, the Safe Drinking Water and Toxic Enforcement Act of 1986, by ballot initiative. This act requires the periodic publication of a list of chemicals known (to the state) to cause cancer or reproductive toxicity. This list draws from many sources, including IARC analyses; because it is precautionary, it is somewhat conservative. It also provides for labeling requirements for any product known to contain such chemicals, unless the release (dose) rate can reasonably be expected to be below a previously determined acceptable level.

---

* Section 301(b)(4) of the Public Health Service Act as amended by Section 262, PL, 95-622.

The most recent version of the Proposition 65 list (12/31/04)* contains the following carcinogenic agents, which could be elements of metallic implants or be released by implant degradation:

- Chromium (hexavalent compounds)
- Cobalt (metal powder; [II] oxide, sulfate heptahydrate)
- Nickel (metallic, acetate, carbonate, carbonyl, oxide, refinery dust, subsulfide), nickelocene

It remains clear that the traditional problem of projecting animal experience to human occupational and clinical situations applies in the consideration of carcinogenesis as a possible consequence of biomaterial implantation. In particular, it should be noted that, despite Brand's comments in his 1983 study, it is only now that significant human populations with implants in place for more than 15 to 20 years are coming into existence. Survivors of these large modern cohorts are now beginning to pass the average latency period for low-concentration chemical carcinogenesis. There are no animal experiments to guide one accurately in what expectations should be. Perhaps Brand's previous remarks might be paraphrased: "despite the rarity of [implant-associated] tumors in [hu]man[s]..." — and more careful attention should be given in the future to the challenging and difficult issues of possible chemical and FB carcinogenesis by clinical implants.

References

Adams, J.E. et al., Prosthetic implant associated sarcomas: a case report emphasizing surface evaluation and spectroscopic trace meta analysis, *Ann. Diagn. Pathol.*, 7(1), 35, 2003.

Alexander, P. and Horning, E.S., Observations on the Oppenheimer method of inducing tumors by subcutaneous implantation of plastic films, in *Carcinogenesis: Mechanisms of Action*, Ciba Foundation Symposium, Wolstenholme, G.E.W. and O'Connor, M. (Eds.), Little, Brown, Boston, 1959, 12.

American Cancer Society, *2004 Cancer Facts and Figures*, American Cancer Society, Atlanta, 2004.

Ames, B.N. and Gold, L.S., Too many rodent carcinogens: mitogenesis increases mutagenesis, *Science*, 249, 970, 1990.

Andrews, E.J. et al., Surface charge in foreign body carcinogenesis, *J. Biomed. Mater. Res.*, 13, 173, 1979.

Arias, E., United States Life Tables, 2002, National Vital Statistic Reports, 53(6), National Center for Health Statistics, U.S. Government Printing Office, Washington, D.C., November 10, 2004.

---

* http://www.oehha.ca.gov/prop65/prop65_list/Newlist.html.

Berenblum, I., A re-evaluation of the concept of co-carcinogenesis, *Prog. Exp. Tumor Res.*, 11, 21, 1969.

Berkel, H., Birdsell, D.C. and Jenkins, H., Breast augmentation: a risk factor for breast cancer? *New Engl. J. Med.*, 326(25), 1649, 1992.

Bischoff, F. and Bryson, G., Carcinogenesis through solid state surfaces, *Prog. Exp. Tumor Res.*, 5, 85, 1964.

Black, J., Systemic effects of biomaterials, *Biomaterials*, 5, 11, 1984.

Black, J., Metallic ion release and its relationship to oncogenesis, in Fitzgerald, R.H., Jr. (Ed.), *The Hip*, Vol. 13, C.V. Mosby, St. Louis, 1985, 199.

Black, J., *Orthopedic Biomaterials in Research and Practice*, Churchill Livingstone, New York, 1988, 292.

Black, J., Metal on metal bearings: a practical alternative to metal on polyethylene bearings? *Clin. Orthop. Rel. Res.*, 329S, S244, 1996.

Boone, C.W. et al. "Spontaneous" neoplastic transformation *in vitro*: a form of foreign body (smooth surface) tumorigenesis, *Science*, 204, 177, 1979.

Bouchard, P.R et al., Carcinogenicity of CoCrMo (F-75) implants in the rat, *J. Biomed. Mater. Res.*, 32, 37, 1996.

Brand, K.G., Foreign body induced sarcomas, in *Cancer: A Comprehensive Treatise*, Vol. 1, Becker, F.F. (Ed.), Plenum, New York, 485, 1975.

Brand, K.G., Human foreign-body carcinogenesis in the light of animal experiments and assessment of cancer risk at implant sites, in *Biomaterials in Reconstructive Surgery*, Rubin, L.R. (Ed.), C. V. Mosby, St. Louis, 36, 1983.

Christensen, H.E. and Fairchild, E.J. (Eds.), *Suspected Carcinogens*, 2nd ed., CDC, National Institute for Occupational Safety and Health, Cincinnati, OH, 1972.

Delgado, E.R., Sarcoma following surgically treated fractured tibia, *Clin. Orthop.*, 12, 315, 1958.

Dube, V.E. and Fisher, D.E., Hemangioendothelioma of the leg following metallic fixation of the tibia, *Cancer*, 30, 1260, 1972.

Friedewald, W.F. and Rous, P., The initiating and promoting elements in tumor formation, *J. Exp. Med.*, 80, 101, 1944.

Furst, A. and Haro, R.T., A survey of metal carcinogenesis, *Progr. Exp. Tumor Res.*, 12, 102, 1969.

Furst, A., An overview of metal carcinogenesis, *Adv. Exp. Med. Biol.*, 91, 1, 1978.

Gaechter, A. et al., Metal carcinogenesis, *J. Bone Joint Surg.*, 59A, 622, 1977.

Gillespie, W.J. et al., The incidence of cancer following total hip replacement, *J. Bone Joint Surg.*, 70B, 539, 1988.

Harrison, J.W. et al., Osteosarcoma associated with metallic implants, *Clin. Orthop. Rel. Res.*, 116, 253, 1976.

Heath, J.C. et al., Carcinogenic properties of wear particles from prostheses made in cobalt–chromium alloy, *Lancet* (March 20), 564, 1971.

Heselson, N.G. et al., Two malignant fibrous histiocytomas in bone infracts, *J. Bone Joint Surg.*, 65A, 1166,1983.

IARC, Surgical implants and other foreign bodies, *IARC Monogr. Evaluation Carcinogenic Risks Hum.*, Vol. 74, WHO, IARC, Lyon, France, 1999.

Innes, J.R.M. et al., Bioassay of pesticides and industrial chemicals for tumorgenicity in mice: a preliminary note, *J. Natl. Cancer Inst.*, 42, 1101, 1969.

Isomäki, H.A. et al., Excess risk of lymphomas, leukemia, and myeloma in patients with rheumatoid arthritis, *J. Chron. Dis.*, 31, 691, 1978.

Jacobs, J.J. et al., Cobalt and chromium concentrations in patients with metal-on-metal total hip replacements, *Clin. Orthop. Rel. Res.*, 329S, S256, 1996.

Li, X.Q. et al., Relationship between metallic implants and cancer: a case-control study in a canine population, *Vet. Clin. Orthop. Trauma*, 6, 70, 1993.

Lipkin, L.E., Cellular effects of asbestos and other fibers: correlations with *in vivo* induction of pleural sarcoma, *Environ. Health Persp.*, 34, 91, 1980.

Madewell, B.R. et al., Osteogenic sarcoma at the site of a chronic nonunion and internal fixation device in a dog, *J. Am. Vet. Med. Assoc.*, 171, 187, 1977.

McDougall, A., Malignant tumor at site of bone plating, *J. Bone Joint Surg.*, 38B, 709, 1956.

Memoli, V.A. et al., Malignant neoplasms associated with orthopedic implant materials in rats, *J. Orthop. Res.*, 4, 346, 1986.

Nyrén, O. et al., Cancer risk after hip replacement with metal implants: a population-based cohort study in Sweden, *J. Natl. Cancer Inst.*, 87(1), 28, 1995.

Oppenheimer, B.S. et al., Further studies of polymers as carcinogenic agents in animals, *Cancer Res.*, 15, 333, 1955.

Rock, M., Cancer, in *Handbook of Biomaterial Properties*, Black, J. and Hastings, G. (Eds.), Chapman & Hall, London, 1998, 529.

Schottenfeld, D. and Haas, J.F., Carcinogens in the workplace, *CA*, 29, 144, 1979.

Sinibaldi, K. et al., Tumors associated with metallic implants in animals, *Clin. Orthop. Rel. Res.*, 118, 257, 1976.

Sky–Peck, H.H., Trace metals and neoplasia, *Clin. Physiol. Biochem.*, 4, 99, 1986.

Stevenson, S. et al., Fracture-associated sarcoma in the dog, *J. Am. Vet. Med. Assoc.*, 180, 1189, 1982.

Sunderman, F.W., Jr., Metal carcinogenesis in experimental animals, *Food Cosmet. Toxicol.*, 9, 105, 1971.

U.S. Department of Health and Human Services, *Report on Carcinogens*, 11th ed., U.S. Department of Health and Human Services, Public Health Service, National Toxicology Program, December 2004.

Vahey, J.W. et al., Carcinogenicity and metal implants, *Am. J. Orthop.*, 24(4), 319, 1995.

Visuri, T. and Koskenvuo, M., Cancer risk after Mckee-Farrar total hip replacement, *Orthopedics*, 14(2), 137, 1991.

Weisburger, J.H. and Williams, G.M., Metabolism of chemical carcinogens, in *Cancer: A Comprehensive Treatise*, Vol. 1, Becker, F.F. (Ed.), Plenum Press, New York, 1975, 185.

Bibliography

Ambrose, E.J. and Roe, F.J.C., *The Biology of Cancer*, D. Van Nostrand, New York, 1966.

Berenblum, I., *Carcinogenesis as a Biological Problem*, North–Holland Pub. Co., Amsterdam, 1974.

Becker, F.F., *Cancer: A Comprehensive Treatise*, Vol. 1: *Etiology: Chemical and Physical Carcinogenesis*, Vol. 4: *Biology of Tumors: Surfaces, Immunology, and Comparative Pathology*, Plenum Press, New York, 1975

Haag, M. and Adler, C.P., Malignant fibrous histiocytoma in association with hip replacement, *J. Bone Joint Surg.*, 71B, 701, 1989.

Kolstad, K. and Högstorp, H., Gastric carcinoma metastasis to a knee with a newly inserted prosthesis, *Acta Scand. Orthop.*, 61, 369, 1990.

Roe, F.J.C., Introduction, in *The Biology of Cancer*, Ambrose, E.J. and Roe, F.J.C. (Eds.), D. Van Nostrand, New York, 1966, 28.

Tait, N.P. et al., Malignant fibrous histiocytoma occurring at the site of a previous total hip replacement, *Br. J. Radiol.*, 61, 73, 1988.

Troop, J.K. et al., Malignant fibrous histiocytoma after total hip arthroplasty, *Clin. Orthop. Rel. Res.*, 253, 297, 1990.

U.S. Department of Health and Human Services, Proceedings of a workshop/conference on the role of metals in carcinogenesis, Atlanta, GA, March 24–28, 1980, *Environmental Health Perspectives*, Vol. 40, 1981.

van der List, J.J.J. et al., Malignant epithelioid hemangioendothelioma at the site of a hip prosthesis, *Acta Orthop. Scand.*, 59, 328, 1988.

14

Mineral Metabolism

14.1 Introduction

The next chapter will deal with the distribution of metallic ions and some simple models for their dispersion. This chapter will consider one well known metal — iron — in detail and a lesser known metal — chromium. This consideration is important in its own right, as well as being an indicator of the complexity of the metabolism of metals. As in the case of most other metals, the details of metabolic pathways and kinetics of these two metals are not fully known. However, the attempt will be to contrast iron metabolism with chromium metabolism.

As discussed in Section 2.2 and Section 2.4, the human body is primarily composed of four nonmetallic elements (in declining order of abundance): oxygen, carbon, hydrogen, and nitrogen, which make up 96.9% of body tissues by weight. Six additional elements, of which only two are metals (calcium and sodium), play major physiological roles and contribute a further ~3.2% of body weight. All other constituents contribute together no more than 30 g and are termed trace elements. These include at least 13 metals, of which 10 are used routinely as nontrace constituents in human implants: iron, copper,* aluminum, vanadium, manganese, nickel, molybdenum, titanium, chromium, and cobalt.

Most of these trace elements (with the possible exception of titanium) play vital physiological roles and thus are termed essential trace elements. The role of each is characterized by three important attributes (Mertz 1981):

- Amplification: all known essential trace elements exert their biological actions through a succession of regulatory and/or synthetic steps that produce a many-fold amplification function and lead to effects on the whole body.
- Specificity: each essential trace element has a specific role as a moiety in a molecule or as an enzyme cofactor. This specificity depends on

---

* Copper is not routinely used in human implants, due to its cytotoxicity, but is a component of some designs of semipermanent intrauterine contraceptive devices (IUDs).

ionic size and valence. Other ions may interfere with the specific role of a trace element but may not replace its function.

- Homeostatic regulation: without exception, for each essential trace element, a panoply of absorption, transport, storage, and excretion mechanisms regulates concentration at the site of action within an optimum range.

Our interest in trace elements is related to this third attribute — to the possibility that the introduction of an endogenous source, i.e., release of material from an implant, may interfere with homeostatic regulation and produce adverse effects at the site of normal action or at other sites, directly or by interference with other trace element-mediated processes.

In discussing the toxic effects of mercury and its organometallic compounds, Schwarz (1977) makes the following point:

> Below a certain threshold [of concentration], the organism can maintain an equilibrium. However, once the threshold level is reached, small increases in doses lead to great increases of toxic effects.... Indeed, this relationship pertains not only to all metals but anything. It is universal, with the possible exception of mutagenicity and carcinogenicity, but even there repair mechanisms are at work which may give a small area of tolerance (p. 3).

The general relationship between metal concentration level and functional effect is shown in Figure 14.1. It should be emphasized that this is only schematic in nature; the details and relative extent of each range depend upon the nature of the metal involved and, probably, upon individual differences between patients. Thus, although calculations may be performed that predict various levels of metallic ions in blood, tissues, etc. (Section 15.4), the real need is to know the details of the metabolic, storage, and excretory pathways. The next two major sections outline iron metabolism, whose details are well known, and chromium metabolism, which is less well known and understood. Until the comparable systems are as well known for the other major metallic components of common implant alloys such as aluminum, chromium, cobalt, nickel, titanium, etc. as they are for iron, great care must be taken in the interpretation of animal and clinical determinations of metallic content *in vivo*.

14.2 Iron Metabolism

14.2.1 Introduction

Iron is a biologically ubiquitous metal that is essential to all higher forms of life owing to its central role in the heme molecule facilitating oxygen and

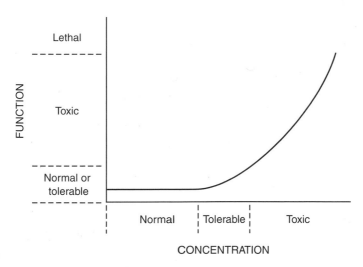

FIGURE 14.1
Relation between metal concentration and its functional consequence.

electron transport. The capacity of porphyrin-Fe–protein complexes to bind large quantities of oxygen reversibly makes hemoglobin and myoglobin well suited to the transport and storage of oxygen in higher organisms. Iron-containing enzymes include the cytochromes, catalase, cytochrome c reductase, succinic dehydrogenase, and fumaric dehydrogenase. Total body iron in an average adult ranges from 2 to 6 g, depending on body weight, hemoglobin concentration, age, sex, and size of the storage compartment. As a trace element, iron's presence in the body is exceeded only by magnesium (see Table 2.3).

On the basis of function, two iron metabolic compartments are recognized:

- An essential compartment containing 70% of the total body iron is composed of hemoglobin, myoglobin, heme enzymes, cofactor, and transport iron.
- A nonessential storage compartment accounts for 30% of the total body iron in a normal individual and consists of iron storage in the form of ferritin and hemosiderin, primarily in the liver, spleen, and bone marrow.

The essential compartment can be further subdivided into the following distribution: 85% in hemoglobin, 5% in myoglobin, 10% in intracellular heme enzymes and iron cofactors in other enzyme systems, and 0.1% as transport iron bound to transferrin.

14.2.2 Absorption

Absorption of iron (see Figure 14.2) represents the single most important factor maintaining the normal balance of iron in the body. It is influenced by age, state of health, current body iron status, and conditions within the gastrointestinal tract, as well as by the amount and chemical form of iron ingested and by the relative iron-chelating nature of other dietary constituents (e.g., phosphates, phytates, ascorbic acid, and amino acids). Dietary intake varies between 10 and 30 mg/day, with a common range of 12 to 5 mg/day. Normally, 0.6 to 1.5 mg/day are absorbed through the gastrointestinal mucosa, representing only 5 to 10% of total dietary iron intake.

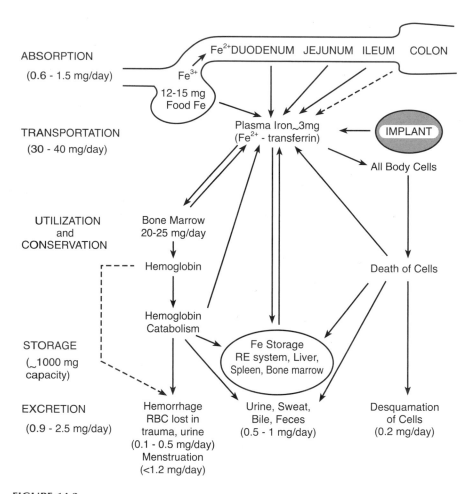

FIGURE 14.2

Iron metabolism in adults. (From Fairbanks, V.F. and Beutler, E., in *Modern Nutrition in Health and Disease,* 7th ed., Shils, M.E. and Young, V.R. (Eds.), Lea & Febiger, Philadelphia, 1988, 193.)

The actual mechanisms of absorption and transport of iron or iron chelates at the mucosal cell level remain unclear; however, it appears that iron enters the mucosal brush border by a passive diffusion process and exits on the serosal surface to the plasma transferrin by an energy-requiring step. Intracellular absorbed iron in excess of immediate physiological needs is combined with a protein, apoferritin, to form ferritin, a water-soluble iron-storage complex. As the mucosal cells become laden with ferritin, further absorption is impeded consistent with diffusion kinetics until ferritin iron is released to the plasma in response to body needs. Most absorbed iron, in the form of intracellular ferritin, is lost into the intestinal lumen when the crypt cells complete their 2- to 3-day maturation and migration to the tips of the villi and are sloughed. Intraluminal factors that decrease iron absorption include rapid gastrointestinal transit time; achylia; malabsorption syndrome; precipitation by alkalinization by phosphates and phytates; and ingested alkaline clays and antacid preparations. Despite intensive research, the systemic factors regulating iron absorption have not been identified. In general, iron absorption increases whenever erythropoiesis (red blood cell production) is stimulated, during pregnancy, and in patients with hemochromatosis; decreased absorption is associated with depressed erythropoiesis and iron overload.

14.2.3   Transportation

After an iron atom enters the physiological system, it is virtually trapped, cycling almost endlessly from plasma to developing erythroblasts. Iron is then released into the circulation for 100 to 160 days, moved to phagocytic cells where it is cleaved from hemoglobin, and finally released into the plasma to repeat the cycle. From the standpoint of distribution of total body iron, the transport compartment is the smallest (~0.008%). However, kinetically, it is by far the most active, turning over as often as 10 times every 24 hours.

The vehicle of this rapid transport and turnover of iron is transferrin, a β_1-globulin of approximately 8.6×10^4 molecular weight, with a half-life of 8 to 10.5 days. Transferrin is synthesized in the liver, and the total body transferrin content of 7 to 15 g is nearly equally distributed between the intra- and extravascular spaces. It functions to accept iron from gut absorption, storage sites, and phagocytic cells and to deliver iron to erythroid marrow for hemoglobin synthesis, to cellular reticuloendothelium for storage, to the developing fetus, and to all cells for incorporation into iron metalloenzymes. Normally, approximately one-third of the total body transferrin (termed total iron-binding capacity; TIBC = 300 to 360 µg/100 ml) is saturated with iron. The remaining transferrin represents a latent or unbound reserve (unbound iron-binding capacity [UIBC]). The degree of saturation (%) and the TIBC are important parameters in the study of iron metabolism and related disease syndromes.

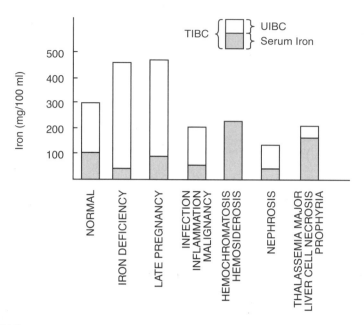

FIGURE 14.3

Serum iron concentration and the specific size of the transport compartment in a variety of clinical conditions. (Adapted from Fairbanks, V.F. and Beutler, E., in *Modern Nutrition in Health and Disease*, 7th ed., Shils, M.E. and Young, V.R. (Eds.), Lea & Febiger, Philadelphia, 1988, 193.)

For example, increased TIBC is characteristically found in iron deficiency, in the third trimester of pregnancy, and in response to hypoxic states, whereas decreased TIBC is evident in infection, protein malnutrition, iron overload conditions, malignancy, cirrhosis of the liver, nephrosis, and protein-losing exteropathies. Figure 14.3 illustrates the relationships between plasma iron and transferrin in a variety of clinical conditions. In general, the level of plasma iron and saturation of TIBC are determined by the sum of factors extracting iron from the blood for storage and utilization balanced against those factors releasing iron into the blood, e.g., absorption, hemolysis, and storage site release.

14.2.4   Utilization

It can be estimated from adult blood volume (typically ~5 l) and erythrocyte lifetime ($t_{1/2} \approx 60$ days) that, although more than 2.5 g of iron exists in hemoglobin within red blood cells, only 20 to 25 mg/day is used in hemoglobin synthesis in bone marrow. This is supplied through the transferrin transport pathway from absorption or release from storage. Defects in absorption, release, and/or transport may produce suppression of hemoglobin synthesis and, over time, lead to an erythrocyte deficiency or anemia.

14.2.5 Storage and Excretion

Iron in excess of metabolic needs is stored intracellularly as ferritin or hemosiderin in various tissues of the body. Ferritin is normally found in many tissues of the body; however, the reticuloendothelial system of the liver and cells in the intestinal mucosa are the most significant metabolic storage sites.

Hemosiderin, a granular water-soluble compound, is thought to be an aggregation of ferritin molecules. It can be seen microscopically in unstained tissue sections of bone marrow as clumps or granules of golden refractile pigment. Similar material is occasionally found *in vivo* in association with iron-bearing implants such as stainless steel device components (Winter 1976) and is thought by some investigators to be locally produced hemosiderin.* Although macrophages adjacent to implants can accumulate hemosiderin from endogenous sources, the source of this particular material is thought to be a combination of iron released from the original hematoma (formed during surgery) and iron oxides and hydroxides formed during corrosion. Primary storage sites are the hepatic parenchymal cells and reticuloendothelial cells of the bone marrow, liver, and spleen.

The relationship governing deposition of iron as ferritin or as hemosiderin is unclear. However, it is postulated that the relative content of iron in either storage form is a function of the total storage iron concentration. By chemically binding or shielding iron from the surrounding intracellular environment, ferritin and hemosiderin serve to reduce its inherent toxicity. Iron in its ionic form in excess of the TIBC of the blood is extremely and instantaneously toxic, as demonstrated by Gitlow and Beyers (1952). Slow intravenous injection of only 10 mg ferric ammonium citrate totally saturated the blood's iron-binding capacity of all patients tested, and the excess randomly diffused into all body tissues. The toxic response was manifested by coughing, sneezing, nausea, and, occasionally, vomiting.

However, the human body tenaciously conserves its content of iron, losing less than 0.01% of the total amount daily through excretory and other mechanisms (see Figure 14.2). Iron loss from the body consists of routine excretion (in urine, bile, feces, sweat), periodic loss (desquammation of cells and menstrual flow [in women]), and occasional loss (hemorrhage secondary to trauma or disease). Iron excretion is essentially passive and increases only very slowly with increases in body stores of iron.

14.2.6 Iron Overload

Considering the precisely regulated intestinal absorption of iron coupled with limited physiological excretory capabilities, one can easily envision the development of an iron overload state if iron, by pathological or iatrogenic route, gained access to the endogenous system. For example, excessive

---

* Titanium-containing hemosiderin-like complexes are seen adjacent to titanium alloy implants, further suggesting that hemosiderin is a nonspecific precipitate.

absorption of iron occurs in idiopathic hemochromatosis, a situation in which iron is continually deposited in the parenchymal cells of various organs, often resulting in arthritis, liver disease, cardiac failure, and diabetes. Excessive intake of iron may lead to hepatic and reticuloendothelial involvement manifesting as portal cirrhosis. This is demonstrated by the Bantu tribesmen of Africa, who have traditionally consumed large quantities of food cooked and stored in iron pots. Additionally, a few reported instances of parenteral iron administration to treat misdiagnosed anemias have resulted in iatrogenic iron overload states with consequent toxic signs indistinguishable from those of hemochromatosis.

Therefore, evidence indicates that excessive amounts of intracellular iron stemming from an iron overload condition may predispose to a variety of liver disorders (Bacon 1998), primarily by causing progressive destruction of parenchymal cells and subsequent fibrotic replacement. The positive relationship of cardiomyopathies and diabetes mellitus in iron overload to the deposition of hemosiderin in the myocardium and the pancreas further substantiates the toxicity of iron even in its bound storage form (Sullivan 2004). In an iron overload state, the serum iron and transferrin saturation are usually increased and the TIBC is somewhat depressed (Figure 14.3).

14.2.7   Iron and Susceptibility to Infectious Disease

For nearly half a century, it has been recognized that an element of host response to bacterial invasion is a reduction in the iron content of the blood serum (reduction in SI; see Figure 14.2) (Weinberg 1974; Ward et al. 1996). The mechanism of this reduction has been identified as a suppression of intestinal absorption of iron concurrent with an increase in storage of iron in the liver and a concomitant reduction in transferrin saturation. The net effect is that growth-essential iron is made less available to microbial invaders, thus producing a so-called "nutritional immunity" (Kochan 1973) for the host.

To illustrate the strength of this argument, patients with infection and inflammation are unable to mobilize iron from reticuloendothelial cell depots irrespective of a normal total body iron content (Shils et al. 1993) and thus experience a transient anemia. This suggests that the physiological system would rather endure a short period of iron deficiency than risk a microbial invasion. In a survey of pathogen–host metal interrelationships, Weinberg (1971) concluded that "…in the contest between the establishment of a bacterial or mycotic disease and the successful suppression of the disease by animal hosts, iron is the metal whose concentration in host fluids appears to be most important."

To acquire iron, microbial cells must often synthesize siderophores, phenolates, or hydroxamates, whose function is to solubilize ferric iron at neutral pH and assimilate the metal. In the presence of small iron-containing metallic particles, such as wear debris from stainless-steel implants up to 10 to 15 µm in major dimension, macrophages may assist this process by attempts to digest or dissolve iron and iron hydroxide. In addition, many microorganisms have the potential to produce powerful iron-binding ligands that compete with the host compounds, e.g., transferrin, for the available iron. Organisms that have the ability to solubilize, assimilate, and bind iron independently are termed autosequesteric.

Because most bacteria and fungi require only 0.3 to 4.0 µM concentrations of iron for growth, human blood plasma with a concentration of 10 to 65 µM would appear suitable to support bacterial growth and multiplication, leading to bacteremia. That bacteremias are the exception rather than the rule illustrates the profound role plasma transferrin plays in resistance to disease by production of "nutritional immunity." Transferrin has an association constant for iron of approximately 10^{30}. This indicates that, in the normal physiological situation in which transferrin is 25% saturated with iron, the equilibrium free, ionic iron concentration is approximately 6×10^{-9} µM or 10^8–fold less than that required for microbial growth. Thus, for microbial invaders to have any chance of survival in a foreign host, they must have evolved the capability to synthesize siderophores with association constants for iron of 10^{30} or greater in order to compete for the available iron.

Indeed, many bacterial invaders have iron-binding ligands capable of extracting iron from host transferrin that is saturated 30% or more. Kochan (1973) has demonstrated the microbiostatic action of various mammalian serums in culture media with respect to bacterial growth of tubercle bacilli (Table 14.1). For example, human serum containing 30% saturated transferrin inhibited bacterial multiplication of the BGG strain of *Mycobacterium tuberculosis*. Addition of 36 µM iron neutralized this bacteriostatic activity.

Similar results were observed for bovine, mouse, and rabbit sera. However, owing to their normally high transferrin saturation, guinea pigs had sera equally susceptible to tuberculosis before and after iron addition. Other microorganisms demonstrating similar behavior include species of Candida,

TABLE 14.1

Correlation of Transferrin Saturation (TR) with Bacterial Growth[a] in Mammalian Sera *in Vitro*

Source of Sera	No. Samples	Fe Concentration in Serum (µm)	Saturation TR (%)	Bacterial Growth[a] No Added Fe	Bacterial Growth[a] 36 µm Added Fe
Human	10	17	30.0	0–1	10–14
Cow	4	34	39.0	0–1	10–14
Mouse	10	41	60.2	1–5	9–15
Rabbit	8	36	64.3	1–5	10–15
Guinea pig	20	49	84.2	9–14	9–14

[a] Bacterial growth expressed as the number of generations of *M. tuberculosis* in 14 days.

Source: Adapted from Kochan, I., *Curr. Top. Microbiol. Immunol.*, 60, 1, 1973.

Clostridium, Escherichia, Pasteurella, Shigella, and Staphylococcus. *In vivo* studies using strains of *Pseudomonas aeruginosa*, *Staphylococcus typhimurium*, *Listeria monocytogenes*, and *E. coli* have corroborated the *in vitro* results.

Weinberg (1974) summarized the role that iron plays in nutritional immunity:

> A very consistent finding is that the intricate checks and balances be-
> tween the iron chelators of the microbes and of hosts are readily and
> markedly upset by changes in the environmental concentration of iron.
> If the metal is added, microbial growth is enhanced; if the metal is
> deleted, host defense is strengthened. This situation obtains not only in
> experimental systems *in vitro* and *in vivo*, but also in clinical disease
> situations.

Weinberg (1974) asks, "Might cryptic disturbances in iron metabolism during the lifetime of individual hosts permit resurgence of latent infections such as tubercular lesions?" In light of a report concerning tuberculosis in dialysis patients (Pradhan et al. 1974), perhaps this question has been unknowingly addressed. Pradhan and colleagues have attributed the 15 times higher incidence of tuberculosis in dialysis patients to an increased susceptibility stemming from the uremic state and a consequently decreased immunological responsiveness. These conditions notwithstanding, it may be possible that sufficient iron (owing to the inherent iron concentration of the dialysate) enters the blood stream during repeated dialysis and constitutes a "cryptic disturbance," thus rendering the patient more susceptible to tubercular infection and/or relapse. Weinberg (1996) and Walter et al. (1997) provide modern reviews of this topic.

14.2.8   Role of Implants in TIBC Saturation

As mentioned previously, Gitlow and Beyers (1952) have shown that 10 mg of intravenous ferric-ammonium citrate was sufficient to saturate the TIBC of the blood and produce immediate signs of toxicity. Weinberg (1974) has expressed the belief that even small additions of iron may increase the transferrin saturation of the blood, rendering an individual more susceptible to infection. The use of stainless steel in joint replacement and fracture fixation applications, coupled with the evidence of Lux and Zeisler (1974) demonstrating the nature and relative proportions of corrosion products in metallotic tissue, would seem at this junction to warrant investigation of the possibility that the well recognized (and accepted) local corrosion may eventually elicit subtle long-term systemic consequences.

A single calculation can illustrate the minute quantities of iron involved in these considerations and, similarly, the amount of corrosion that these quantities represent. For a standard 316L stainless steel orthopaedic total hip replacement prosthesis with a total surface area of approximately 200 cm^2, corrosion equivalent to 10 mg of iron release would constitute a general surface dissolution to a depth of 625 Å — an amount beyond light microscopic resolution. In terms of local corrosion, a pit of 1 mm depth would release 10 mg of iron. Naturally, for bilateral hip implantation or for devices with a porous sintered stainless-steel surface, the increased surface area would mean that proportionately less iron would need to corrode per unit area for equivalent effects. As suggested in Figure 14.2, the most likely mode of release is into the transferrin transport system.

It is clear, however, that such corrosion would not be equivalent to the clinical experiment of Gitlow and Beyers (1952). Corrosion would release iron over a period of time rather than in a single "dose." Furthermore, other implant-derived metals such as chromium and aluminum can also bind to transferrin, further reducing the UIBC and contributing to a higher apparent transferrin saturation (TR).

14.3 Chromium Metabolism*

14.3.1 Introduction

Chromium differs from iron by only two atomic numbers (24 vs. 26) and by less than 7% in average atomic weight. Both elements can form divalent and trivalent ions, although chromium can additionally form a hexavalent ion. However, there are profound differences in their biological roles. Iron is well known for its primary role in hemoglobin, the primary oxygen transport molecule in mammals; chromium plays a no less vital role in regulating metabolism. These differences in biological roles and metabolic pathways are an excellent example of the principle of specificity in essential trace element function. Figure 14.4 compares and contrasts these roles and also illustrates the principle of amplification of function: extremely small daily intakes of each element have led to vital physiological roles in the whole organism.

It would be desirable to be able to depict a complete and systemic overview of chromium uptake, transportation, utilization and conservation, storage, and excretion, as shown in Figure 14.2 for iron; however, this is not possible. Based in part on estimates, Table 14.2 summarizes the overall picture of the situation.

14.3.2 Absorption

Absorption of Cr^{+3} takes place in the gastrointestinal tract. Although the diet may contain Cr^{+2} and Cr^{+6} as well as Cr^{+3}, the latter valence is the predominant form in the acidic conditions of the stomach and upper digestive tract (Mertz 1983). Because Cr^{+3} is essentially excluded from cellular contents due

---

* This section draws strongly on the work of Langård and Norseth (1986).

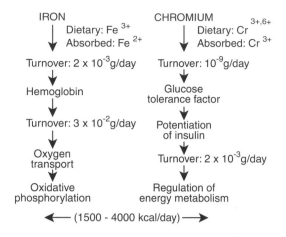

FIGURE 14.4

Comparison of iron and chromium amplification. (Adapted from Mertz, W., *Science*, 213, 1332, 1981.)

TABLE 14.2

Chromium Metabolism

Daily intake	
Dietary supply[a]	200 µg
Absorbed (@1.5% absorbance)[b]	3 µg
Transport	
Serum content (3.2 L @ 0.16 ppb[c])	0.5 mg
Daily utilization	Unknown, leads to 2 mg insulin synthesis/day[d]
Storage	
Daily addition	1 µg
Total body burden (70-kg individual)	7 mg
Daily excretion	
Urinary (1.5 l @ 0.2 ppb[e])	0.3 µg
Fecal, desquammation, etc. (balance)	~ 1.7 µg

[a] *Source*: Table 14.3, maximum recommended.
[b] *Source*: Table 14.3, mean value.
[c] *Source*: Versieck, J. and Cornelis, R., *Anal. Chim. Acta*, 116, 217, 1980.
[d] *Source*: Mertz, W., *Science*, 213, 1332, 1981.
[e] *Source*: Cornelis, R. and Wallaeys, B., in *Trace Element — Analytical Chemistry in Medicine and Biology*, Vol. 3., Walter de Gruyter & Co., Berlin, 1984, 219.

to an inability to cross cellular membranes (Sanderson 1976), it is very poorly absorbed. However, chromium can be found within cells in nonimplanted individuals, suggesting that mechanisms exist *in vivo* to oxidize dietary Cr^{+3} to Cr^{+6} (Rogers 1984). Detection of chromium in nonparticulate form, especially in nonphagocytic cells such as erythrocytes, must be considered as strong evidence of the presence of Cr^{+6}.

Although daily absorption of chromium is very small compared to that of iron (3 μg vs. 1 to 2 mg), the serum concentration is even lower (5 μg [0.16 ppb] vs. 3 mg [0.94 ppm]). As in the case of iron, serum chromium is primarily bound to transferrin (Hertel 1986), although it can also be nonspecifically bound to albumin. The turnover of biosynthetic chromium as an element in a glucose tolerance factor (GTF) leads to the synthesis of insulin and to the ability to metabolize carbohydrates (Schroeder 1966).

14.3.3   Storage and Excretion

About one third of the daily absorption (perhaps that portion reduced to Cr^{+6}) is stored in the reticuloendothelial structures in cells and nonspecifically in other cells, such as erythrocytes. The balance is excreted, primarily fecally and through desquammation of cells. In comparing chromium metabolism to iron metabolism, the overall picture is one of radical differences, despite the similarity of the elements, even in the absence of implants. This should highlight the difficulties in understanding release, storage, and excretion of metals from implants in which less knowledge of the metabolic pathways is involved.

14.3.4   Biological Consequences of Excess Chromium

As indicated elsewhere in this work, chromium has historically been viewed benignly, due to its essential role in sugar metabolism and the widely held belief that the dietary form, Cr^{+3}, was the only or predominant form encountered *in vivo*, no matter what the route of release. More recent views suggest roles for chromium and chromium-bearing molecules in a wide variety of toxic, carcinogenic, and allergenic effects. The latter two phenomena are discussed in Chapter 13 and Chapter 12, respectively; see Dayan and Paine (2001) for a comprehensive historical review of all three effects.

14.4   Human Dietary Metal Intake

The only significant source of essential trace elements, including metals, for human metabolic processes is through the gastrointestinal tract. Transdermal absorption and inhalation, although capable of causing local host responses, rarely can be shown to contribute to internal metal concentrations or remote storage. Primarily, humans depend upon dietary sources for essential trace elements. Table 14.3 lists the recommended dietary allowances (RDAs) and suggested safe and adequate intakes (SAIs) for two physiological and ten essential trace elements, as determined by the U.S. National Research

TABLE 14.3

Daily Recommended and Safe Mineral Intake

Mineral	Dietary Content	Absorbed (%)	Internal[c]
Recommended dietary allowances (RDA)[a,b]			
Phosphorus	800 mg	50–70	400–560 mg
Calcium	800 mg	20–40	160–320 mg
Magnesium	315 mg	40–60	125–190 mg
Zinc	14.5 mg	2–38	0.3–5.1 mg
Iron	10 mg	Heme: 20[d]	
		Nonheme: 6–18	0.5–1.0 mg
Iodine	150 μg	30–50	45–75 μg
Selenium	62.5 μg	80	50 μg
Safe and adequate intake (SAI)[a]			
Fluorine	1.5–4.0 mg	35–100	0.5–4.0 mg
Manganese	2.0–5.0 mg	?	<5.0 mg
Copper	1.5–3.0 mg	36	0.5–1.1 mg
Molybdenum	75–250 μg	?	<250 μg
Chromium	50–200 μg	0.5–2[e]	0.25–1.0 μg

[a] *Source*: National Research Council, *Recommended Dietary Allowances*, 11th ed., National Academy Press, Washington, D.C., 1992.

[b] Adjusted for average of male (79 kg) and female (63 kg), 25 to 50 years old.

[c] Calculated; presumably equal to loss by all routes.

[d] Decreases with increasing nonheme iron in meal.

[e] Decreases with increasing daily chromium intake.

Council.* Note that, because of its strong action in preventing tooth decay, fluorine is included, although its natural concentration in the body is very low and despite the absence of a known normal biological role in mammals. This table also lists ranges of percent absorption and resulting internal availability. It is against this latter amount that release by an implant should be judged.

Three final points deserve to be made to complete this discussion of normal mineral metabolism. In the first place, even in the absence of the routine common consumption of the "one-a-day" type of vitamin and mineral supplements (which usually contain 50 to 150% of the RDA or SAI of all essential trace elements), modern diets in the developed nations generally provide all essential minerals required for normal physiological functions in healthy individuals. The widespread "enrichment" of foodstuffs such as milk, bread, and breakfast cereals; the increasing amounts of fresh foods consumed; and

---

* The roles of trace metallic elements in human nutrition are coming under much more scrutiny than in previous years. Perhaps this is a partial explanation for a more recent replacement of RDAs and SAIs with the concept of daily adequate intake (DAI) (Vincent 2004).

modern food-preservation and -preparation techniques virtually guarantee this result.* Furthermore, the homeostatic systems that control metal absorption, transport, storage, and excretion render the occasional practice of consuming "megadoses" of essential trace elements meaningless: in the general case, the excess will not be absorbed and will simply be excreted directly. For some easily absorbed minerals, excess consumption may lead to transient toxicity. If defects in regulation exist, excessive intakes may lead to one or another of various metal storage diseases (Underwood 1977; Mertz 1988). Fortunately, these are rare and, in many cases, have familial, presumably genetic, predispositions.

In the second place, it must be emphasized that concern about *in vivo* metal released from implants centers primarily on two situations:

- The possibility of very elevated (10- to 100-fold normal) concentrations occurring near implants or in remote storage sites
- The possibility of release of metal in a different valence state than normally occurs in the body with subsequent formation of biologically active organometallic species

As will be discussed at further length in Chapter 15, measurements of serum concentrations and urinary excretion of metals, although useful, do not provide a true picture of either of these effects. Unfortunately, with the advent of modern, highly sensitive techniques for determining metal content of biological materials (atomic absorption spectroscopy, neutron activation analysis, inductively coupled plasma-mass spectroscopy, etc.), a number of commercial concerns have become involved in diagnostic studies of trace element profiles in patients and in normal individuals. Homeostasis permits a broad range of concentrations about the optimal concentration for any essential trace element (see Figure 14.1); thus, in the absence of a metallic implant, which could produce elevated concentrations and/or different valence states, small changes in serum metal concentrations within a normal range may only reflect daily variations in intake, utilization, etc.

It is highly unlikely that such studies can lead to primary diagnosis of actual metal deficiencies or overloads, with a concomitant need for corrective therapy, that have not already been detected by clinical indications (Kruse–Jarres 1987). Thus, the validity of such studies in healthy individuals or in nonimplant patients for other than verification of prior diagnoses must be viewed with great skepticism. In current practice, the appropriate use of such studies is for large-scale, prospective epidemiology to determine whether relationships exist between group mean values and incidence or severity of metal induction or storage diseases.

---

* One exception to this assertion may be chromium; increasing dietary use of refined (white) sugar, which contains less chromium than raw sugars but requires insulin for metabolic conversion (Mertz 1983), may lead to progressive chromium deficiency. See Baran (2004) for a more complete discussion.

Finally, because implants can release metal in various forms, including inorganic ions, organometallic soluble complexes, and fine particles, primarily or secondarily by precipitation (Jacobs et al. 1995), the mere presence of metal in a biological fluid or tissue cannot be placed in context without an understanding of the bioavailability of that metal. That is, the discussion of the role of bacterial access to iron (Section 14.2.8) can and should be generalized to address the question of which cells encounter metals in their pericellular environment and whether the form permits chemical and biochemical interaction with extra- or intracellular process. Unfortunately, traditional approaches to the issue of bioavailabilty (see Caussy et al. 2003) neglect release from implants. Thus, the question raised by MacDonald (2003) as to whether a safe level of metal ions is released from a particular class of orthopaedic implants simply cannot be answered at this time.

Notwithstanding these caveats, the next chapter will take up in detail more general issues of release, distribution, and excretion of ions from implants for which some data and models exist.

References

Bacon, B.R., Metabolic liver disease. Iron overload states, *Clin. Liver Dis.*, 2(1), 63, 1998.

Baran, E.J., Trace elements supplementation: recent advances and perspectives, *Mini Rev. Med. Chem.*, 4(1), 1, 2004.

Caussy, D. et al., Lessons from case studies of metals: investigating exposure, bioavailability, and risk, *Ecotox. Environ. Safety*, 56, 45, 2003.

Dayan, A.D. and Paine, A.J., Mechanisms of chromium toxicity, carcinogenicity, and allergenicity: review of the literature from 1985 to 2000, *Hum. Exp. Toxic.*, 20, 439, 2001.

Fairbanks, V.F. and Beutler, E., Iron, in *Modern Nutrition in Health and Disease*, 7th ed., Shils, M.E. and Young, V.R. (Eds.), Lea & Febiger, Philadelphia, 1988, 193.

Gitlow, S.E. and Beyers, M.R., Metabolism of iron, *J. Lab. Clin. Med.*, 39, 337, 1952.

Hertel, R.F., Sources of exposure and biological effects of chromium, in *Environmental Carcinogens: Selected Methods of Analysis*, Vol. 8, O'Neill, I.K., Schuller, P. and Fishbein, L. (Eds.), IARC Scientific Publication 71. International Agency for Research on Cancer, Lyon, 1986, 63.

Jacobs, J.J. et al., Local and distant products of modularity, *Clin. Orthop. Rel. Res.*, 319, 94, 1995.

Kochan, I., The role of iron in bacterial infections with special consideration of host-tubercle bacillis interaction, *Curr. Top. Microbiol. Immunol.*, 60, 1, 1973.

Kruse–Jarres, J.D., Clinical indications for trace element analysis, *J. Trace Elem. Electrolytes Health Dis.*, 1, 5, 1987.

Langård, S. and Norseth, T., Chromium, in *Handbook on the Toxicology of Metals*, 2nd ed. Vol. II: *Specific Metals*, Friberg, L., Nordberg, G.F. and Vouk, V.B. (Eds.), Elsevier, Amsterdam, 1986, 185.

Lux, F. and Zeisler, R., Investigations of the corrosive deposition of components of metal implants and the behavior of biological trace elements in metallosis tissue by means of instrumental multielement activation analysis, *J. Radioanal. Chem.*, 19, 289, 1974.

MacDonald, S.J., Can a safe level for metal ions in patients with metal-on-metal total hip arthroplasties be determined? *J. Arthropol.*, Suppl. 3, 19(8), 71, 2004.

Mertz, W., The essential trace elements, *Science*, 213, 1332, 1981.

Mertz, W., Chromium: an ultra-trace element, *Chemica Scripta*, 21, 145, 1983.

Mertz, W. (Ed.), *Trace Elements in Human and Animal Nutrition*, 5th ed. Academic Press, New York, 1988.

National Research Council, *Recommended Dietary Allowances*, 11th ed., National Academy Press, Washington, D.C., 1992.

Pradhan, R.P. et al., Tuberculosis in dialyzed patients, *JAMA*, 229, 798, 1974.

Rogers, G.T., *In vivo* production of hexavalent chromium, *Biomaterials*, 5, 244, 1984.

Sanderson, C.J., The uptake and retention of chromium by cells, *Transplantation*, 21, 526, 1976.

Schroeder, H.A., Chromium deficiency in rats: a syndrome simulating diabetes mellitus and retarding growth, *J. Nutrition*, 88, 439, 1966.

Schwarz, K., Essentiality vs. toxicity of metals, in *Clinical Chemistry and Chemical Toxicology of Metals*, Brown, S.S. (Ed.), Elsevier/North–Holland, Amsterdam, 1977, 3.

Shils, M.E., Olson, J.A. and Moshe, S. (Eds.), *Modern Nutrition in Health and Disease*, 8th ed., Lea & Febiger, Philadelphia, 1993.

Sullivan, J.L., Is stored iron safe? *J. Lab. Clin. Med.*, 144(6), 280, 2004.

Underwood, E.J., *Trace Elements in Human and Animal Nutrition*, 4th ed., Academic Press, New York, 1977.

Vincent, J.B., Recent developments in the biochemistry of chromium (III), *Biolog. Trace Elem. Res.*, 99, 1, 2004.

Walter, T. et al., Iron, anemia, and infection, *Nutr. Rev.*, 55(4), 111, 1997.

Ward, C.G., Bullen, J.J. and Rogers, H.J., Iron and infection: new developments and their implications, *J. Trauma*, 41(2), 356, 1996.

Weinberg, E.D., Roles of iron in host–parasite interactions, *J. Infect. Dis.*, 124, 401, 1971.

Weinberg, E.D., Iron and susceptibility to infectious disease, *Science*, 184, 952, 1974.

Weinberg, E.D. Iron withholding: a defense against viral infections, *Biometals*, 9(4), 393, 1996.

Winter, G.D., Wear and corrosion products in tissues and the reactions they provoke, in *Biocompatibility of Implant Materials*, Williams, D. (Ed.), Sector Publications, London, 1976, 28.

Bibliography

Brown, S.S. and Savory, J. (Eds.), *Clinical Chemistry and Chemical Toxicology of Metals*, Academic Press, Amsterdam, 1984.

Burrows, D., *Chromium: Metabolism and Toxicity*, CRC Press, Boca Raton, FL, 1983.

Cohen, M.D. et al., Mechanisms of chromium carcinogenicity and toxicity, *Crit. Rev. Toxicol.*, 23(3), 255, 1993.

Cornelis, R. and Wallaeys, B., Chromium revisited, in *Trace Element — Analytical Chemistry in Medicine and Biology*, Vol. 3., Walter de Gruyter & Co., Berlin, 1984, 219.

Crichton, R.R. and Ward, R.J., Iron homeostasis, *Met. Ions Biol. Syst.*, 35, 633, 1998.

Davies, I.J.T., *The Clinical Significance of the Essential Biological Metals*, Charles C Thomas, London, 1972.

Ducros, V., Chromium metabolism. A literature review, *Biol. Trace Elem. Res.*, 32, 65, 1992.

Friberg, L., Nordberg, G.F. and Vouk, V.B. (Eds.), *Handbook on the Toxicology of Metals*, 2nd ed. Vol. I: *General Aspects*. Vol. II: *Specific Metals*. Elsevier, Amsterdam, 1986.

Gibson, R.S., Essential trace elements and their nutritional importance in the 1990s, *J. Can. Diet. Assoc.*, 51, 292, 1990.

Goldenberg, H.A., Regulation of mammalian iron metabolism: current state and need for further knowledge, *Crit. Rev. Clin. Lab. Sci.*, 34(6), 529, 1997.

Mertz, W., Chromium in human nutrition: a review, *J. Nutr.*, 123(4), 626, 1993.

Mu, Y. et al., Causes of titanium release from plate and screws implanted in rabbits, *J. Mater. Sci.: Mater. Med.*, 13, 583, 2002.

Okazaki, Y. et al., Comparison of metal concentrations in rat tibia tissues with various metallic implants, *Biomaterials*, 25, 5913, 2004.

Schroeder, H.A., *The Trace Elements and Man: Some Positive and Negative Aspects*, Devin–Adair, Old Greenwich, CT, 1973.

da Silva, J.R.R.F. and Williams, R.J.P., *The Biological Chemistry of the Elements*, 2nd ed., Oxford University Press, Oxford, 2001.

Theil, E.C., Iron, ferritin, and nutrition, *Annu. Rev. Nutr.*, 24, 327, 2004.

Versieck, J. and Cornelis, R., Normal levels of trace elements in human blood plasma or serum, *Anal. Chim. Acta*, 116, 217, 1980.

Von Schroeder, H.P. et al., Titanemia from total knee arthroplasty, *J. Arthropol.*, 11, 620, 1996.

Wang, Y.T. and Shen, H., Bacterial reduction of hexavalent chromium, *J. Ind. Microbiol.*, 14(2), 159, 1995.

Williams, D.R., *The Metals of Life: The Solution Chemistry of Metal Ions in Biological Systems*, Van Nostrand Reinhold, London, 1971.

Xiu, Y.M., Trace elements in health and diseases, *Biomed. Environ. Sci.*, 9(2–3), 130, 1996.

Zaffe, D. et al., Accumulation of aluminium in lamellar bone after implantation of titanium plates, Ti-6Al-4V screws, hydroxyapatite granules, *Biomaterials*, 25, 3837, 2004.

15

Systemic Distribution and Excretion

15.1 Introduction

The traditional approach to consideration of biological performance has been to focus on the implant–host interface. Thus, material response studies have dealt with degradation of implant properties and host response studies have focused on formation of a capsule and other events within the adjacent tissue. More modern considerations recognize that a mammal, such as a test animal or a human patient, is an interconnected structure with various mechanisms permitting exchange between all of its tissues and organs. The systemic and remote site results of such exchanges involving implants and implant degradation products will be dealt with in Chapter 16.

Chapter 3 through Chapter 5 and Chapter 7 have considered mechanisms that can modify native proteins or release materials from implants. This chapter examines some aspects of the distribution and excretion of these implant-related products. Their distribution through the various systems of the body can take place in a number of different ways:

- Movement of solid bodies
- Movement of particulate materials, passively or actively (cell mediated)
- Movement of dissolution or corrosion products by passive diffusion or by active circulatory transport
- Movement of modified cells or native proteins

15.2 Movement of Solid Bodies

15.2.1 Large Particles

Large particles or portions of implants can move through soft tissue if they possess a certain degree of structural asymmetry. A sphere, such as a shotgun* pellet, will stay in its initial position for an indefinite time. An asymmetric "needle," such as a sewing needle or a porcupine quill, will move point first and may travel for long distances due to the action of muscle forces on it.

It is also possible for large material particles to become involved in blood circulation. Wear particles from vascular prostheses will move "downstream" until they are trapped in reduced vessel diameters on the arterial side of capillary beds or in the lungs on the venous side of the circulatory path. Much larger particles can also be transported. A report of four cases of shell fragments transported into the cerebral circulation is a dramatic illustration of this possibility (Kapp et al. 1973).

More common is the finding of extracellular particles too large to be phagocytosed, such as some wear debris, precipitated corrosion products, or fibrillar fragments from tendon prostheses, in the lymphatic drainage, in regional lymph nodes, or in remote medullary locations or organs. Such observations have been made in animals (Margevicius et al. 1996) as well as in patients (Case et al. 1994; Jacobs et al. 1995; Urban et al. 2004) with functioning implants of various types. Note that all "foreign" particles found in remote sites in patients with implants may not have been released from implants (Gatti and Rivasi 2002), so care should be taken in their identification and analysis.

Pins, wires, and other implants used for internal fixation of fractures and for adjunctive tissue immobilization during placement of permanent implants can also become dislodged and migrate. Lyons and Rockwood (1990) reviewed reports of 47 such occurrences after surgery in the vicinity of the shoulder. Smooth pins and wires were more likely to be reported as migrating than threaded ones; screws and staples were not reported as migrating. Eight of the patients died (six of them suddenly) due to damage to heart and blood vessels near the heart by the migrating implants. In a majority of the reports (35 of 39) in which a postoperative time course could be determined, migration apparently occurred within 8 months of implantation, although the mean time to diagnosis was 22 months.

Migrating device fragments are no respecter of organs; they have been reported to enter the lungs (Aalders et al. 1985) and the heart (Lyons and Rockwood, 1990) and to move as far as from the shoulder to the spleen (Potter et al. 1988). Therefore, thoughtful design of materials and the implants using them should minimize or eliminate the possibility of release of macroscopic fragments.

---

* It was once a reasonable assumption that such pellets were composed primarily of lead; however, since 1981 lead shot has been illegal for use by hunters over wetlands in the U.S. Thus, pellets that have been *in situ* for less than 25 years may be copper- or nickel-coated lead or made of copper-coated steel, tungsten, or bismuth. This should be taken into account when host response is considered.

15.2.2 Phagocytic Transport

As Section 8.2.3 discussed, particles that are sufficiently small are phagocytosed by a variety of cells. Cellular phagocytosis has four possible results:

- The phagocytic cell (PC)* can successfully digest the particle. Partial digestion and externalization (exocytosis) of the particle may also occur, but rarely so.
- The PC attempts to digest the particle but the degradation products prove to be cytotoxic. Then the PC dies, its phagosomes and cell membrane lyse, and another PC may attempt to phagocytose the particle and digest it. If this progression continues through many repetitions, dead PCs accumulate, resulting in caseation; the resulting mass of dead cells resembles cheese.
- The PC may transport the particle by passing into the blood or lymphatic circulation, but most usually to regional lymph nodes where particle-loaded cells accumulate and may produce granulomas, such as the "teflonomas" reported by Charnley (1961) after the use of a poly(tetrafluoro)ethylene as a bearing surface in total hip replacement. In some cases, this may lead to a secondary histiocytic response in the vessels or lymph nodes (Albores–Saavedra et al. 1994).
- The PC may be able to transport the particle to the lungs. There it is possible for the particle to be extruded through the lung wall and exhaled through the airway (Styles and Wilson 1976).

It should additionally be noted that all of these outcomes may result in activation of the PC (Schnyder and Baggiolini 1978), with concomitant release of biologically active agents, which may alter local host response to the implant (see Section 8.2.3)

In the context of this chapter, it would be very desirable to make some statements about the rates of transport of particles by phagocytes in the third and fourth situations listed previously. It is probably not possible to generalize, but some extension of the comments in Section 8.2.3 is desirable.

The transport of particles by phagocytic cells (primarily macrophages because neutrophils are short lived and FBGCs tend to remain near the implant site) consists of at least two major steps: uptake and transport. Very little is known about transport rates in the lymphatic system, primarily because most uptake studies have been done *in vitro* or by systemic injection of a colloid of particles *in vivo* followed by sequential sampling of the PC population in the arteriovenous circulatory system.

---

* The term phagocytic cell (PC) is used here for generality, rather than the more common term phagocyte, because it now appears that a number of different cell types may display phagocytic behavior.

Some details are known about the first step, uptake. Two general approaches have been taken to describe the uptake process. The first is to fit the kinetics of phagocytic removal of particles to the Michaelis–Menten model used in studies of enzyme activity (Normann 1974). In this approach, uptake is considered to have two phases: attachment to the PC and engulfment.

Attachment is modeled as consisting of a reversible attachment step and an irreversible engulfment step:

$$P + PC \underset{k_2}{\overset{k_1}{\longleftrightarrow}} \underset{\text{attachment}}{\left[PC - P \right]} \xrightarrow[\text{engulfment}]{k_3} PCp \tag{15.1}$$

where P is an extracellular particle, and p is an intracellular one. Previous studies have shown that, for a wide variety of animal species, V, the velocity of clearance of circulating particles (uptake), follows a first-order proportional absorption law dependent upon particle concentration, C (Normann 1974):

$$V = \frac{dC}{dt} = -kC \tag{15.2}$$

The following equation is typical of the results of this approach:

$$\frac{1}{V} = \frac{1}{k_3 E_o} + \left[\frac{K_c}{k_3 E_o} \right] \frac{1}{[C]} \tag{15.3}$$

where
    V = clearance velocity (uptake rate of particles by PCs)
    C = concentration of extracellular particles
    E_o = total available attachment sites
    K_c = overall kinetic constant = $(k_2 + k_3/k_1)$

A saturation effect (presence of a fixed maximum rate) is attributed to the fact that the number of sites on the phagocyte membrane that can initiate invagination and engulfment (E_o) is limited.

This result faces two major criticisms. The first is that the uptake velocity is not a first-order process for all particle concentrations, and the second is that it seems unlikely that specific limited numbers of membrane loci exist.

The second approach (Stiffel et al. 1970) is to describe the observed kinetics as exponential in the general form given by Equation 15.4:

$$C = C_o 10^{-Kt} \tag{15.4}$$

where

K = total body phagocytic index (essentially, the particle clearance velocity)

C_o = initial particle concentration

t = time

The major difficulty with this result is that, once again, it is not a good description of the kinetics of phagocytic behavior. What is actually observed is a complex uptake velocity behavior with three domains, provided that the particles are within a defined size range and that the initial concentration is high enough so that the kinetics are not dictated by flow processes (Vernon–Roberts 1972). The initial phase seems to be first order and dictated by the adsorption of serum opsonins to the particles or the adsorption of the coated particles to the phagocyte. The second phase is exponential, dictated by the dose (concentration of particles) as in any other dose–response situation. The third phase is a slowly disappearing component seen when a heterogeneous distribution of particles is injected. What this "tail" actually represents is the removal of smaller particles.

The possible explanation for this strange kinetic pattern is that there are two opposing effects. One is a saturation effect attributed to a limited number of binding sites by some and, more appropriately, to a limited concentration of serum opsonins by others (Jenkin and Rowley 1961). The second, countervailing effect is the increased efficacy of clearance as the blood (or presumably tissue) concentration of particles goes down. The limit on the particle size range mentioned in Chapter 8 restricts these investigations to particles on the order of the size of leukocytes, approximately 4 to 7 μm.

A somewhat more pragmatic approach (Korn and Weisman 1967; Weisman and Korn 1967) has led to the conclusion that the kinetics of uptake are determined by a constant (absorption) vesicle volume. Careful studies with well controlled particle size ranges led to the conclusion that, in an amoeba model, although larger particles are taken up singly, small particles are accumulated external to the cell until a critical volume is reached, whereupon the "cemented" mass is absorbed simultaneously. Typical results obtained by earlier investigators in a mammalian model that also lead to this conclusion are given in Table 15.1. In this table, it is also useful to note that oxygen consumption is required during phagocytosis by PMNs (because the process requires energy and PMNs are aerobic cells) and that it increases with particle size.

There are however, additional difficulties. All particles are not equal: composition, morphology, and surface charge may play a role in uptake velocity. As discussed in Section 8.4.1, a variety of dissolved metal ions, such as Ni^{+2} and Cr^{+3}, suppress phagocytic efficiency (Graham et al. 1975). Therefore, one might expect a slower uptake of nickel- or chromium-bearing particles, due to high local metal concentrations, than of polymeric particles of the same size, tissue concentration, etc. Kawaguchi et al. (1986) have shown additionally that phagocytosis of polystyrene (as measured by cellular oxygen

TABLE 15.1

Effect of Particle Size on Phagocytosis by Guinea Pig PMNs

Diameter of Particles (μm)	Polystyrene Uptake (μg/mg wet wt. PMNs)	O$_2$ Consumption (μl/mg PMN/min)	No. Particles/PMN
0.088	7.4	0.0144	24,000
0.264	30.1	0.0372	3,600
0.557	28.1	0.0412	360
0.871	36.9	0.0396	102
1.305	34.3	0.0427	34
3.04	35.9	0.0422	3
>7	0	<0.012	0
No polystyrene	0	0.0124	0

Source: Adapted from Roberts, J. and Quastel, J.H., *Biochem. J.*, 89, 150, 1963.

consumption) depends strongly upon surface potential and thus upon fixed surface charge. Kapur et al. (1996) have also shown that surface charge heterogeneity can greatly affect phagocytic ability.

Although these models, calculations, and experiments tell something about the relatively likelihood of uptake (clearance velocity) as a function of particle size and properties, they shed little light upon the question of net removal rates from implant sites. This remains an area for further investigation. Far more is known about active and passive removal of dissolved species.

15.3 Transport of Dissolved Species

15.3.1 Leaching of Monomers

Leaching or dissolution of polymers into circulatory system fluids results in rapid dispersion throughout the body. This is a result of an arteriovenous circulatory rate of approximately 1 min^{-1}. That is, the normal blood volume (about 6 to 8% of body weight or about 5 l) passes through the lungs once a minute. An illustration of the rapidity of this circulation is the study of Homsy et al. (1972) concerning release of monomer from poly(methyl)methacrylate bone cement upon its insertion into the body. In a canine model, insertion of a dose of freshly mixed cement as a femoral transcortical plug in a dose of less than 2 g/kg body weight produced monomer levels of up to 1 mg/100 ml in the inferior vena cava within 2 min of implantation. The peak concentration was reached in 3 to 4 min, followed by a decline ascribed to monomer clearance by evaporation through the lungs as well as progression of polymerization of the cement that reduced the source concentration. Similar results were obtained in patients receiving PMMA-cemented femoral endoprostheses: peak monomer concentrations occurred in the vena cava by

2 minutes postimplantation and 99%+ of (integrated) exhaled monomer was detected in the airway within 6 min.

15.3.2 Corrosion of Metals

15.3.2.1 Local Effects

The corrosion of metals has been discussed in Chapter 4. It is appropriate to inquire how metallic corrosion and dissolution products are distributed in the body.

It is clear that, usually, an accumulation of corrosion products is found around a metal implant. These products include membrane-bound ions, particles released by intergranular and fatigue processes, locally precipitated products resembling hemosiderin, and insoluble reaction products such as metal hydroxides. The combination of these leads to the familiar tissue discoloration termed metallosis, particularly in older reports. In addition to tissue discoloration, consequences of passive diffusion and distribution adjacent to an implant may also be seen histologically as a varying degree of cell reaction. Figure 15.1 shows the variation of effect with material "reactivity" — that is, corrosion and/or dissolution rate combined with tissue response — for needles inserted in the cerebral cortex of rabbits for periods of up to 1 to 1.5 years. Typical materials used were aluminum; platinum (nonreactive); molybdenum; tantalum (reactive); and silver, iron, and cobalt (highly reactive and toxic).

The picture presented by Figure 15.1 reflects corrosion and diffusion of metal; however, it is complex and difficult to analyze because the breadth and type of response about each implant depend upon the rate of corrosion, the valence (speciation) of released metal, its diffusion constant, and its toxicity. Furthermore, the release may be affected by anatomical location

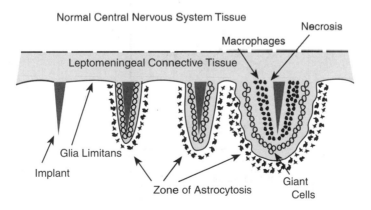

FIGURE 15.1
Histological changes around implants of increasing reactivity (left to right) in the rabbit cerebral cortex. (Adapted from Stensaas, S.S. and Stensaas, L.J., *Acta. Neuropath. (Berl.)*, 41, 145, 1978.)

because local physicochemical conditions vary (see Section 2.2), resulting in different rates of corrosion (Oron and Alter 1984). Implant site infection may also affect the corrosion rate (Hierholzer et al. 1984) as well as tissue response to the corrosion products.

A more accurate view of passive diffusion may be obtained by direct analysis of the tissues in and near the implant site. Energy-dispersive microanalysis has been widely used to study situations such as metal diffusion into bone from implanted dental devices (Arvidson and Wroblewski 1978). One of the more graphic studies is that of Lux and Zeisler (1974), who used neutron activation analysis to examine the spatial distribution of corrosion products in soft tissues adjacent to a steel fracture fixation device. Their results, obtained by analysis of tissues obtained at device retrieval, are shown in Figure 15.2.

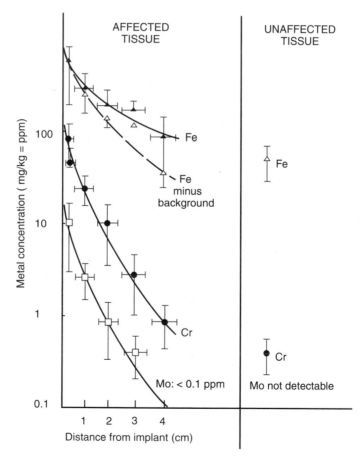

FIGURE 15.2

Tissue metal content surrounding an implant. (Adapted from Lux, F. and Zeisler, R., *J. Radioanal. Chem.*, 19, 289, 1974.)

In a study of 38 patients with histologically diagnosed metallosis at retrieval of fracture fixation hardware, Lux and Zeisler found mean concentrations of iron, chromium, and molybdenum near a stainless-steel–tissue interface to be two orders of magnitude above background values previously determined in tissues from patients without metallic implants. These concentrations declined logarithmically with distance from the implant, reaching background ("normal") levels at distances of greater than 4 cm from the implant. The ratio of Fe:Cr:Mo in the alloy (V4A) was 66:17.5:2.3 ($\cong$ 29:7.5:1) and typical tissue concentration ratios were 56.5:8:1 (at the tissue–implant interface) and 117:9:1 (1 cm away from the interface). Nickel, which formed 12% of the implant alloy, was detected at the interface but not in the surrounding tissue.

A number of conclusions may be drawn from these results:

- Ion concentrations (and persuadably leachate concentrations from polymeric materials) may be very high in the vicinity of implants when compared to systemic and remote site concentrations.

- The local accumulation of released products depends upon the nature of their reactions with surrounding tissues and their diffusion concentrations. In this example, nickel diffuses away rapidly and is seen only at the interface, chromium and molybdenum diffuse less rapidly, and iron is accumulated locally, presumably due to the formation of precipitates that contribute to the discoloration of metallosis.

- Tissue concentrations do not necessarily reflect alloy proportions. Finding metals near implants in their alloy constituent proportions is more evidence of wear debris accumulation than of burdening of tissues with soluble or precipitated corrosion products (Michel 1987).*

- Finally, it should be pointed out that the mere detection of metal in tissues does not reflect its biological availability. Metal may be present as free ions (unlikely), bound to specific carrier molecules (e.g., Fe–transferrin), nonspecifically bound (e.g., to albumin), in the form of a wear particle, or as a precipitate. Any of these forms may be extracellular or intracellular.

This pattern observed by Lux and Zeisler (1974) reflects the end stage of an equilibrium between the implant and the tissue. In a later study utilizing a rabbit implant model, Lux et al. (1976) reported a nonspecific decrease in

---

* One of the difficulties in understanding such results arises in distinguishing among corrosion products in solution, local precipitates, and insoluble particles, whether intra- or extracellular. If the local composition matches the composition of the implant, then the evidence is fairly reliable that the material is present in particulate form (as Michel, 1987, suggests), even if not resolvable by light microscopy. However, the reverse is not true because selective corrosion may change the apparent composition of small particles.

transport rate with time for all detectable corrosion products; this was ascribed to maturation of the fibrous capsule about the implant. Furthermore, they showed an inverse correlation between tissue iron and zinc content, even though zinc was not released by the implant. These findings underline the great complexity of consideration of release and distribution of implant degradation products, even in the near vicinity of the implant.

In a traditional sense, as would be observed in an *in vitro* corrosion study, equilibrium would nevertheless be reached when an equilibrium concentration of ions was reached in the surrounding fluid. However, *in vivo*, the bathing medium is dynamic, and a fractional excretion process is always in competition with corrosion processes as they approach equilibrium.

15.3.2.2   Distribution of Body Water

If maximum implant corrosion rates (as determined by formation of soluble species) can be measured, then equilibrium times should depend only upon the volume of the medium and the fractional excretion rates. The medium under discussion, water, has the relative volumes and distribution in the human body as shown in Figure 15.3.

If no input/output of fluid occurs, a volume of 42 l would be under consideration. Similarly, if no compartmental exchange took place, smaller volumes of fluid might be considered — as small as 3.2 l in the case of an implant bathed in blood. However, the situation is dynamic, as shown in Figure 15.4. In this figure, note that some water entering the gastrointestinal tract never exchanges directly with the internal water compartments but passes straight through as a portion of fecal excretion (dashed line to right of plasma pool). The 1.3 l/day excretion identified as "other" includes this volume as well as sweat (lost from the fast interstitial pool) and the water content of sloughed or desquammated cells (lost from the intracellular pool).

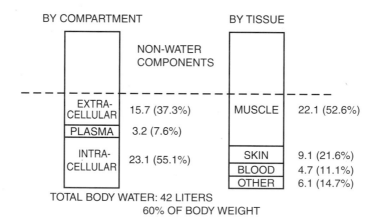

FIGURE 15.3
Water content of the human body (70 kg).

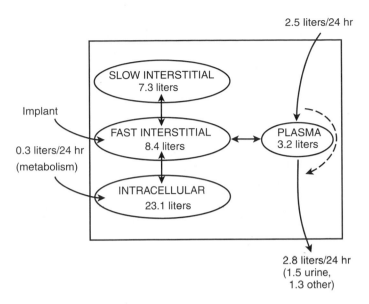

FIGURE 15.4
Daily water input/output/exchange for the human body (70 kg).

One can now see that volumes vary considerably depending upon the details of consideration. An implant placed in soft or hard tissue is directly in contact with a fast interstitial pool of 8.4 l, as shown. This contacts slower exchange pools of 7.3 l (interstitial) and 23.1 l (intracellular). It also contacts a fast exchange pool of 3.2 l (plasma water). This pool passes through the kidneys at a rate of 180 l/24 h and experiences a net throughput (intake = output) of 2.5 to 2.8 l/24 h. Thus, on an annual basis, an implant is in contact with a pool size exceeding 1000 l. The point of equilibrium of corrosion or leached products depends on the overall kinetics of release from the implant, exchange, and excretion. These kinetics are difficult to analyze. The previous chapter considered the details of one system, the iron system, in some depth.

15.4 Distribution and Excretion of Dissolved Species

15.4.1 Metallic Ion Distribution

However, some of the elements of these distribution systems can be studied in more detail. One factor to examine is urinary excretion, which is probably the major route for clearance from the body of metals released from implants, although biliary excretion may also play a role for some metals (Brauer 1959). Of the metals of interest as components of implants, only iron is known to be excreted (incorporated in porphyrins, which are degradation products of hemoglobin) predominantly through a biliary route (Ishihara and

Matsushiro 1986). Biliary excretion is mediated by concentration in and/or excretion by the liver of low molecular weight (<10,000) organometallic species known collectively as metallothioneins (Cherian and Goyer 1978; Klaassen 1976). These are released through the bile duct, stored in the gall bladder, and released as bile at a rate of 0.4 to 1.2 l/day into the jejunum. A significant proportion of the ionic content of bile, perhaps as much as 95%, is reabsorbed in the ileum, with only 200 mg/day excreted. Biliary excretion serves primarily to aid in digestion of fats and metal excretion appears to be a secondary role (Ganong 1989).

Urine, on the other hand, is formed primarily to regulate plasma composition and pH. It is formed in the mammalian kidney by a combination of three processes: glomerular filtration, tubular reabsorption, and tubular secretion. In the glomeruli, all formed cellular elements of blood and any molecules with a molecular weight above approximately 5000 are retained while all small molecules and a considerable amount of water are filtered into the proximal renal tubules. In a 70-kg person, between 115 and 125 ml/min of plasma are filtered. Normally nearly all of the water is also filtered out. If this were excreted, it would result in a 24-h urine volume of as much as 180 l.

This does not happen because over 99% of the water is reabsorbed in the proximal renal tubules, resulting in a nominal rate of urine production near 1 ml/min. In addition, other materials such as the physiological metal ions (Na^+, K^+, etc.), essential anions (Cl^-, OH^-, etc.) and organic molecules (glucose, urea, etc.) are reabsorbed. Some reabsorption processes are passive but others are active (energy requiring). As shown in the left portion of Figure 15.5, each active reabsorption process — for example, for glucose — has an asymptotic limit (different for each reabsorbed species) termed the tubular reabsorption limit (T_m). This has the effect of limiting and controlling the maximum concentration of that particular species in plasma.

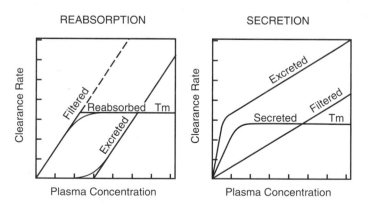

FIGURE 15.5

Renal reabsorption and secretion. (Adapted from Pitts, R.F., in *Physiology of the Kidney and Body Fluids, An Introductory Text,* Year Book Medical Pub. Inc., Chicago, 1963, 69, 116.)

TABLE 15.2

Urinary Secretion of Implant Alloy Components[a]

Element	Plasma Conc. (μg/l)	Urine Conc. (μg/l)	Permeability Ratio (K_x)	Excretion Ratio (E_x)
Al	2.2	6.4	2.9	0.040
Co	0.05	0.33	6.6	0.092
Cr	0.06	0.13	2.2	0.030
Ni	0.2	1.0	5.0	0.069
Ti	3.3	0.41	0.12	0.006
V	0.16	0.61	3.8	0.053
Reference: creatinine	10 mg/l	1.5 g/l	150	2.08

[a] These data differ considerably from those in the first edition due to significant improvements in collection and analysis techniques. However, it is widely believed that urine collection, especially from female subjects, is subject to contamination. Therefore, K_x and E_x may be too high; values should be considered in relative rather than absolute terms.

[b] Reconstructed, assuming 1.5 g creatinine/liter.

Sources: Al, Ti, V: Jacobs, J.J. et al., *J. Bone Joint Surg.*, 73A, 1475, 1991; Co, Cr, Ni[b]: Sunderman, F.W., Jr. et al., *J. Orthop. Res.*, 7, 307, 1989; creatinine: Ganong, W.F., in *Review of Medical Physiology*, 14th ed., Appleton & Lange, Norwalk, CT, 1989, 593.

Finally, materials may be removed from plasma by secretion through the walls of the distal renal tubules. This process may be passive or active; in the latter case (right portion of Figure 15.5), the effect is also to demonstrate a limit. Metals in plasma are bound specifically to transferrin or other carrier proteins (nickeloplasm, etc.) or nonspecifically to albumin, all of which have too high a molecular weight to be filtered in the glomeri. Therefore, urinary excretion of essential and trace metals must be primarily through a tubular secretion pathway.* Because this represents an interaction between post-glomerular plasma and distal tubule urine, it is instructive to look at the relative concentrations of metal in these fluids (Table 15.2).

The permeability ratio, K_x, is the ratio of concentration in urine to that in plasma. Values greater than 1 suggest positive secretion, values near 1 indicate simple equilibrium between urine and plasma, and values less than 1 suggest a barrier to secretion. The permeability ratio times the relative volumes of urine and plasma (= 0.78) is the proportion of normal plasma content secreted in 24 h. The *excretion ratio*,** E_x, based upon a 24-h urine volume of 2.5 l and a renal filtration of 180 l/24 h, reflects the efficiency of secretion or the proportion of the renal filtrate secreted in 24 h. The higher the value of E_x is, the greater is the probability of secretion of an ion in any one pass through the kidneys. The clearance rate, C_x, of a substance, x, is given by:

---

* However, some metal–protein dissociation may occur, leading to direct excretion; tubular reabsorption is also possible (Araki et al. 1986a).

** The term "excretion ratio" is used irrespective of renal mechanism involved.

$$C_x = K_x V \text{ (ml/min)} \tag{15.5}$$

where V = rate of urinary output.

Creatinine is a degradation product released by cell death and is widely used as a concentration marker for studying ionic concentration in urine. Urine may be more or less concentrated, depending on fluid intake, perspiration loss, etc., but the serum concentration and amount of urinary creatinine excretion in 24 h remains remarkably constant in normal individuals (Ganong 1989; Araki et al. 1986b).

15.4.2   Distribution Models: One Compartment

Projections of the equilibrium accumulations of metals in the body have been made using this type of data (Taylor 1973). Taylor proposed that, for a given rate of continuous release of corrosion products, R, per day, the increase in an organ or the total body content of a metal can be given as

$$Q_t = Q_o + \frac{R}{k}\left(1 - e^{-kt}\right) \tag{15.6}$$

where

Q_o = the normal metal content
Q_t = the content after "t" days
k = the fractional rate of excretion of the metal

That is, in a given day, R metal is released and kQ_t is excreted. Letting t go to infinity (when equilibrium is presumably achieved), one then finds that

$$Q_e = Q_o + \frac{R}{k} \tag{15.7}$$

where Q_e is the equilibrium metal content. Note that this is a first-order analysis that treats the body as a single homogeneous compartment. For a hypothetical cobalt–chromium implant (60% Co, 30% Cr, 8% Mo, 1% Ni, 1% Fe) with a surface area of 200 cm^2 and a corrosion rate of 30 mg/cm^2/day, Taylor obtains the results given in Table 15.3. Taylor concluded that modest elevations of cobalt and nickel and large elevations of chromium content should occur in this case. Similar calculations for implantation of stainless steel predict a modest elevation of nickel and a large increase in chromium content.

Taylor's calculations are probably in error on two fundamental grounds. Although admittedly using high corrosion rates, he does not point out that these rates are high by at least an order of magnitude. Second, the fractional excretion rates used are based upon urine/plasma concentration ratios and do not take into account exchange with slower compartments, particularly situations in which precipitated storage is possible, as in the liver. Reducing

TABLE 15.3

Secretion and Accumulation Rates of Alloy
Components of a Cobalt–Chromium Alloy

Element	Q_o (mg)	k (day⁻¹)	R (mg/day)	Q_e (mg)	Q_e/Q_o
Co	3	0.07	3.6	54	18
Cr	6	0.0011	1.8	1636	273
Mo	5	0.139	0.48	8	1.7
Fe	4000	0.0010	0.06	4060	1.02
Ni	10	0.0010	0.06	70	7

the corrosion rate by an order of magnitude and, continuing to use his
assumption, calculating fractional excretion rates based upon whole-body
content (Q_o) and urine concentrations (Sunderman et al. 1989) for Co, Cr,
and Ni yields the results given in Table 15.4. The very large Q_e/Q_o ratios for
Co and Cr suggest that concentrations of these elements would never come
to equilibrium but should be observed to increase steadily with time postimplantation. Such effects have been reported in animals (Woodman et al. 1983)
and humans (Michel et al. 1991) for long periods of time.

The fundamental error in all of these considerations is the idea that the
metals distribute freely and do not concentrate or bind preferentially in any
site. In perhaps the first attempt to study systemic distribution of metals
released from implants in animals, Ferguson and his coworkers (1962a, b)
observed the following patterns:

- A large regional variation of metal ion concentration can be found
  in normal rabbit and human tissue. Furthermore, different metals
  have different patterns. Thus, the nickel concentration is higher in
  the liver than in other tissues, and the molybdenum concentration
  is higher in liver and kidney than in lung or spleen.

- After implantation of metals, organ concentrations of ions rise. The
  spleen has a broad ability to retain metals; nickel and cobalt are
  preferentially retained by the kidney.

TABLE 15.4

Recalculation of Secretion and Accumulation Rates of Alloy
Components of Cobalt–Chromium Alloy of Table 15.3

Element	Q_o (mg)	Secretion (24 h, μg)	k (day⁻¹)	R (mg/day)	Q_e (mg)	Q_e/Q_o
Co	3	0.82	0.00027	0.36	1336	445
Cr	6	0.32	0.00005	0.18	3606	601
Ni	10	2.5	0.00025	0.006	34	3.4

Continuing studies of accumulation and distribution of corrosion products released by implants up to and including autopsy studies on patients with long-term implants (Michel et al. 1991) support these observations.

15.4.3 Distribution Models: Multicompartment

For technical and ethical reasons, it is extremely difficult to perform whole-body studies of metal metabolism in humans. However, a methodology has been developed that involves study of the distribution and excretion of a single dose of radioactive metal ions administered intravenously in animals. It is possible that this method may be applied selectively to humans in the future.

Although the technique was originally developed by Sunderman at the University of Connecticut, Greene et al. (1975) provide the best early report. An experimental animal, such as the rat or rabbit, is used as a model. A single intravenous injection of nickel as $^{63}NiCl_2$ is given at a dose of 0.24 mg/Ni/kg body weight. The animals are housed in metabolic cages so that urine and feces can be collected, and serum specimens are obtained periodically over a period of time.

For nickel in the rabbit, an expression for the concentration of nickel in serum takes the form of:

$$S(\mu g \,/\, liter) = A_1 e^{-a_1 t} + A_2 e^{-a_2 t} \qquad (15.8)$$

The first term is large, corresponding to an early rapid disappearance rate, and the second term is small, corresponding to a reduced disappearance rate from 3 to 7 days after injection. This can be interpreted in terms of a large, fast exchange compartment (the intercellular space) exchanging with a smaller, slower compartment of undetermined identity. The four constants assume different values for rats and rabbits.

Greene et al. (1975) made the following extrapolations:

> From what is known about nickel corrosion, one can estimate that in humans who have implants made of a nickel-containing alloy, the rate of nickel release from the device can range between 5 and 500 mg/year per individual. This corresponds to a range of 0.81 to 0.0081 µg/h per kg body weight on the basis of 70 kg for humans. The following table gives the estimated steady state values of nickel concentration in plasma resulting from three different input rates within that range.

Infusion Rate (µg/h per kg of Body Weight)	Steady State Ni Concentration (µg/l)	
	Rabbit	Rat
0.81	45	19.9
0.081	4.5	1.99
0.0081	0.45	0.20

These figures have to be compared with the normal range of nickel concentration in human plasma...2.6* ± 0.08 µg/l.

Taylor's calculations (Taylor 1973) for an alloy that released 22 mg per year predict a 7× increase (3.4× corrected calculation based upon his secretion data) in total body burden of nickel. Because Greene made no assumption on the partitioning of metallic ions between various compartments, the elevation that he predicts for plasma must be taken as the total body elevation. For a 2 mg per year release rate, Greene would predict a 1.76× increase (by rabbit data) or a 1.34× increase (by rat data). These are somewhat smaller than Taylor's original calculations (but near to the corrected calculations of Table 15.3); however, they lend credence to the idea that net concentrations of metal ions will rise in the presence of an endogenous source of ions, such as a corroding implant.

Sunderman's approach has a number of difficulties, including the partition question and the inability to identify internal compartments except by inference from calculations. This work has been extended and is reported by Onkelinx (1977). He has developed a more general multicompartment model, as shown in Figure 15.6. Here, V_1 represents the intracellular compartment, and V_2 and V_3 represent other compartments with net (reversible) interchange flow rates f_2 and f_3, respectively. Again, the assumption of a partition coefficient of 1 is made so that ion fluxes can be represented as fluid flow rates at constant concentration. Excretion is represented by a flow

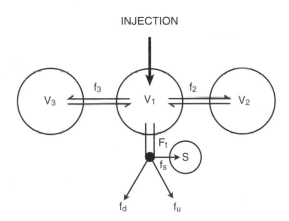

FIGURE 15.6
General multicompartment model for metal metabolism. (Adapted from Onkelinx, C., in *Clinical Chemistry and Chemical Toxicology of Metals*, Brown, S.S. (Ed.), Elsevier North–Holland, Amsterdam, 1977, 37.)

---

* Note that this is significantly higher than typical modern values; see, for instance, Table 15.2. The probably lower true value makes the predicted increases even more striking.

TABLE 15.5

Comparison among Compartment Volumes, Interchange, and Excretion for Ni, Co, and Cr in Rats

	$^{63}Ni^{2+}$	$^{57}Co^{2+}$	$^{51}Cr^{3+}$
Age (days)	85	60	60
Compartment volumes (ml/100 g body wt.)			
V_1	36.1	46.4	30.8
V_2	4.0	78.2	16.7
V_3	—	65.6	7.7
Apparent excretory flow rates (ml/h)			
F_t	3.91	7.29	1.42
f_u	3.07	5.97	0.91
f_d	0.62	0.72	0.07
f_s	0.22	0.60	0.44
Ratios of excretory flow rates			
f_u/F_t	0.79	0.82	0.64
f_d/F_t	0.16	0.10	0.05
f_s/F_t	0.06	0.08	0.31
Compartment net interchange flow rates (ml/h)			
f_2	0.06	13.11	2.47
f_3	—	0.56	0.13

Source: Adapted from Onkelinx, C., in *Clinical Chemistry and Chemical Toxicology of Metals,* Brown, S.S. (Ed.), Elsevier North–Holland, Amsterdam, 1977, 37.

rate, F_t, composed of collection in irreversible sinks (f_s), urinary excretion (f_u), and fecal excretion (f_d). Loss of tissue, desquammation, etc. are lumped with f_s.

Table 15.5 reports some results obtained by injection of nickel, cobalt, and chromium into rats between 2 and 3 months old. Onkelinx (1977) reported results for other ages, suggesting age dependence, especially for chromium. Examination of this table graphically shows the differences in metal metabolism for these ions. Although it is difficult to apply physical identities to compartment volumes, the differences are obvious. Nickel does not penetrate V_3, as previously pointed out, and the relative penetration of each ion is quite different. Of particular interest is the ratio f_s/F_t. Here, modest amounts of nickel and cobalt are trapped in a tissue sink, but over 30% of chromium is retained. Again, with reference to Taylor (1973), if this material is bound irreversibly, the effect would be to lower transient tissue concentrations and lengthen the time until steady state is reached, but raise the final body burden above that originally predicted.

It is inviting to equate secondary compartments (in this case, V_1, V_2, and S), as derived from Onkelinx' analysis with specific tissue types or organs, on the basis of apparent volumes. This is simplistic; metabolic pools and storage depots can only be identified by following the course of metal, in the form of a suitable radioactive isotope, from the implant site to its eventual destination. Unfortunately, such studies may not ethically be performed in humans, so compartment identities may remain unclear for a long time to come.

15.4.4 Equilibrium Models

Another experimental approach to this problem (Smith and Black 1977; Smith 1982) is to implant metallic devices with varying surface areas and track the plasma levels as a function of time. In these reports, an experiment was performed in a short-term rabbit model to investigate whether implantation of 316L stainless steel is accompanied by elevated plasma levels of iron and chromium.

For a given alloy system with a uniform processing history, the parameter that would appear to govern the rate of corrosion product delivery to the body in any particular implant site is the ratio of implant surface area to body weight (SA/BW). For a 70-kg patient receiving a typical total hip joint replacement (surface area = 200 cm^2), this ratio is approximately 2.86 cm^2/kg. This value is termed "1×" and multiples of it reflect higher relative exposures. Note that the use of such a ratio probably underestimates the exposure in small-animal models. Renal clearance is roughly proportional to basal metabolic rate (per kilogram of body weight). Because individual metabolic rate in adult mammals, including humans, is proportional to (BW)$^{0.734}$ (Brody 1945), a 1.5-kg rabbit has a basal metabolic rate/kg 2.78 times that of a 70-kg patient. Thus, 100× for the patient is approximately 36× for the rabbit, if adjusted to reflect basal metabolic rates, or, conversely, 100× for the rabbit is 278× for the patient. The concept of SA/BW ratio can be extended to *in vitro* studies by recognizing that a 70-kg patient has a water content of 42 l (Figure 15.4), forming the ratio of surface area to body fluid volume (SA/BFV) and assigning a value of 4.76 cm^2/l.

In Smith and Black's (1977) studies, New Zealand white rabbits received implants of passivated surgical grade 316L stainless steel (ASTM F 55, type B) in two forms (Steinmann pin segments and 40-µm spherical powders) at two anatomic sites (paraspinal musculature and femoral medullary canal) as shown in Table 15.6. Blood specimens were obtained at intervals of up to 7 months, and tissue specimens were obtained at sacrifice. The serum was analyzed for chromium, free (nonheme) iron (PI), total iron-binding capacity (TIBC), and percent of TIBC saturation (% sat.). The tissues were analyzed for iron and chromium.

No significant differences (experimental vs. control) were detected in PI, TIBC, or % sat. until 20 weeks postoperative. Group V plasma iron concentration was 14% elevated ($p < 0.05$) by 20 weeks postoperative. None of the groups exhibited significant changes in TIBC or % sat.; however, the latter showed a "tendency" toward elevation, particularly in Group V. The kidney

TABLE 15.6

Animal Groups for Evaluation of SA/BW Effects

Group	N =	Implant	Site	SA/BW (Unadjusted)
I	10	Pin	Muscle	1
II	10	Pin	Bone	1
III	15	Microspheres	Bone	1
IV	10	Microspheres	Bone	10
V	15	Microspheres	Bone	100
VI	14	None	—	0

showed an ability to accumulate iron; however, Group V liver iron concentrations were elevated 30% on dry weight and total protein basis.

The results for chromium are shown in Table 15.7. Plasma iron elevations in Group V at 20 and 28 weeks indicated that iron release (corrosion into the blood circulation) exceeded the inherent iron turnover rate of the Fe–transferring-binding system. The consequent trend toward elevation in % sat., if observed in humans, might occasion a reduction in a patient's disease resistance (see Section 14.2.8). Plasma iron and, especially, plasma chromium concentrations appear to reflect the duration of implantation and the SA/BW ratio. Sporadic elevations in plasma chromium in Groups I through IV toward the last 2 months of the study may suggest periods of

TABLE 15.7

Serum and Tissue Chromium Content after Stainless Steel Implantation as a Function of Implantation Time and SA/BW Ratio in Rabbit

Sample (ng/ml)	Control (Group VI) Group I	% Change from Control (Significance)[a]			
		Group II	Group III	Group IV	Group V
Serum					
Pre-op	13.1 ± 0.9		$-11.4\ (p < 0.05)$		
4 wk PO	11.4 ± 0.4				$+16.7\ (p < 0.001)$
8 wk PO	12.9 ± 0.1	Lost group			$+12.8\ (p < 0.08)$
20 wk PO	11.2 ± 0.4		$+6.2\ (p < 0.05)$		$+21.4\ (p < 0.01)$
24 wk PO	10.3 ± 0.7	$+15.5\ (p < 0.01)$	$+17.5\ (p < 0.01)$	$+24.3\ (p < 0.01)$	$+23.3\ (p < 0.01)$
28 wk PO	15.3 ± 0.7	$+17\ (p < 0.01)$			$+10.4\ (p < 0.01)$
Tissue (ng/mg dry wt.)					
Kidney	1.97 ± 0.5				
Liver	1.07 ± 0.7			$+64.2\ (p < 0.02)$	$+85\ (p < 0.01)$

[a] Only significant changes are shown.

Source: Adapted from Smith, G.K., Ph.D. thesis, University of Pennsylvania, Philadelphia, 1982.

accelerated corrosion or release into the circulation. Because plasma chromium concentrations are probably not in equilibrium with storage compartments, these chromium elevations are not likely to be an indicator of body stores but rather a dynamic measure of serum transport at the moment of sampling. The kidney demonstrated no capacity to accumulate iron or chromium.

On the other hand, the liver exhibited elevated iron and chromium accumulations, which were apparently a function of SA/BW ratio, in contrast to Ferguson's study (Ferguson et al. 1962a, b), which reported no elevations in iron or chromium in the liver or kidney. From persistently elevated plasma iron and chromium concentrations, it can be expected that liver accumulations would have continued beyond the experimental period and that, with time, groups I through III may have exhibited elevations.

One of the weaknesses of this approach is that it is impossible to distinguish the metal released from the implant from that available from dietary sources or storage depots. The presence of the implant may alter the binding and storage mechanisms that normally handle metal (Woodman et al. 1983). An alternate approach would be to use radioactive isotopes as injected materials (Bergman et al. 1980) or, preferably, as components of implant alloys, followed by periodic sacrifice and autoradiography. However, the rarity of appropriate isotopes, difficulties in fabricating suitable implants, and safety concerns about handling the animals and their waste products severely handicaps this approach.

It is clear from these equilibrium studies that trace metal metabolism is highly complex and that detailed studies of each metal of implant importance should be carried out in the future.

15.5 Final Comment

Systemic distribution, storage, and excretion of corrosion and degradation products from implants has not attracted great attention as a subfield of study within biomaterials science and engineering. Initially, this was due to an inability to detect normal or elevated levels of such materials, especially metal-bearing ions, and a parallel failure to recognize their biological importance. More recently, studies of host response have continued largely to focus on circumimplant effects and have continued to equate low corrosion/elution rates and small plasma concentration elevations with absence of accumulation of degradation products and, thus, absence of biological effects. The weakness of this assumption may be illustrated by the following argument.

A proposal may be to establish how many cars are in a particular turnpike rest area by only examining the flow of traffic on the roadway. First considerations suggest a possible positive correlation between the number of cars passing a marker nearby on the main roadway and the number to be found in the rest area. However, the rest area might be closed for repairs (large number on roadway, none in rest area) or the driving conditions may have recently become treacherous, perhaps due to icing, causing drivers to decide to delay their further travel (small number on roadway, large number in rest area). Thus, on second consideration, the conclusion is that the only way reliably to determine the number of cars in a turnpike rest area at any one time is to count them. The situation for detection of debris and corrosion products in remote tissues and organs is parallel by analogy.

What is required is the recognition that any implant, whether designed specifically for that purpose or not, acts as a slow-release system *in vivo*. Thus, the appropriate approach to understanding the total host response to implants must parallel that of biological fate studies in pharmacology and environmental fate studies in ecology.

From this viewpoint, three important questions should be answered when a new implantable biomaterial is evaluated:

- What is the nature of the degradation products released from the implant *in vivo*?
- Where do they go within the body?
- What is the host response to release, distribution, remote concentration, and excretion of these degradation products?

These are extremely difficult questions to answer. Although there are theoretical bases for the answers to the first and second questions, the third remains conjectural until actual human clinical data can be obtained. This can only be done within the context of carefully controlled prospective studies in well identified cohorts of patients with implants and suitable controls. Jacobs et al. (1991) offer an example of this approach in a study that has now extended some 15 years and is gradually being correlated with studies of retrieved tissues and fluids as patients reach the end of life.

Previously, some aspects of local host response have been considered. The next chapter will take up the more global issue of systemic and remote site host response produced by the transport phenomena discussed in this chapter.

References

Aalders, G.J. et al., An exceptional case of pneumothorax — "a new adventure of the K wire," *Injury*, 16, 564, 1985.

Albores–Saavedra, J. et al., Sinus histiocytosis of pelvic lymph nodes after hip replacement. A histiocytic proliferation induced by cobalt–chromium and titanium, *Am. J. Surg. Pathol.*, 18, 83, 1994.

Araki, S. et al., Filterable plasma concentration, glomerular filtration, tubular balance, and renal clearance of heavy metals and organic substances in metal workers, *Arch. Environ. Health*, 41, 216, 1986a.

Araki, S. et al., Comparison of the effects of urinary flow on adjusted and nonadjusted excretion of heavy metals and organic substances in "healthy" men, *J. Appl. Toxicol.*, 6, 245, 1986b.

Arvidson, K. and Wróblewski, R., Migration of metallic ions from screwposts into dentin and surrounding tissues, *Scand. J. Dent. Res.*, 83, 200, 1978.

Bergman, B. et al., The distribution of nickel in mice, an autoradiographic study, *J. Oral Rehabil.*, 7, 319, 1980.

Brauer, R.W., Mechanisms of bile secretion, *JAMA*, 169, 1462, 1959.

Brody, S., *Bioenergetics and Growth, with Special Reference to the Efficiency Complex in Domestic Animals*, Reinhold, New York, 1945, 352.

Case, C.P. et al., Widespread dissemination of metal debris from implants, *J. Bone Joint Surg.*, 76B, 701, 1994.

Charnley, J., Arthroplasty of the hip. A new operation, *Lancet*, 1, 1129, 1961.

Cherian, M.G. and Goyer, R.A., Minireview, metallothioneins and their role in the metabolism and toxicity of metals, *Life Sci.*, 23, 1, 1978.

Ferguson, A.B. et al., Trace metal ion concentration in the liver, kidney, spleen, and lung of normal rabbits, *J. Bone Joint Surg.*, 44A, 317, 1962a.

Ferguson, A.B. et al., Characteristics of trace ions released from embedded metal implants in the rabbit, *J. Bone Joint Surg.*, 44A, 323, 1962b.

Ganong, W.F., Renal function and micturation, in *Review of Medical Physiology*, 14th ed., Appleton & Lange, Norwalk, CT, 1989, 593.

Gatti, A.M. and Rivasi, F., Biocompatibility of micro- and nanoparticles. Part I: in liver and kidney, *Biomaterials* 23(11), 2381, 2002.

Graham, J.A. et al., Effect of trace metals on phagocytosis by alveolar macrophages, *Infect. Immunol.*, 11, 1278, 1975.

Greene, N.D. et al., Engineering and biological studies of metallic implant materials, in *Biomaterials*, Horowitz, E. and Torgesen, J.L. (Eds.), NBS Special Publication 415, U.S. Government Printing Office, Washington, D.C., 1975, 45.

Hierholzer, S. et al., Increased corrosion of stainless steel implants in infected plated fractures, *Arch. Orthop. Trauma Surg.*, 102, 198, 1984.

Homsy, C.A. et al., Some physiological aspects of prosthesis stabilization with acrylic polymer, *Clin. Orthop. Rel. Res.*, 83, 317, 1972.

Ishihara, N. and Matsushiro, T., Biliary and urinary excretion of metals in humans, *Arch. Environ. Health*, 41, 324, 1986.

Jacobs, J.J. et al., Local and distant products from modularity, *Clin. Orthop. Rel. Res.*, 319, 94, 1995.

Jacobs, J.J. et al., Release and excretion of metal in patients with titanium-base alloy total hip replacement components, *J. Bone Joint Surg.*, 73A, 1475, 1991.

Jenkin, C.R. and Rowley, D., The role of opsonins in the clearance of living and inert particles by cells of the reticuloendothelial system, *J. Exp. Med.*, 114, 363, 1961.

Kapp, J.P. et al., Metallic fragment embolization to the cerebral circulation, *J. Trauma*, 13, 256, 1973.

Kapur R. et al., Human monocyte morphology is affected by local substrate charge heterogeneity, *J. Biomed. Mater. Res.*, 32, 133, 1996.

Kawaguchi, H. et al., Phagocytosis of latex particles by leukocytes, I, Dependence of phagocytosis on the size and surface potential of particles, *Biomaertials*, 7, 61, 1986.

Klaassen, C.D., Biliary excretion of metals, *Drug Metab. Rev.*, 5, 165, 1976.

Korn, E.D. and Weisman, R.A., Phagocytosis of latex beads by *acanthamoeba*. II. Electron microscopic study of the initial events, *J. Cell. Biol.*, 34, 219, 1967.

Lux, F. and Zeisler, R., Investigations of the corrosive deposition of components of metal implants and of the behavior of biological trace elements in metallosis tissue by means of instrumental multi-element activation analysis, *J. Radioanal. Chem.*, 19, 289, 1974.

Lux, F. et al., A mechanistic model for the metabolism of corrosion products and of biological trace elements in metallosis tissue based on results obtained by activation analysis, *J. Radioanal. Chem.*, 32, 229, 1976.

Lyons, F.A. and Rockwood, C.A., Current concepts review. Migration of pins used in operations on the shoulder, *J. Bone Joint Surg.*, 72A, 1262, 1990.

Margevicius, K.J. et al., Identification and distribution of synthetic ligament wear particles in sheep, *J. Biomed. Mater. Res.*, 31, 319, 1996.

Michel, R., Trace metal analysis in biocompatibility testing, *CRC Crit. Rev. Biocompat.*, 3, 235, 1987.

Michel, R. et al., Systemic effects of implanted prostheses made of cobalt–chromium alloys, *Arch. Orthop. Trauma Surg.*, 110, 61, 1991.

Normann, S.J., Kinetics of phagocytosis. II. Analysis of *in vivo* clearance with demonstration of competitive inhibition between similar and dissimilar foreign particles, *Lab. Invest.*, 31, 161, 1974.

Onkelinx, C., Whole-body kinetics of metal salts in rats, in *Clinical Chemistry and Chemical Toxicology of Metals,* Brown, S.S. (Ed.), Elsevier North–Holland, Amsterdam, 1977, 37.

Oron, U. and Alter, A., Corrosion in metal implants embedded in various locations of the body in rats, *Clin. Orthop. Rel. Res.*, 185, 295, 1984.

Pitts, R.F., Tubular reabsorption; tubular secretion, in *Physiology of the Kidney and Body Fluids, An Introductory Text,* Year Book Medical Pub. Inc., Chicago, 1963, 69, 116.

Potter, F.A. et al., The migration of a Kirschner wire from shoulder to spleen: a brief report, *J. Bone Joint Surg.*, 70B, 326, 1988.

Schnyder, J. and Baggiolini, M., Role of phagocytosis in the aviation of macrophages, *J. Exp. Med.*, 148(6), 1449, 1978.

Smith, G.K., Systemic transport and distribution of iron and chromium from 316l stainless steel implants, Ph.D. thesis, University of Pennsylvania, Philadelphia, 1982.

Smith, G.K. and Black, J., Elevation of Fe and Cr concentrations in blood plasma after stainless steel implantation, *Trans. ORS*, 2, 281, 1977.

Stensaas, S.S. and Stensaas, L.J., Histopathological evaluation of materials implanted in the cerebral cortex, *Acta. Neuropath. (Berl.)*, 41, 145, 1978.

Stiffel, C. et al., Kinetics of the phagocytic function of reticuloendothelial macrophages *in vivo*, in *Mononuclear Macrophages*, van Furth, R. (Ed.), Academic Press, New York, 1970, 335.

Styles, J.A. and Wilson, J., Comparison between *in vitro* toxicity of two novel fibrous mineral dusts and their tissue reactions *in vivo*, *Ann. Occup. Hyg.*, 19, 63, 1976.

Sunderman, F.W., Jr. et al., Cobalt, chromium, and nickel concentrations in body fluids of patients with porous-coated knee or hip prostheses, *J. Orthop. Res.*, 7, 307, 1989.

Taylor, D.M., Trace metal patterns and disease, *J. Bone Joint Surg.*, 55B, 422, 1973.

Urban, R.M. et al., Accumulation in liver and spleen of metal particles generated at nonbearing surfaces in hip arthroplasty, *J. Arthroplasty*, 19 (8 Suppl. 3), 94, 2004.

Vernon–Roberts, B., The kinetics of phagocytosis stimulation and depression of the phagocytic activity of macrophages, in Vernon–Roberts, B., *The Macrophage*, Cambridge University Press, Cambridge, 1972, 92.

Weisman, R.A. and Korn, E.D., Phagocytosis of latex beads by *acanthamoeba* I. Biochemical properties, *Biochemistry*, 6, 485, 1967.

Woodman, J.L. et al., Release of cobalt and nickel from a new total finger joint prosthesis made of vitallium, *J. Biomed. Mater. Res.*, 17, 655, 1983.

Bibliography

Anderson, J.M. and Miller, K.M., Biomaterial biocompatibility and the macrophage, *Biomaterials*, 5, 5, 1984.

Friedman, M.H., *Principles and Models of Biological Transport*, Springer–Verlag, Berlin, 1986.

Guyton, A.C., The kidneys and body fluids, in *Textbook of Medical Physiology*, 8th ed., Guyton, A.C. (Ed.), W.B. Saunders, Philadelphia, 1991, 273.

Harrison, P.M. and Treffry, A., Storage and transport of transition-metal ions, in *Inorganic Biochemistry, A Review of the Recent Literature Published up to Late 1977*, Vol. 1, H.A.O. Hill (Ed.), The Chemical Society, London, 1979, 120.

Ingham, E. and Fisher, J., The role of macrophages in osteolysis of total joint replacement, *Biomaterials*, 26, 1271, 2005.

Iyengar, G.V., Review: reference values for the concentrations of As, Cd, Co, Cr, Cu, Fe, I, Hg, Mn, MO, Ni, Pb, Se, and Zn on selected human tissues and body fluids, *Biol. Trace Elem. Res.*, 12, 263, 1978.

Koushanpour, E. and Kriz, W., *Renal Physiology, Principles, Structure, and Functions*, 2nd ed., Springer–Verlag, New York, 1986.

Langkamer, V.G. et al., Systemic distribution of wear debris after hip replacement. A cause for concern? *J. Bone Joint Surg.*, 74B, 831, 1992.

Lote, C.J., *Principles of Renal Physiology*, 4th ed., Chapman & Hall, London, 2000.

Pitts, R.F., *Physiology of the Kidney and Body Fluids, An Introductory Text*, 3rd ed., Year Book Medical Pub. Inc., Chicago, 1974.

Roberts, J. and Quastel, J.H., Particle uptake by polymorphonuclear leucocytes and Erlich ascites-carcinoma cells, *Biochem. J.*, 89, 150, 1963.

da Silva, J.J.R.F. and Williams, R.J.P., *The Biological Chemistry of the Elements*, 2nd ed., Clarendon Press, Oxford, 2001.

Solomon, A.K., Compartmental methods of kinetic analysis, in *Mineral Metabolism*, Vol. 1A, Comar, C.L. and Bronner, F. (Eds.), Academic Press, New York, 1960, 119.

Valtin, H. and Schafer, J.A., *Renal Function*, 3rd ed., Little, Brown and Co., Boston, 1994.

16

Effects of Degradation Products on Remote Organ Function

16.1 Introduction

This chapter will complete the discussion of the effects of materials on biological systems (host response). With the exception of a number of recognized systemic effects, this chapter will simply recapitulate and emphasize areas already discussed in Chapter 8 through Chapter 15.

Systemic effects of foreign materials, such as implants, are now well recognized. It is more correct to distinguish between remote effects (involving actions, perhaps secondary to deposition and concentration of degradation products) on a target tissue or organ and systemic effects (those affecting large-scale systems such as the cardiovascular or neurological systems) However, for the sake of brevity, they will be grouped together here under the common title of systemic effects.

The effects of drugs, collectively pharmacological effects, are by and large necessarily systemic or remote effects. Drugs are given or injected in one portion of the body and directly or indirectly affect cellular and systemic physiology in other areas, even if a purely local or topical effect is intended. Discussion of such effects is beyond the scope of this book; however, many of the effects that have been discussed are essentially pharmacological effects secondary to the primary or intended effect. Nonetheless, drug release materials provide a hypothetical example that illustrates the complexity of possible host response to an implant:

- The drug and/or carrier material is designed to evoke a local (implant site) response, such as alleviation of pain or reduction of fibrosis.
- The drug and/or degradation products from the carrier may evoke desirable or undesirable systemic effects, such as alteration of arterial pressure.
- The drug may have a specific remote organ target, such as the heart.

- The degradation products of the carrier might produce adverse effects in other remote organs, such as the kidney.

16.2   Examples of Systemic Effects

16.2.1   Polymers

An example of these types of effects is that associated with release of methyl methacrylate monomer during the polymerization of PMMA-type cements *in vivo*. Homsy et al. (1972) (see Section 15.3.1) were attracted to this problem not by the observation of the rapid transport of the monomer to the lungs, but by the observed systemic effects. Early in the use of these cements, it was observed that systemic hypotension developed immediately after the insertion of the cement into the prepared bone cavity. Arterial pressure drops of more than 15 mmHg were observed associated with transient cyanosis, and a number of cardiac arrests drew medical attention to the effect (Keret and Reis 1980). Further studies in dogs showed that this problem is accentuated by marked fluid and/or blood loss (McMaster et al. 1974).

The corrective therapy now used to prevent the development of centrally mediated hypotension after PMMA insertion is maintenance of the patient in a state of positive hydration. In addition, it has been shown that venting the bony (medullary) cavity with a drain line during device insertion reduces the driving pressure differential that aids in monomer take-up by blood and may reduce the embolization of fat to the lungs as encountered in intramedullary fixation of fractures (Giannoudis et al. 2002). Polymers released from implants have few if any known systemic effects beyond this hypotensive effect. The rates of release and the normal routes of molecular catabolism apparently combine to keep concentrations of products from common polymeric implants below levels required for direct pharmacological activity.

This is not to suggest that elevated blood levels of polymer degradation products do not exist or that they may be harmless in the long term. In the short term, host responses may be indistinguishable from disturbances of homeostasis associated with surgery (Dahl 1997). However, in cases of high surface area and/or repetitive exposure, as in hemodialysis (as a treatment for renal insufficiency or failure), significant deviations from normal conditions may be encountered. Lewis et al. (1977) examined the blood of individuals undergoing chronic hemodialysis, looking explicitly for breakdown products or plasticizers that might be released from the polyvinyl chloride (PVC) polymer used as a blood conduit material. Significant levels, up to a mean level of 751 ng/ml serum of *bis* (2-ethylhexyl) phthalate, a common PVC plasticizer, were found in these patients after dialysis. Although the catabolism of this material was rapid and thus led to its being undetectable in blood 5 to 6 hours after completion of dialysis, the yearly dose for the chronic dialysis patient was estimated to be 150 to 250 mg. The long-term effects of this are unknown, as is the case for the majority of long-term, low-level exposures to foreign materials and their degradation products.

A final interesting example is provided by the early (now abandoned) practice of using injected fluid silicone materials for cosmetic tissue augmentation. In addition to producing local fibrosis, these fluids can migrate through tissue and produce a variety of remote effects, including tissue mass formation, adenopathy, and, possibly, pulmonary failure (Kossovsky and Heggers 1987). However, broader claims of connective tissue and immune disorders associated with silicone gel-filled breast augmentation devices appear to have no firm basis (Gabriel 1998; Noone 1997).

16.2.2 Metals

The situation with metals is somewhat different. In addition to the "physiological" metals (Ca, Na, K, and Fe) and despite very low normal plasma and tissue concentrations, a large number of metals, including Co, Cr, Mg, Zn, and Cu, have normal roles in metabolism and are thus classified as essential trace elements. Therefore, it should come as no surprise that naturally occurring diseases of inherited as well as acquired etiology involve imbalances in the metabolism of these metals.

In addition to anemia (iron deficiency), iron overload diseases also exist. One such disease, hemochromatosis (Elinder 1986), results in the accumulation and deposit of iron in the form of the compound hemosiderin in tissues with rough endoplasmic reticulae. This accumulation has a number of physiological effects. One example is the development of diffuse arthritis in widely separated joints. This also occurs secondarily to the internal bleeding associated with hemophilia. Hemochromatosis involves skin pigmentation, liver failure, and diabetes. Elinder (1986) points out that although iron is a physiological element, it is potentially toxic in all doses and forms and is capable of producing a variety of local and systemic toxic effects in animals and humans.

A less well-known disease is Wilson's disease (Aaseth and Norseth 1986), or the so-called copper man syndrome. This is an accumulation disease, primarily hereditary, in which copper accumulates in a variety of tissues, including liver, cornea, and skin, instead of being maintained in balance. A green skin color develops and a high incidence of mortality due to intravascular hemolysis and liver failure results from the cytotoxicity of copper and its compounds.

Metals that are normally foreign to the body, such as Pb, Be, and As, can combine competitively with enzymes that normally use other trace metals as cofactors. Even normally present metals, such as Al and Cr, may do so, if present in sufficiently high concentrations. The abnormal cofactor–enzyme combinations may have higher stability than the normal cofactor bonds. Thus, the effect is to inactivate a portion of the enzyme pool without stimulating additional enzyme production. In low concentrations, the net effect will be to inhibit enzyme activity. This can be seen in a reduction of the efficiency or effectiveness of an enzyme process. Examples of this are the peripheral neuropathy observed in the case of long-term, low-level ingestion of lead and the suppression of hemoglobin synthesis by chromium. At higher concentration levels, metals can be highly toxic poisons through enzyme inactivation as in the familiar case of arsenic.

Beyond these specific mechanisms, a wide variety of systemic medical problems has been suggested as associated with imbalances in trace metal levels. As noted in Section 14.4, care must be taken in dealing with this literature because a less than totally scientific nutritional school of thought ascribes virtually all unexplained physical and mental disabilities to such effects. The mere detection of a foreign metal with adverse biological effects, such as mercury, is insufficient to reach conclusions concerning possible clinical problems; for example, recent studies associate autoimmunity in patients with dental amalgam more with the silver content of the restoration than with mercury or its compounds (Enestrom et al. 1995). There are, however, legitimately recognized associations, such as the increased incidence of cardiomyopathy associated with elevated cobalt intake (Alexander 1972) and the recognized association of arteriosclerosis with hardness (primarily Ca content) of ground water (Perry 1973).*

Consideration of the effects of metals must address all aspects of physiology. Perhaps one should be more observant of systemically detectable deviations from mean values of clinical parameters, such as liver transaminase serum concentrations in patients with chronic implants (Chopra 1988), even when they remain within "normal" limits. Concentrations of metals well below those needed to produce externally measurable changes in such physiological variables can produce profound behavioral abnormalities and mental disorders (Weiss 1978).

16.2.3   Ceramics

As noted in Section 4.11, ceramics used in implants may be insoluble or soluble. Insoluble ceramic biomaterials, such as alumina, titania, zirconia, etc., pose no systemic challenge, at least in nonparticulate form. To avoid unwanted local site responses, resorbable ceramics, such as tricalcium phosphate, etc., are chosen so that their elemental cations and anions (including Cl^-, SO_4^{-2}, CO_3^{-2}, and PO_4^{-3}) lie primarily within the range of physiological compositions. However, the possibility of soluble mineral components such as Sr^{**} in the latter generally argues for the use of fully defined (synthetic)

---

* As well as, presumably, the general levels of trace element intake.
** ^{90}Sr, a radioactive element with a half-life of 29 years, was present as a natural impurity in zirconium and zirconia in their early use as biomaterials (Burger et al. 1997). Although they are now fully removed from such materials, its presence presented an early example of an unwanted source of systemic effects.

materials rather than those obtained from natural sources to avoid possible systemic effects caused by their dissolution products.

16.3   A Review of Systemic Aspects of Host Response

Host responses will now be reviewed briefly in terms of systemic or remote site effects.

16.3.1   Interaction of Molecules with Surfaces

Proteins and enzymes released from surfaces in an irreversibly denatured state will possibly elicit remote effects directly or indirectly through the action of the immune system. Depletion of pools of unactivated coagulation or complement factors, as frequently occurs during hemodialysis or blood oxygenation, may suppress coagulation effects at remote sites of injury. Conversely, the increased circulating concentration of surface-activated factors may also have systemic or remote sequelae. It is also possible that denatured molecules bound to wear debris subject to passive or active transport can elicit systemic or remote effects.

16.3.2   Inflammation

Inflammation would be expected to be a local effect restricted to the vicinity of the implant. It is possible that an implant can release pyrogenic agents directly or produce them indirectly through denaturation processes. Some evidence indicates that denatured molecules or released products of unknown identity may produce long-term systemic hallmarks of inflammation, as in the chronic erythrocyte sedimentation rate elevation observed by Shih et al. (1987) in patients after PMMA-cemented total hip replacement. In addition, friction, wear, and some dissolution processes that release particulate material may result in an inflammatory response at a site of remote accumulation. An example of this is the abdominal "teflonoma" frequently seen after use of poly(tetrafluoro) ethylene as the material for fabrication of acetabular cups in Charnley's early efforts at hip replacement (Charnley 1979). More subtle may be the effects associated with particulate transport and accumulation through venous or lymphatic return pathways (Langkamer et al. 1992). Precipitation/redissolution of corrosion products in remote sites may also be expected to produce inflammation due to response to the resulting particulate material or to increased local concentrations of ions.

16.3.3 Coagulation and Hemolysis

Similarly, one can expect that primary coagulation problems would be localized to the vicinity of a cardiovascular system implant or external blood conduit or treatment device. The ability of implants to surface activate factors in the coagulation cascade (as noted earlier), as well as to shed thrombi, renders this a systemic effect with remote site manifestations. Similarly, whether through blood–surface interactions, turbulent shear, or by direct mechanical damage in valves, pumps, etc., hemolysis is a systemic problem due to the reduction in viable erythrocytes and the rapid dispersion of hemoglobin and cell fragments. It is clear that the current factors limiting successful long-term left ventricular assist and total (artificial) heart replacement are remote effects (primarily cerebral and pulmonary infarcts) secondary to systemic distribution of shed thrombi.

16.3.4 Adaptation

The discussion of adaptation emphasized the effects at the biomaterial–tissue interface. This is certainly the most important adaptive remodeling site, and it is expected that systemic or remote effects would be secondary to this and thus not directly related (if they occur at all). However, one should not rule out, *a priori*, the possibility of cytokines, growth factors, etc. released from sites of adaptive remodeling having effects on remote tissues or organs.

16.3.5 Chemical Carcinogenesis

Of necessity, chemical carcinogenesis must be considered a systemic problem because of the variable sensitivity of cells to chemically induced neoplastic transformation and the possibility of metastases. If chemically mediated carcinogenesis occurs in humans due to the use of implant materials, it can thus be expected to have a significant systemic manifestation. It is worth pointing out again that possibilities of systemic and remote-site tumorgenesis associated with implants tend to be overlooked in patient populations for two reasons:

- The tumor types expected are no different from those that would already exist in a comparable patient population without implants.
- The specialization of medicine makes the connection of a tumor in a remote tissue or organ system to the presence of an implant in another tissue or organ system unlikely (Black 1984).

16.3.6   Foreign-Body Carcinogenesis

One would expect foreign-body carcinogenesis that occurs in patients to be a local problem. However, the ability of particulate materials to move in the body and the inherent ability of many neoplasms to metastasize render it a potential systemic problem. It must be emphasized that this is a putative consideration because the presence of primary foreign body neoplasias (at the implant site) has not been reliably detected in humans (see Section 13.3).

16.3.7   Infection

Acceptance of Weinberg's (1974) arguments concerning nutritional immunity (see Chapter 14) means that it is necessary to recognize the possibility of problems associated with elevated iron concentrations in the vicinity of implants and with elevated concentrations in remote storage sites. Furthermore, suppression of the immune system may also predispose to infection at distant sites as well as at the implant–tissue interface.

The possibility of the inverse — that is, of hematogenous "seeding" of an implant site infection from a distant site such as a dental abscess or urinary tract infection — must not be discounted, although clinical data remain equivocal at this time (Thyne and Ferguson 1991). In most surgical specialties, pre- and perioperative precautions are now employed for implantation procedures when there is foreknowledge of infection present at a remote site, particularly in the oral cavity (Carmona et al. 2002).

16.3.8   Allergic Foreign-Body Response

The discussion of this subject (Chapter 12) emphasized the systemic nature of the response. Therefore, in addition to possible problems in the vicinity of the implant such as pain, loosening, etc., a wide variety of allergic responses at remote sites can potentially be associated with the presence of metallic, and possibly polymeric, implants as sensitizing or challenge agents. Sensitization is a matter of particular concern because it may evoke a later local or systemic response apparently spatially unrelated to the original site of implantation.

16.4   A Final Comment

It is important to re-emphasize that studies of host response have focused primarily on the implant site and adjacent tissues. In the future, a much broader view must be taken and the response of the entire host, whether experimental animal or human patient, must be studied in detail.

However, a major pitfall in such considerations must be avoided. Much is made in the lay press about individuals who develop an apparent "environmental allergy": an elevated sensitivity, with immune response symptoms, to a very broad variety of agents that have in common only that they are man-made. An analogous situation exists in the field of clinical application of biomaterials with lay concern over the relationship between release of mercury from mercury-based dental amalgams and a broad variety of patient symptoms. Without passing judgment on either of these situations,* I would like to suggest, somewhat in the spirit of Furst's requirements for accepting the carcinogenicity of a metal in animal models (see Section 13.2.4), that the following criteria should be met before the existence of a remote or systemic effect in humans is taken as proven:

- The basic mechanism of the biological response must be demonstrated in at least one *in vitro* situation or in an animal biological model.

- After the causative implant-related species has been identified, its release by a functional implant and systemic distribution in an animal model or in patients (preferably both) must be shown.

- The putative biological response must be identified in an animal model or in patients (preferably both) with functional implants.

- If it is demonstrated in patients, the biological response must be recognized on the basis of a statistically sound epidemiological study, with suitable nonexposed controls and, unless the response is of a threshold type, must demonstrate a dose–response or exposure–incidence relationship.

In my mind, these are the necessary and sufficient conditions to conclude that an implant-related systemic (and/or remote site) effect exists in patients. Their presence does not settle the issue of the clinical importance of the effect; this depends upon other considerations such as treatment alternatives (including no treatment) and the benefit of the use of the device in which the biomaterial is incorporated.

However, I would suggest that if the first criterion is met — that is, a biological mechanism leading to a putative systemic or remote site effect is identified — then an index of suspicion should be attached to the biomaterial in question. Similarly, isolated case reports of local or distant adverse implant-related responses should also arouse a degree of suspicion; what they lack in numbers they make up for to a degree in specificity. A lack of sound knowledge in any of the latter three areas should not lead to an inference of safety; this would be morally equivalent to the statement that "What I don't know can't hurt me."

---

* See Section 12.4 for a more complete discussion of immune responses to implants and Section 14.4 for a critique of environmental allergy and related issues.

For this reason, I have suggested that a biomaterial can never be considered safe or unsafe, but merely biocompatible (or not) in a specific application (Black 1995). Rather, satisfaction of the first criterion should lead to changes in behavior in consideration of that biomaterial for specific current device designs (Black 1988) and in planning future basic and applied studies of the biomaterial's safety and efficacy in present as well as proposed applications.

References

Aaseth, J. and Norseth, T., Copper, in *Handbook on the Toxicology of Metals*, Vol. II., Friberg, L., Nordberg, G.F. and Vouk, V.B. (Eds.), Elsevier, Amsterdam, 1986, 233.

Alexander, C.S., Cobalt-beer cardiomyopathy, *Am. J. Med.*, 53, 395, 1972.

Black, J., Systemic effects of biomaterials, *Biomaterials*, 5, 11, 1984.

Black, J., Does corrosion matter? *J. Bone Joint. Surg.*, 70B, 517, 1988.

Black J., "Safe" biomaterials, *J. Biomed. Mater. Res.*, 29, 791, 1995.

Burger, W. et al., New Y-TZP powders for medical grade zirconia, *J. Mater. Sci. Mater. Med.*, 8, 113, 1997.

Carmona, I.T. et al., An update on the controversies in bacterial endocarditis of oral origin, *Oral Surg. Oral Med. Oral Pathol. Oral Radiol. Endod.*, 93, 660, 2002.

Charnley, J., *Low Friction Arthroplasty of the Hip*, Springer–Verlag, Berlin, 1979, 6.

Chopra, S., *Disorders of the Liver*, Lea & Febiger, Philadelphia, 1988.

Dahl, O.E., Cardiorespiratory and vascular dysfunction related to major reconstructive orthopedic surgery, *Acta Orthop. Scand.*, 68, 607, 1997.

Elinder, C.-G., Iron, in *Handbook on the Toxicology of Metals*, Vol. II., Friberg, L., Nordberg, G.F. and Vouk, V.B. (Eds.), Elsevier, Amsterdam, 1986, 276.

Enestrom, S. and Hultman, P., Does amalgam affect the immune system? A controversial issue, *Int. Arch. Allergy Immunol.*, 106(3), 180, 1995.

Gabriel, S.E., Soft tissue response to silicones, in *Handbook of Biomaterial Properties*, Black, J. and Hastings, G. (Eds.), Chapman & Hall, London, 1998, 556.

Giannoudis, P.V. et al., Review: systemic effects of femoral nailing: from Kuntscher to the immune reactivity era, *Clin. Orthop. Rel. Res.*, 404, 378, 2002.

Homsy, C.A. et al., Some physiological aspects of prosthesis stabilization with acrylic polymer, *Clin. Orthop. Rel. Res.*, 83, 317, 1972.

Keret, D. and Reis, D.R., Intraoperative cardiac arrest and mortality in hip surgery. Possible relationship to acrylic bone cement, *Orthop. Rev.*, IX(7), 51, 1980.

Kossovsky, N. and Heggers, J.P., The bioreactivity of silicone, *CRC Crit. Rev. Biocompat.*, 3, 53, 1987.

Langkamer, V.G. et al., Changes in the proportions of peripheral blood lymphocytes in patients with worn implants, *J. Bone Joint Surg.*, 74B, 831, 1992.

Lewis, L.M. et al., Determination of plasticizer levels in serum of hemodialysis patients, *Trans. Am. Soc. Artif. Intern. Organs*, XXIII, 566, 1977.

McMaster, W.C. et al., Blood pressure lowering effect of methylmethacrylate monomer, *Clin. Orthop. Rel. Res.*, 98, 254, 1974.

Noone, R.B., A review of the possible health implications of silicone breast implants, *Cancer*, 79(9), 47, 1997.

Perry, H.M., Jr., Minerals in cardiovascular disease, *J. Am. Diet. Assoc.*, 62, 631, 1973.

Shih, L.-Y. et al., Erythrocyte sedimentation rate and C-reactive protein values in patients with total hip arthroplasty, *Clin. Orthop. Rel. Res.*, 225, 238, 1987.

Thyne, G.M. and Ferguson, J.W., Antibiotic prophylaxis during dental treatment in patients with prosthetic joints, *J. Bone Joint Surg.*, 73B, 191, 1991.

Weinberg, E.D., Iron and susceptibility to infectious disease, *Science*, 184, 952, 1974.

Weiss, B., The behavioral toxicology of metals, *Fed. Proc.*, 37(1), 22, 1978.

Bibliography

Davies, I.J.T., *The Clinical Significance of the Essential Biological Metals*, Charles C Thomas, Springfield, IL, 1972.

Debelian, G.J. et al., Systemic diseases caused by oral microorganisms, *Endod. Dent. Traumatol.*, 10, 57, 1994.

DiCarlo, E.F. and Bullough, P.G., The biological responses to orthopedic implants and their wear debris, *Clin. Mater.*, 9(3–4), 235, 1992.

Friberg, L., Nordberg, G.F. and Vouk, V.B. (Eds.), *Handbook on the Toxicology of Metals*, Vols. I and II. Elsevier, Amsterdam, 1986.

Ling, R.S.M., Systemic and miscellaneous complications, in *Complications of Total Hip Replacement*, Ling, R.S.M. (Ed.), Churchill–Livingstone, London, 1984, 201.

McCall, J.T. et al., Implications of trace metals in human diseases, *Fed. Proc.*, 30(3), 1011, 1971.

Pier, S.M., The role of heavy metals in human disease, *Tex. Rep. Biol. Med.*, 33(1), 85, 1975.

Rothman, R.H. and Hozack, W.J., *Complications of Total Hip Arthroplasty*, W.B. Saunders, Philadelphia, 1988.

Schroeder, H.A., Trace metals and chronic diseases, *Adv. Intern. Med.*, 8, 259, 1956.

Schierholz, J.M. and Beuth, J., Implant infections: a haven for opportunistic bacteria, *J. Hosp. Infect.*, 49(2), 87, 2001.

Webb, M., Metabolic targets of metal toxicity, in *Clinical Chemistry and Chemical Toxicology of Metals*, Brown, S.S. (Ed.), Elsevier North–Holland, Amsterdam, 1977, 51.

Williams, D.F. (Ed.), *Systemic Aspects of Biocompatibility*, Vols. I and II, CRC Press, Boca Raton, FL, 1981.

Interpart 2

Implant Materials: Clinical Performance*

I2.1 Introduction

Elaine Duncan (1990) once posed the question of whether biomaterials are at risk of becoming endangered species. Her query was motivated, in part, by a letter distributed by Dow Corning, Inc. (Midland, MI) warning of the company's intention of withdrawing an old standby polyurethane biomaterial, Pellethane™, from the market — at least for applications intended to last longer than 30 days *in vivo*. Citing published reports of cracking of the material after longer times *in vivo* (Stokes and Chem 1988), a company representative, J.R. Stoppert (1989), asserted that no data support long-term use of the material.

My immediate reaction to this statement was incredulity. The use of materials similar to Pellethane had been reported by Boretos and Pierce (1968) more than 20 years earlier. Discussing such materials, Boretos (1973) said that "[they] possess a combination of properties not available in other materials, outstanding of which [is]...excellent stability over long implant period." So, how can there be no data to support long-term human implantation of Pellethane?

I believe that what Stoppert (1989) meant is that there were, literally, *no* data. That is, there was evidence neither to support nor to contradict biomedical device designers' decisions to use Pellethane™ in long-term applications. Boretos' (1973) comments are not data and neither are the majority of papers published about this material or, for that matter, about virtually any other biomaterial in use in long-term clinical applications.** Most of these papers, especially those dealing with clinical observations, are not studies in the strict scientific sense, and the failure to conduct studies results in the absence of data, whether positive or negative.

---

* An earlier version of this interpart was published in Black (1990). Table I2.1 is adapted from Table 14.2 in Black (1988).
** The first competent study that I am aware of documenting *in vivo* stress-related degradation of such materials, albeit in an animal model, did not appear until 1990 (Zhao et al. 1990).

What has happened is that workers in the field of biomaterials have been blinded by success. The techniques used in the 1960s to qualify materials (limited *in vitro* studies, 12- to 104-week animal studies, 2-year human clinical studies; see Chapter 18 and Chapter 19) are still current practice in the early 2000s. This is despite the widespread use of biomaterials in long-term clinical applications that, in at least one device type (total hip replacement; Malchau et al. 2002), exceed 25 years in individual and group patient experience. It appears that two critical aspects of the study of biomaterials have been neglected: the epidemiology and human physiology of biomaterials.

I2.1.1   Epidemiology of Biomaterials

Continuing to study the success and failure of implanted materials in experiments with animals numbering in the tens and twenties, biomaterials researchers have largely overlooked the vast clinical "experiments" under way in which thousands, in many cases tens or hundreds of thousands, of human patients receive virtually identical biomaterials as chronic implants. A Center for Disease Control survey performed in 1988 (Moss et al. 1991)* suggests that as many as 14.5 million people, or nearly 1 in 20 in the U.S., had permanent implants. With the exception of occasional reports of clinical failures and studies of the materials aspects of retrieved devices, almost nothing is known about biomaterials' performance in these implants in the human clinical environment. Dependable incidence and prevalence data on the devices are hard to obtain; such data on the materials from which they are made, including their exact (not merely specified) composition and processing, are still essentially nonexistent.

Today, making the same mistake as certain penologists who, wishing to know about crime, study only failed criminals (that very small nonrandom proportion of the criminal population actually apprehended, convicted, and incarcerated), one persists in studying only random device failures. Even these limited studies, based upon clinical or postmortem retrievals, are frequently incomplete, focusing on the clinical features of the failure or upon the physical attributes of the failed device, depending upon the background and interests of the principal investigator, but rarely dealing with both aspects in a balanced way.

Recent increased interest in studying outcomes of surgical procedures (change in patient lifestyle, satisfaction level, relative cost, etc.) rather than merely the success of the procedure (rated as excellent, good, etc. on largely subjective bases) may improve matters, but only if accurate information on the implant and its materials of construction is made part of the permanent

---

* As this is written in 2005, it is odd, bordering on the bizarre, that Moss et al. 1991, which is based upon data that is now 17 years old (!), remains the most reliable source of such data for the U.S. experience with permanent implants. This stands in stark contrast to many other countries in which device registries and resultant up-to-date statistics are now available for periods exceeding two decades of clinical use.

clinical record. Suggestions have been repeatedly made concerning the need for registration systems for implants in the U.S. so that this information may follow patients as they move from place to place. Countries with national health services, such as the U.K., have had some success in developing such national registries. National systems exist for registration of certain classes of implants such as hip replacements — for example, in Sweden (from 1979) and Norway (from 1987).

However, countries with predominantly private health care systems, such as the U.S., have encountered difficulties in establishing such systems. Numerous proposals have been made for a national system for all permanent implants in the U.S. (Black 1996; see also Chapter 22). An important contemporary effort is one sponsored by the American Academy of Orthopedic Surgeons (Maloney 2001), but it has been very slow to get under way, even on a pilot basis, due to concerns about protection of patient confidentiality (Maloney 2004). Some medical device manufacturers maintain registries of their products, but access to these is severely restricted. Efforts by profit and nonprofit private concerns have floundered after a few years due to their voluntary and incomplete nature.

12.1.2 Human Physiology of Biomaterials

One would be quick to discount the knowledge of a nephrologist who based his or her entire understanding of human renal function on the study of healthy rats, rabbits, dogs, and an occasional human autopsy specimen. Fortunately, professional nephrologists have a vast armamentarium of *in vivo* tests that permit them to study the physiology of the functioning human kidney in health and in disease. The biomaterials scientist, when addressing functioning human implants, lacks all but the most rudimentary of these capabilities: clinical imagining, using primarily single-plane x-rays. The pH, pO_2, interfacial stresses, etc. in the vicinity of a functioning implant and the ranges of values that assure long-term success or predict imminent failure cannot be stated with any certainty.

However, it is possible to obtain such data, at least in animal models. Baranowski and Black (1987) reported repetitive *in vivo* measurement of pH and pO_2, associated with successful and unsuccessful stimulation of bone growth, near active and inactive implanted stainless steel electrodes in the tibial medullary canal of rabbits. With care and well-designed protocols, such techniques could be extended to studies in human subjects, especially with the increasing development of microcatheters and arthroscopes. Already, as discussed in Chapter 15, studies are being performed to detect and quantify metal-bearing species associated with implants in human patients. Early studies even suggest a correlation between elevations in serum concentrations and loosening of implants (Jacobs et al. 1991), although the relationships between cause and effect remain unclear.

I2.2   An Example: Total Hip Replacement

Even in the absence of clinical epidemiology and the development of clinical tests of biomaterials' performance, it is still possible to gain some knowledge from current clinical experience. A clinical internship and, if possible, continuing contact with a clinical population can be extremely valuable for a biomaterials scientist or engineer, especially if he or she is prepared to be observant and analytical in approach. It is probably possible in any clinical implant application to produce a list of symptoms (radiographic, clinical, or histological findings) and associated putative mechanisms leading to implications or conclusions concerning the clinical performance of the implanted materials. Table I2.1 presents such a triple listing for a frequent orthopaedic procedure: total replacement of the hip. Note that other device-related clinical findings are possible; those listed are believed to be directly referable to the biomaterials used in or in conjunction with the device rather than to device design, surgical technique, or patient use factors.

TABLE I2.1

Materials-Associated Findings in Total Hip Replacement

Finding	Mechanism	Implication
Radiographic		
PMMA fragments (early)	Operative debris	Third-body wear; single-cycle fracture
PMMA fragments (late)	Fatigue	Third-body wear; cup loosening
PMMA mantle fracture (early)	Inadequate bony support; single-cycle fracture	Stem subsidence; loosening
PMMA mantle fracture (late)	Inadequate bony support; fatigue	Stem subsidence; loosening
Broken cerclage wire	Fatigue	(early) Trochanteric dislodgement, nonunion, wire migration; (late) wire migration
Stem deformation	Plastic deformation	Change in bony support; inadequate stem size or yield point; impending failure
Stem, cup, or cup screw fracture	Fatigue	Manufacturing defect; chronic mechanical overload; (early) inadequate bony support; (late) change in bony support
Eccentric cup-head centers	Plastic deformation; wear	UHMWPE creep; uniform wear; spalling?
Loose metallic debris	Wear	Third-body wear; fretting (loose component)
	Fatigue ± corrosion	Inadequate processing of porous coating

(continued)

TABLE 12.1 (CONTINUED)

Materials-Associated Findings in Total Hip Replacement

Finding	Mechanism	Implication
Loose ceramic debris	Cracking	Component impingement, subluxation, recurrent dislocation
Focal lytic lesion[a]	Particle phagocytosis	Excessive wear debris; endotoxin?
	Immune response?	Metal sensitivity? (both) Progressive failure?
Progressive dissecting lesion[a]	Osteoclasis	Excessive wear debris; metal sensitivity? Neoplasm?
Clinical		
Intraoperative hypotension	Central control	Methyl methacrylate (monomer) sensitivity? Fat embolism?
Hip pain[a]	Immune response	Metal sensitivity?
	Venous blockade	Excessive wear
Bursa formation	Local inflammation	Metal sensitivity?
Ectopic calcification	Wear debris nucleation?	Excessive wear
Dermatitis	Delayed hypersensitivity?	Metal sensitivity?
Eczema	Delayed hypersensitivity?	Metal sensitivity?
Bronchospasm	Delayed hypersensitivity?	Metal sensitivity?
Histologic		
Fibrous capsule	Local host response	Normal response
Histiocytosis with multinuclear cells	Chronic inflammation	Manufacturing defect; inappropriate material; excessive wear
Lymphocytic infiltration with plasma cells	Delayed hypersensitivity?	Metal sensitivity? Polymer sensitivity?
Fibrosarcoma	Neoplastic transformation	Chemical neoplasia?
Lymphoma	Neoplastic transformation	Chemical neoplasia?
Rhabdomyosarcoma	Neoplastic transformation	Chemical neoplasia?
Malignant fibrous histiocytoma	Neoplastic transformation	Chemical neoplasia?
Osteosarcoma	Neoplastic transformation	Chemical neoplasia?

[a] In absence of infection.

Note: ? = possible mechanism or implication.

Source: Adapted from Black, J., *Orthopedic Biomaterials in Research and Practice*, Churchill–Livingstone, New York, 1988, 319.

I2.3   A Final Word

Many of the basic sciences underlying the field of biomaterials science and engineering have been neglected. When issues of long-term survival of biomaterials *in vivo* are considered, the lack of attention to epidemiology and physiology still remains a key issue. Unless researchers become more careful and observant of clinical performance, biomaterials may, indeed, as Elaine Duncan suggested, become endangered species and one will hear more often, "'And there are no data,' he said."

References

Baranowski, T.J., Jr. and Black, J., The mechanism of faradic stimulation of osteogenesis, in *Mechanistic Approaches to Interactions of Electric and Electromagnetic Fields with Living Systems*, Blank, M. and Findl, E. (Eds.), Plenum Press, New York, 1987, 399.

Black, J., *Orthopedic Biomaterials in Research and Practice*, Churchill–Livingstone, New York, 1988, 319.

Black, J., "And there are no data, he said," *Biomater. Forum*, 12(4), 9, 1990.

Black, J., Overview of PMS in an international perspective: global developments and global cooperation, *Int. J. Risk Safety Med.*, 8, 3, 1996.

Boretos, J.W., *Concise Guide to Biomedical Polymers: Their Design, Fabrication, and Molding*, Charles C Thomas, Springfield, IL, 10, 1973.

Boretos, J.W. and Pierce, W.S., Segmented polyurethane: a polyether polymer, *J. Biomed. Mater. Res.*, 2, 121, 1968.

Duncan, E., Editorial: endangered species? *Biomater. Forum*, 12(3), 4, 1990.

Jacobs, J.J. et al., Release and excretion of metal in patients who have a total hip-replacement component made of titanium-base alloy, *J. Bone Joint Surg.*, 73A, 1475, 1991.

Malchau, H. et al., The Swedish Total Hip Replacement Register, *J. Bone Joint Surg.*, 84A Suppl 2, 2, 2002 (Erratum: *J. Bone Joint Surg.*, 86A, 363, 2004).

Maloney, W.J., National Joint Replacement Registries: has the time come? *J. Bone Joint Surg.*, 83A, 1582, 2001.

Maloney, W.J., Personal communication, 2004.

Moss, A.J. et al., *Advance Data No. 191*, (PHS) 91-1250. U.S. Government Printing Office, Washington, D.C., 1991.

Stokes, K.B. and Chem, B., Polyether polyurethanes, biostable or not? *J. Biomater. Appl.*, 3, 228, 1988.

Stoppert, J.R. (1989), Letter cited in Duncan, E., *Biomater. Forum*, 12(3), 4, 1990.

Zhao, Q. et al., Cellular interactions with biomaterials: *in vivo* cracking of prestressed Pellethane 2363-80A, *J. Biomed. Mater. Res.*, 24, 621, 1990.

Bibliography

Finerman, G.A.M. et al. (Eds.), *Total Hip Arthroplasty Outcomes*, Churchill–Livingstone, New York, 1998.

Fraker, A.C. and Griffin, C.D. (Eds.), *Corrosion and Degradation of Implant Materials: Second Symposium*, ASTM Special Technical Publication 859, American Society for Testing and Materials, Philadelphia, 1985.

Hench, L.L. and Wilson, J. (Eds.), *Clinical Success of Skeletal Prostheses*, Chapman & Hall, London, 1995.

Improving medical implant performance through retrieval information, *Current Bibliographies in Medicine*, 99-5, National Library of Medicine, Washington, D.C., 2000.

Improving medical implant performance through retrieval information: challenges and opportunities, National Institutes of Health Technology Assessment Conference Summary, Technology Assessment Statement 19, 2000.

Leir, H.K., *Casebook: Alien Implants*, Dell, New York, 2000.

Syrett, B.C. and Acharya, A. (Eds.), *Corrosion and Degradation of Implant Materials*, ASTM Special Technical Publication 684 American Society for Testing and Materials, Philadelphia, 1979.

Weinstein, A., Horowitz, E. and Ruff, A.W. (Eds.), *Retrieval and Analysis of Orthopedic Implants*, NBS Special Publication 472, U.S. Government Printing Office, Washington, D.C., 1977.

Weinstein, A. et al. (Eds.), *Implant Retrieval: Material and Biological Analysis*, NBS Special Publication 601, U.S. Government Printing Office, Washington, D.C., 1981.

Part IV

Methods of Testing for Biological Performance

17

In Vitro Test Methods

17.1 Test Strategies

Biological performance, as defined in Chapter 1, has two aspects: material response and host response. Because the traditional approach has been to define biological performance in terms of biocompatibility (host response), and then to observe evidence of material degradation that arises during *in vitro* and *in vivo* testing, the development of tests has concentrated upon those that measure host response. In practice this has not been a bad course of events. Despite the uncertainties in both areas, it is still easier to predict material response than to predict host response. Thus, it remains a good strategy to proceed through the following five steps in early biomaterial qualification studies:

- Select candidate materials based upon engineering properties and previous material and host response information.
- Experimentally determine whether the host response is satisfactory (acceptable) for the intended application.
- Carefully watch for evidence of unacceptable material response during the conduct of host response studies.
- Verify satisfactory material response (for the material selected) during long-term *in vivo* implant studies if it is relevant to the application.
- Be responsive to clinical reports that may reflect changes in material response in actual service.

That is, given an adequate *a priori* level of expected material response, it is still more appropriate to expend a larger effort on determining host rather than material response. The selection of *in vitro* host response tests for materials qualification will be dealt with in Chapter 19.

17.2 *In Vitro* Test Types

A broad range of materials is available and only a very small percentage has been used in biological environments; thus, there has been a continual need for quick screening methods that can be used *in vitro*. These can be divided into two general classes:

- Tissue culture methods
- Blood contact methods (for blood contact applications)

Within each of these classes are a wide variety of tests and variations of test methods. Some variations are traditional for particular applications and others are the practice of a particular laboratory. Thus, these types of methods can only be considered in a general way.

17.3 Tissue Culture Tests

17.3.1 Generic Methods

Tissue culture refers collectively to the practice of maintaining portions of living tissue in a viable state *in vitro*. There are three generic methods:

- Cell culture: the growth of initially matrix-free, disassociated cells. This method closely parallels the methods used to grow bacteria *in vitro*. Cells may be grown in solution or on agar or other media substrates. Exposure to biomaterials may be through direct contact with bulk materials, diffusional contact through an agar (or other gel) intermediate layer, or by inclusion of particles or extracts or elutants from materials in the culture media.
- Tissue culture: the growth of portions of intact tissue without prior cellular dissociation. This method usually utilizes a substrate rather than a suspended technique. Exposure to biomaterials is similar to that for true cell culture.
- Organ culture: the growth of intact organs *in vitro*. This may vary from the use of fetal bone explants that can survive without external support systems to the use of whole, adult, perfused organs such as the kidney or heart. Again, a variety of exposures to biomaterials is possible.

As Rae (1980) has pointed out, each of these generic methods involves compromises and deviations from *in vivo* conditions. These problems will be discussed further in the next section.

17.3.2 Problems Inherent in Tissue Culture

Several key points concern the use of tissue culture techniques. The principal difference between *in vivo* and *in vitro* conditions, after noting the obvious humoral one (lack of access to pathways to and from remote locations in the intact animal) is the failure of local blood circulation and lymphatic drainage. Tissue in culture media can interchange materials only by diffusion. Diffusion distances must be quite short or otherwise toxic effects will be seen; this is obvious because cells *in vivo* are never more than a few hundred microns distant from a capillary. Even quite modest volumes of tissue will show central or focal necrosis due to a diffusional limit on nutrients or waste products. For this reason, tissue culture as a field is often referred to as a study of cell death. The use of cell culture (rather than tissue or organ culture) minimizes these effects until cell densities rise to levels associated with frequent intercellular contact.

Associated with diffusional problems and lack of humoral components is the general observation that, perhaps as a consequence, metabolic rates *in vitro* are always lower than those *in vivo*. Even in the absence of necrosis, cell, tissue, and organ culture conditions are inhibitory, with an initial maximum effect and a significant residual effect. Some of this inhibition may be an accidental result of growth in 21% oxygen because many cells *in vivo* are acclimated to much lower oxygen tensions. Although less active *in vitro* than *in vivo*, all cells display cell type specific growth rates. Unfortunately, fibroblasts retain quite high replication rates *in vitro*, so even a small contamination of specimen with a slower replication rate, such as a neural cell culture, may result in a "weedy" overgrowth of these unwanted cells.

Most tissue culture models attempt to maximize cell metabolism by growing cells in monolayers (to provide easy exchange with large fluid volumes) and by adding various stimulatory agents (fetal or neonatal serum, vitamin C, etc.) and preservation agents (α-tocopherol [vitamin E]), antibiotics, fungicides, etc.). Fortunately, most cells are contact inhibited and thus form monolayers easily in culture; this condition is called confluence and is characterized by a relatively constant cell number. Cell monolayers are not, in general, subject to diffusion limits. Although these agents improve the viability and longevity of tissue culture models, their formation produces still greater differences between *in vitro* and *in vivo* conditions.

The morphology and the function of cells *in vivo* depend to a degree on the chemistry of the pericellular environment and the nature of the substrate (matrix) supporting and surrounding the cells (see Section 11.3). Lack of these environmental factors may cause cells to become inactive or to revert, at least functionally, to more primitive (less committed) types. An example is the chondrocyte; if it is grown in an agar gel, it retains its appearance and biosynthetic function, but if it is cultured on a typical matrix-free surface, it rapidly takes on fibroblastic shape and synthetic function. Related to this problem is the previously noted recognition that cells frequently exist *in vivo* in regions of mixed interdependent cell types, such as in bone marrow or the cerebral cortex. In such situations, cell shape and function may depend in part on interaction with other cell types; this may be reproduced in cell culture by coculture: growing more than one cell type in a common container — in some cases, with permeable barriers to isolate individual cell types geographically but not diffusionally.* Such coculture may be necessary to demonstrate *in vitro* complex processes such as bone matrix mineralization.

Another, less well appreciated difference from *in vivo* conditions is the absence of external mechanical strain on cells. Particularly in the musculo-skeletal, respiratory, and cardiovascular systems, *in vivo* cells are subjected to a broad spectrum of mechanical forces and deformations, which may be transduced directly or perhaps through electromechanical intermediate signals. It is possible to reproduce the effects of these mechanical stimuli in a limited way by culturing cells on membranes subject to various cyclic deformations. This is now a common enough practice that commercial devices have been developed.

Finally (and this cannot be overemphasized), cell culture results cannot be useful or relevant, even in preliminary screening for local host response, unless care is taken in selection of the biomaterial samples being evaluated. Earlier (Section 2.6), I pointed out the need to replicate processing, cleaning, and sterilization conditions expected in the clinical application. However, in designing tissue culture studies, one must include other important considerations. These include:

- Selection of the appropriate cell type (especially for implants intended to be placed internal to specific organs such as heart, liver, etc.)
- Consideration of the dosage aspect of exposure because cells may tolerate materials at low exposures but be adversely affected at high dosages (Shanbhag et al. 1994)
- Usage of appropriate forms of the biomaterial and its expected degradation products in the proposed application

17.3.3   Cell Types and Observations

Cell types may vary in activity and properties between species — within species, between individuals, and within a specific cell line — between generations. In the scientific literature, one finds references to cell types with designations such as "P1534 leukemic cells." These citations refer to cells from established cell lines available from the American Type Culture Collection (ATCC)** (Hay 1983) or similar sources. These organizations isolate, characterize, and preserve (by ultrafreezing) uniform cell populations. One may order specimens from particular generations (passages) of these cells

---

* Although such arrangements vary widely between experimenters, they are referred to generically as Boyden chambers, after their original developer (Boyden 1962).
** http://www.atcc.org/.

and grow them in the laboratory for use in testing. In general, the lower the generation number is (often referred to as the passage number), the more the cells will resemble those *in vivo* in appearance and function. With care, the use of established cell line techniques screens out a large component of biological variability.

An alternate approach is to use freshly derived cells or so-called primary cultures. Such cultures are more vigorous than maintained cell lines; however, they are difficult to prepare in a repeatable manner, are usually poorly characterized, and (as previously noted) may suffer from overgrowth of faster growing or "weed" cells, such as fibroblasts.

Tissue culture techniques, as a group, may be used to study the following aspects of host responses:

- Cell survival: toxicity; organelle and membrane integrity
- Cell reproduction: growth inhibition
- Metabolic activity: energetics, synthesis, and catabolism
- Affective activity: inhibition of locomotion, chemotaxis, and phagocytosis; alteration of cellular size, shape, and appearance
- Cell damage: chromosomal aberration, mutagenicity, and carcinogenicity

Tissue culture techniques for screening materials may use one or more normal mammalian cell lines such as murine macrophages, abnormal cells such as HeLa or lymphoma cells, or bacterial cell lines such as *Staphylococcus aureus* or *Escherricia coli*. Each test that has been developed uses selected cells suitable for the particular questions posed.

17.3.4 Examples of the Use of Tissue Culture in Materials Evaluation

A classic example of such studies (Galin et al. 1975) illustrates the general approach. In this case, cultures of rabbit kidney cells were used to investigate the toxicity of several types of ocular implants. The implants were exposed to the cells directly by placement on a gel-supported cell monolayer and indirectly by inclusion in media in which the cells were cultured. Toxicity was assayed by observations of progressive cell death in the monolayer and by cellular changes in culture.

Galin's study examined the host response to a fabricated implant. Similar tests may be used to study biomaterials in unfabricated forms or to observe host response to degradation products such as wear debris. An early example of the latter is the work of Cohen and coworkers, who examined tissue culture response to finely divided particles of implant alloys as models for wear debris and corrosion product release. A number of cell lines were used and the effects of the metallic debris and debris supernatant on cell counts in the replication phase (Pappas and Cohen 1968) and in the lag phase (Mital and Cohen 1968) were obtained. The authors concluded that using lag phase cell counts to detect direct toxicity was more sensitive than lumping toxicity and growth and replication inhibition together.

It has been suggested that the primary effects seen in the exposure of polymeric biomaterials to cells in tissue culture are due to low molecular weight species that diffuse out of the biomaterial. Thus, many techniques use the material as well as extracts of the material prepared with various hydrophilic and hydrophobic solvents. A study by Homsy et al. (1970) examined this issue by autoclaving a number of specimens in a pseudoextracellular fluid (PECF) for 62 hours at 115° and then using the PECF supernatant as a challenge for cultures of cells derived from newborn mouse hearts. In addition, specimens of the supernatant were analyzed quantitatively to determine the total concentration of $-CH_3$, $-CH_2$, and $-CH$ radicals present. A total of 22 polymers were studied (Table 17.1). A comparison of cellular toxicity of the supernatant with the concentration of organic radicals eluted from the polymer showed a strong positive correlation that apparently overwhelms the details in differences between the chemistries of individual polymers. Thus, Homsy and colleagues suggested that this tissue culture method and/or an analysis of a PECF supernatant may be used as rapid, reliable screening techniques for new polymers.

17.3.5   Use of Tissue Culture for Host Response Screening

As previously noted, Rae (1980) discussed the pros and cons of various approaches to cell, tissue, and organ culture methods in the general determination of biocompatibility of implant materials. The present consensus is that these techniques are best used to measure early, acute response to materials.

However, the real utility of *in vitro* culture techniques depends to a great degree on their correlation with *in vivo* local host response. Many attempts have been made to correlate *in vitro* cell culture studies with results of animal exposure studies. For example, Wilsnack (1976) used an ATCC human fibroblast cell line, WI-38, to examine the *in vitro* cytotoxicity of a large number of polymeric materials and compared the results with responses in rabbits to systemic and local injections of soluble material eluted with saline solution and with cottonseed oil, according to USP methods (see Section 20.2.1). He concluded that the *in vitro* test was more sensitive than the *in vivo* one selected (yielding more examples of cytoxicity); however, correlation between *in vitro* and *in vivo* results was poor when both were positive. In this case, one can point to reasons other than inherent inadequacies in cell culture to explain disparities between *in vitro* and *in vivo* results: different species, single cell line vs. multiple cell types, solid materials vs. eluted materials, etc. This example illustrates the difficulties in extrapolation from *in vitro* biological tests. However, Johnson and Northup (1983) attempted a similar correlation, but with fewer differences between techniques: they

TABLE 17.1

Correlation between Tissue Culture Response to PECF and PECF Chemical Analysis[a]

Polymer[b]	Tissue Culture Response[c]	Total -CH$_3$, -CH$_2$, and -CH in PECF by IR Analysis (mpm[d] equivalent n-hexanol)
Silicone (Silastic™ 372)	+1	5
Polyethylene (U. of Texas)	+1	17
Fluorinated ethylene propylene (type 1)	+1/+2	nd[e]
Polyphenylene oxide (type 1)	+1/+2	27
Polyethylene (type 1)	+2	nd[e]
Acrylic molding powder	+2	nd[e]
Polyphenylene oxide (type 2)	+2	17
Polyethylene (type 2)	+2	17
Fluorinated ethylene propylene (type 1)	+2	23
Ionomer (type 1)	+2	142
Polypropylene (food grade)	+2	198
Vinylidene fluoride	+2/+3	3
Nylon™(grade 101)	+2/+3	14
Ionomer (type 2)	+2/+3	30
Cellulose proprionate	+3	81.7
Polystyrene	+3	168
Nylon™ (grade 38)	+4	12
Poly(vinyl)chloride	+3/+4	277
Polyurethane (type 1)	+4	89
Polyurethane (type 2)	+4	328
Poly(vinyl)chloride (U. of Texas)	+4	514
Acrylonitrile, butadiene, styrene (ABS)	+4	516

[a] Polymer exposed to PECF for 62 h @ 115°C, 30 psia.
[b] See Homsy, C.A. et al., *J. Macromol. Sci.-Chem.*, A4(3), 615, 1970, for a more complete description of polymers.
[c] Scale: +1 = some vacuolization, morphological changes, and growth inhibition; +2 = moderate vacuolization, morphological changes; +3 = severe growth inhibition and vacuolization; +4 = total growth inhibition.
[d] Moles per million.
[e] Not detected.

conducted a "battery" of four *in vitro* tests using an ATCC murine fibroblast cell line, L-929, and compared the results with the local response to 7-day rabbit intramuscular implantation. Each test outcome was ranked 1+ to 4+ and pass/no pass (fail) criteria were established. The results of several of their test series are summarized in Table 17.2.

Wieslander et al. (1990) extended these studies and examined the effects of elution conditions. They suggested that testing using a combination of water extracts obtained at elevated temperatures and physical contact between cells and material produced the most reliable results.

In vitro tests have come to be seen as screening tests serving as precursors for more involved, costly, and time-consuming animal implantation. A secondary use, resulting from extensive correlative investigations such as those

TABLE 17.2

Correlation between *In Vitro* Screening
Tests and Short-Term Implantation

		Implantation	
		Pass	Fail
In vitro:	Pass	94.7%	—
	Fail	—	5.3%

$N = 687$.

Source: Adapted from Johnson, H.J. and North-up, S.J., in *Cell-Culture Test Methods, ASTM STP 810*, Brown, S.A. (Ed.), American Society for Testing and Materials, Philadelphia, 1983, 25.

of Johnson and Northup (1983), is for batch-to-batch quality control by materials or device manufacturers.

These three studies and similar ones make use of a single *in vitro* cell line. In fact, the ATCC L-929 cell line has come to be a *de facto* standard for *in vitro* testing of biomaterials and is used in several ASTM *in vitro* host response test methods, such as F-813 and F-895 (see Chapter 20). However, a more favored approach is that of generating a cell culture spectrum (CCS). In this technique, a number of different cell lines are used and are challenged by the biomaterial (or extracts of the biomaterial) being studied in one or more standard exposure techniques. The cell types are selected to represent a variety of origins and sensitivities. The response of each of perhaps six cell types is then quantified. An index based upon these quantitative findings is thus a CCS reflection of relative acute host response. A consensus CCS would be more sensitive in revealing differences between acute host response of different materials. It can be hoped that, in the future, this method can be fully developed, tested, and adopted by the ASTM and CCS indices developed for all current biomaterials. Then new materials can be compared, insofar as acute response is concerned, by application of this test protocol and reference to a table of standard results.

Although not reflecting consensus, a number of screening protocols in use today utilize cell culture methods, with biomaterials or eluted materials as the challenge, in evaluation of a quantitative host response to implant materials. For instance, primary testing (level 1) as utilized by Autian (1977) uses five tissue culture tests as a portion of a 14-test initial battery that results in the derivation of a cumulative toxicity index (CTI). The culture tests involve one direct exposure model and four tests using extracts. Dillingham (1983) has shown that these five tests produce significant degrees of correlation with the *in vivo* tests incorporated in the CTI.

Northup (1986) has provided a useful summary of early efforts to use cell culture techniques for the study of the generalized features of local host response.

17.3.6 Delayed Hypersensitivity Tests

Immune system (specific) response to biomaterials is extremely difficult to evaluate *in vitro*. Numerous claims have been made about the ability to screen individuals for hypersensitivity to foreign materials by challenging cell-free serum with foreign materials and detecting the resulting antigen–antibody complexes. These claims are probably groundless in a biomaterials host response context for two reasons: first, freely circulating antigens are associated with humoral rather than the expected T-cell-mediated response to foreign nonproteinaceous materials (see Section 12.3); second, any response that occurs *in vivo* is to a complexed or opsinized material rather than to the material itself.

In vitro testing for T-cell-mediated type 4 delayed hypersensitivity is possible, again depending upon use of an appropriate challenge agent. The most reliable technique is the leukocyte migration inhibition factor (MIF) test (Merritt and Brown 1980) (Section 12.4.2). Like the supposed humoral response tests, however, this test is more a test of the prior sensitization of a test animal or individual subject than of the ability of a specific material to induce immune sensitization. Hallab et al. (2000) have summarized the use of *in vitro* tests based upon leukocyte migration and concluded that those based upon the transmembrane cell migration, as in the Boyden (1962) chamber approach, appear best suited for studies in which multiple comparisons need to be made among subjects and/or materials and involving sequential repetitions of measurements.

Proper conduct of this type of *in vitro* test requires considerable care and the availability of known nonsensitive, nonimplanted animals or individuals as longitudinal control donors. Care must be taken with all of these tests to avoid spurious results due to possible inhibitory and/or cytotoxic properties of the challenge agents used (see also Chapter 12). Other *in vitro* tests have been used to examine immune sensitivity to biomaterials with varying degrees of success (Merritt 1986).

17.3.7 Mutagenicity and Carcinogenicity Tests

The use of tissue culture in evaluation of biomaterials has centered on studies of acute toxicity and of inhibition of growth or activity. Considerations of carcinogenic potential of materials discussed in Chapter 13 suggest the need for a rapid screening test for neoplastic transformation. Such tests exist, but are quite controversial.

It is now generally accepted that chemical carcinogenesis proceeds by a mutagenic route, with the neoplastic attributes heritable. Thus, any confirmed carcinogens are expected to be mutagens as well. However, because the converse is not yet proven — that is, that all mutagens have the potential of being carcinogens — the controversy over tests for carcinogenicity tends to focus on interpretation of the results.

TABLE 17.3

Results of Validation of Ames Test

Status of Agent	Number Tested	Number Mutagenic (%)
Reported Animal carcinogens	176	158 (90)
Reported Human carcinogens	18	16 (89)
Reported Animal noncarcinogens	108	13 (12)

Source: Adapted from Ames, B.N., *Science*, 204, 587, 1979.

The most widely used test method depends upon evidence of mutagenesis as an index of carcinogenic potential. This test, the Ames test (Ames et al. 1975), is conducted in the following way. A culture is prepared with a mutant bacterial cell line (usually *Salmonella typhimurium*) that requires histidine for growth. It is grown in histidine-free culture with the material to be tested and a fresh preparation of rat liver cell homogenate. This provides enzyme systems that will detect potential mutagenic materials that require metabolic conversion to mutagens. Only cells that then mutate back to the more normal histidine-independent state can multiply.

This test has been used widely and its results have been shown to have very strong correlations with carcinogenic potential. Ames (1979) reported on a study of 302 chemicals; the results are summarized in Table 17.3. The finding of 12% "false" positives was discussed by Ames, who suggested that a number of these may be weak carcinogens that were not previously detected by (less sensitive) animal tests. This high degree of correlation between mutagenicity and carcinogenicity (McCann et al. 1975) has suggested to many workers that the Ames test has a useful role in early material screening.

The Ames test has a number of attractive attributes. It is inexpensive, quick, and relatively safe. By exposing approximately 10^6 organisms to a mutagen, it can detect transformation rates far below those possible in any reasonable animal test. Furthermore, it has been shown to be able to detect any of the recognized mutagenic mechanisms. However, it has been strongly criticized. Ashby and Styles (1978) had difficulty in reproducing Ames' results, especially at low mutagen concentrations. They suggest that the sensitivity of the test is lower than Ames asserted and also feel that correlations between mutagenic potency and carcinogenic potency should be viewed with extreme caution.

More recent general criticism of this and other tests of potential neoplastic transforming agents has focused on the practice of the use of high doses of challenge materials, which may also be directly cytotoxic. High doses are frequently used to improve statistical response and reduce cost, followed by extrapolation of effects to low doses. Many workers have suggested that cytotoxicity encourages unnaturally elevated rates of cell replication, thus artificially enhancing the rate of production of transformed cells and leading to a too high risk after extrapolation (Epstein and Swartz 1988).

It is clear that the Ames test, in common with other tissue culture tests, must be done with great care. Precautions (DeSerres and Shelby 1979) should include the use of multiple bacterial strains, multiple suspension systems, a wide range of doses of material under evaluation, and use of positive and negative controls in each study. The need for careful control of the form and chemical composition of the material being studied was demonstrated by Abbracchio et al. (1982), who showed that crystallinity plays a key role in the biological response to particulate metal sulfides.

The need for great care in conducting the test in order to duplicate Ames' results, as well as more fundamental criticisms concerning the relationship between mutagenicity and carcinogenicity, led Purchase et al. (1978) to compare six *in vitro* and *in vivo* tests for carcinogenic potential of organic compounds. They concluded that the Ames type of test is highly accurate (93% accurate in predicting animal carcinogenesis in their study vs. 90% for Ames, 1979) (Table 17.3); however, they also concluded that

> The inclusion of the [other] four tests in a screening battery predictably resulted in a great increase in overall inaccuracy and loss of discrimination, even though the detection of carcinogens is increased. All tests were shown to generate both false positive and false negative results, a situation which may be controlled by the use, where possible, of chemical-class controls, to identify the test which is optimal for the class of chemical under test.

That is, they suggest that the use of compounds of similar structure as positive and negative controls permits validation and selection of specific tests from a battery of tests.

Forster (1986) has reviewed *in vitro* mutagenicity testing with special reference to evaluation of biomaterials. Despite the inherent shortcomings of the test methods and the need to adapt them to the material in question and the potential application, he suggests that *in vitro* mutagenicity tests should play a role in any screening study of biomaterials. The strategy, then, should be much the same as that for the use of tissue culture tests of toxicity.

17.4 Blood Contact Tests

17.4.1 General Comments

Materials problems in cardiovascular devices are primarily those of initial or short-term inadequate biological performance due to the acute nature of the host response to foreign materials in the cardiovascular system. Chapter 9 previously considered the principal problems of coagulation of blood and lysis of blood-borne cells. These problems not only are intrinsic to materials but also are extrinsically related to design features such as the presence of interfaces, inappropriate flow rates, and localized turbulence conditions, as well as overall device function.

Thus, it is hard to divorce the problems of determining host response to materials for blood contact applications from the details of device design and qualification. Materials testing, insofar as host response is concerned, can be separated into three types of tests: *in vitro* static, *ex vivo* dynamic, and *in vivo* dynamic. These are usually applied sequentially to a new material or to a material being considered for a new application. It is important to note with regard to this last comment that considerable regional variations exist in environment in the cardiovascular system. It is well recognized that a material that works well in a high-flow arterial application often fails in a static venous site.

Initial testing for host response to blood contact materials is usually done *in vitro*. Despite the wide recognition of the inadequacy of these tests, they continue to be used on a screening basis for two reasons:

- They are relatively inexpensive compared with *in vivo* tests.
- They are not known to yield false negatives; that is, a material that does poorly in these screening tests will not be a satisfactory implant material in cardiovascular applications.

These tests are generally of a comparative type and examine coagulation times or hemolysis rates in static or dynamic systems during or after contact with foreign materials.

17.4.2   Static Tests

Of the static tests, the Lee–White and the Lindholm tests are best known (Lindholm et al. 1973; Mason 1973; Mason et al. 1974). The reference material is usually silicone-coated soft glass. Although this is not a satisfactory material for implant use due to its mechanical properties, it is perhaps the best inexpensive test material with a low and reproducible host response. Few materials in use as cardiovascular implant materials exceed the biological performance of this material *in vitro*. Repeated efforts have been made to develop and widely distribute standard reference materials, such as low-density polyethylene (LDPE) and polymethylsiloxane (PDMS) (Bélanger et al. 2001), but they have generally been unsuccessful. Thus, the tests described in this and the next section are more useful for comparing new materials with older materials within a single study, using selected positive and negative "reference" materials, rather than providing intrinsic measurements of host response.

The thrombotic potential of a surface is usually evaluated by timing the development of clot in a static situation and comparing this time for clot development, to the same point of maturity, for blood drawn simultaneously from the same source (donor) and exposed to one or more reference surfaces.

Adequate testing requires considerable replication in specimens in a single test and in repetition of tests on different days, with different donors, etc. A canine donor is usually used, although some investigators have used human volunteer donors.

Hemolysis can be determined simultaneously in such a static test by centrifugation of the clotted blood followed by optical spectrophotometric measurement of the hemoglobin content of the supernatant serum. Again, it is usual to compare the results obtained with a test material and reference materials using blood drawn at one time (ASTM International [2004]: F756-00). If the hemolysis rate is deemed acceptable for the intended application on an *in vitro* screening basis, then more detailed static testing may be performed, such as determination of complement activation (ASTM International [2004]: F1984-99 ; F2065-00) and alteration of leukocyte morphology (ASTM International [2004]: F2151-01) by biomaterial contact. Unfortunately, like all blood response studies, these are effectively restricted to evaluation of materials in solid (nonparticulate, nonsoluble) form.

17.4.3   Dynamic Tests

It is extremely difficult to evaluate coagulation effects of biomaterials on blood *ex vivo* because the growth of the thrombus interferes with flow dynamics in the system external to the donor and may have potential lethal effects on the donor. A short-term solution to this problem that is only applicable to relatively thromboresistant materials is to determine the density of adhered platelets after a brief exposure under controlled flow conditions (Skarja et al. 1997). Arguing from knowledge of the role of platelets in the intrinsic and common pathways (Figure 9.1), one can then predict relative coagulation rates (Grabowski et al. 1977).

A further sophistication can be afforded by the wide variety of standard *in vitro* quantitative assays available for the vast majority of factors involved in the coagulation cascade. Such a study is performed by obtaining a blood specimen, testing it for the presence of a clotting factor, and retesting after brief, timed exposure to the test material (and a reference material), in much the same manner as testing for complement activation (see previous section). Although these tests are very precise, their specificity is unclear because it is difficult to predict coagulation outcomes from the change in concentration of any one factor.

If the material to be evaluated does not promote significant coagulation, hemolysis can be quantified by exposing the surface to blood briefly, in a transient mode, or over a longer period, in a stable *ex vivo* system. Erythrocyte damage is determined by direct analysis of released hemoglobin or by counting the percentage of erythrocyte "ghosts" in a blood smear. In animal *ex vivo* models, this test can be improved by prelabeling erythrocytes with $^{51}Cr^{+6}$. This method takes advantage of the easy penetration of Cr^{+6} through cell membranes and its intracellular conversion to Cr^{+3} that is then only released if the cell wall is disrupted. Then, the ^{51}Cr activity in cell-free serum samples is a direct measure of hemolysis. Again, adequate testing requires comparison with a standard surface and repetition of the test with a number of donors. This approach is based on historic use of ^{51}Cr^{+6} in clinical determination of blood volumes; however, modern concerns about the biological activity of Cr[VI] now limit it to animal subjects.

In vitro and *ex vivo* tests share a number of problems. The biggest of these is the nonstandard nature of blood. Blood is an extremely variable material. Its coagulation and lytic response depend upon species, health of the individual donor, diet, medication, and age, among other factors. Even the act of drawing blood may change the host response capabilities of the donor's blood, thus rendering the use of a standard donor extremely misleading. Therefore, all *in vitro* tests for blood–biomaterial interactions must lean heavily on isochronal comparisons of the test material with a widely used negative reference material such as siliconized glass and repeated tests using different donors.

Another problem is the inability to reproduce implant site blood dynamics *ex vivo*. Even the use of reasonable vessel sizes and flow rates based on study of the planned implant site may prove misleading. The details of the properties of the vascular intima near the implant site have a profound influence on the actual flow conditions, as do the features of the final implant/host configuration. Thus, although some success is encountered in static and single, or one-pass, *in vitro* tests, those based upon continued flow and observations over a period of hours show poor correlation with *in vivo* performance.

Nonetheless, these one-pass and continued-flow tests, in which a direct connection between an animal's or patient's circulatory system is created, are collectively termed *ex vivo* tests and, as the second type of test, are becoming increasingly popular. *In vitro* or *ex vivo* tests for screening purposes are no more than screening tests. They must be followed up by well-designed *in vivo* testing, which is the subject of the next chapter.

A major effort to evaluate and compare *in vitro* (as well as *ex vivo* and *in vivo*) tests was made by a working group originally assembled by the National Heart Lung Blood Institute in 1985 (Harker et al. 1993).

17.5 Final Comments

The tone of this chapter may seem overly pessimistic, especially when read against the background of the previous interpart on clinical study of biomaterials. Certainly, all biomaterials workers wish for the ease and precision of the medical diagnostic tools seen on StarTrek but then return to the laboratory to struggle with the inadequacies of established *in vitro* test methods. It is probably the case that development and improvement of test methods for *in vitro* or *ex vivo* prediction of host response has continued to be neglected in recent years because this topic is not especially novel or attractive to public or private funding agencies. Courtney et al. (1994), Charissoux et al. (1996), and Kirkpatrick et al. (1998) have discussed these general issues in more detail; Hanks et al. (1996) and Schmalz (1997) have addressed issues specific to applications in the oral cavity.

However, even the crude methods presently available have much to commend them due to low cost, relative speed and ease of conduct, and low risk to participants. Therefore, I suggest — especially given an increased societal sensitivity to the use of animals in medical research — that renewed interest and effort in this area might be richly rewarded.

References

Abbracchio, M.P., Heck, J.D. and Costa, M., The phagocytosis and transforming activity of crystalline metal sulfide particles are related to their negative surface charge, *Carcinogenesis*, 3, 175, 1982.

ASTM International, Standard practice for assessment of hemolytic properties of materials, F756-00, in *2004 Annual Book of ASTM Standards*, Vol. 13.01: *Medical Devices; Emergency Medical Services*, ASTM International, West Conshohocken, PA, 2004.

ASTM International, Standard practice for testing for whole complement activation in serum by solid materials, F1984-99, in *2004 Annual Book of ASTM Standards*, Vol. 13.01: *Medical Devices; Emergency Medical Services*, ASTM International, West Conshohocken, PA, 2004.

ASTM International, Standard practice for testing for alternate pathway complement activation in serum by solid materials, F2065-00, in *2004 Annual Book of ASTM Standards*, Vol. 13.01: *Medical Devices; Emergency Medical Services*, ASTM International, West Conshohocken, PA 2004.

ASTM International, Standard practice for assessment of white blood cell morphology after contact with materials, F2151-01, in *2004 Annual Book of ASTM Standards*, Vol. 13.01: *Medical Devices; Emergency Medical Services*, ASTM International, West Conshohocken, PA, 2004.

Ames, B.N., Identifying environmental chemicals causing mutations and cancer, *Science*, 204, 587, 1979.

Ames, B.N., McCann, J. and Yamasaki, E., Methods for detecting carcinogens and mutagens with the salmonella/mammalian-microsome mutagenicity test, *Mutat. Res.*, 31, 347, 1975.

Ashby, J. and Styles, J.A., Does carcinogenicity potency correlate with mutagenic potency in the Ames assay? *Nature*, 271, 452, 1978.

Autian, J., Toxicological evaluation of biomaterials: primary acute toxicity screening program, *Artif. Organs*, 1(1), 53, 1977.

Bélanger, M.-C. et al., Hemocompatibility, biocompatibility, inflammatory, and *in vivo* studies of primary reference materials low-density polyethylene and polydimethylsiloxane: a review, *J. Biomed. Mater. Res. (Appl. Biomater.)*, 58, 467, 2001.

Boyden, S., The chemotactic effect of mixtures of antibody and antigen on polymorphonuclear leukocytes, *J. Exp. Med.*, 115, 453, 1962.

Charissoux, J.L. et al., Development of *in vitro* biocompatibility assays for surgical material, *Clin. Orthop. Rel. Res.*, 326, 259, 1996.

Courtney, J.M. et al., Biomaterials for blood-contacting applications, *Biomaterials*, 15, 737, 1994.

DeSerres, F.J. and Shelby, M.D., The Salmonela mutagenicity assay: recommendations, *Science*, 203, 563, 1979.

Dillingham, E.O., Primary acute toxicity screen for biomaterials, in *Cell-Culture Test Methods, ASTM STP 810*, Brown, S.A. (Ed.), American Society for Testing and Materials, Philadelphia, 1983, 51.

Epstein, S.S. and Swartz, J.B., Carcinogenic risk estimation, *Science*, 240, 1043, 1988.

Forster, R., Mutagenicity testing and biomaterials, in *Techniques of Biocompatibility Testing*, Vol. II, Williams, D.F. (Ed.), CRC Press, Boca Raton, FL, 1986, 137.

Galin, M.A., Chowchuvech, E. and Galin, A., Tissue culture methods for testing the toxicity of ocular plastic materials, *Am. J. Opthalmol.*, 79, 665, 1975.

Grabowski, E.F. et al., Platelet adhesion to foreign surfaces under controlled conditions of whole blood flow, *Trans. Am. Soc. Artif. Intern. Organs XXIII*, 141, 1977.

Hallab, N. et al., Hypersensitivity to metallic biomaterials: a review of leukocyte migration inhibition assays, *Biomaterials*, 21, 1301, 2000.

Hanks, C.T. et al., *In vitro* models for biocompatibility, *Dent. Mater.*, 12(3), 186, 1996.

Harker, L.A., Ratner, B.D. and Didisheim, P. (Eds.), *Cardiovascular Materials and Biocompatibility, Cardiovas. Pathol.* 2(3) (Suppl.), 1993.

Hay, R.J., Availability and standardization of cell lines at the American Type Culture Collection, in *Cell-Culture Test Methods, ASTM STP 810*, Brown, S.A. (Ed.), American Society for Testing and Materials, Philadelphia, 1983,114.

Homsy, C.A. et al., Rapid *in vitro* screening of polymers for biocompatibility, *J. Macromol. Sci.-Chem.*, A4(3), 615, 1970.

Johnson, H.J. and Northup, S.J., Tissue-culture biocompatibility testing program, in *Cell-Culture Test Methods, ASTM STP 810*, Brown, S.A. (Ed.), American Society for Testing and Materials, Philadelphia, 1983, 25.

Kirkpatrick, C.J. et al., Current trends in biocompatibility testing, *Proc. Inst. Mech. Eng.*, 212(H), 75, 1998.

Lindholm, D.D., Klein, E. and Smith, J.K., Relative thrombogenicity of blood interface materials: methods and results, *Proc. Dialysis Transplant Forum*, 3, 39, 1973.

Mason, R.G., Blood compatibility of biomaterials: evaluation of a simple screening test, *Biomater. Med. Dev. Artif. Organs*, 1(1), 131, 1973.

Mason, R.G. et al., Blood compatibility of biomaterials: further evaluation of the Lindholm test, *Biomater. Med. Dev. Artif. Organs*, 2(1), 21, 1974.

McCann, J. et al., Detection of carcinogens as mutagens in the Salmonella/microsome test: assay of 300 chemicals, *Proc. Nat. Acad. Sci.*, 72(12), 5135, 1975.

Merritt, K., Immunological testing of biomaterials, in *Techniques of Biocompatibility Testing*, Vol. II, Williams, D.F. (Ed.), CRC Press, Boca Raton, FL, 1986, 123.

Merritt, K. and Brown, S.A., Tissue reaction and metal sensitivity, *Acta Orthop. Scand.*, 51, 403, 1980.

Mital, M. and Cohen, J., Toxicity of metal particles in tissue culture. Part II: a new assay method using cell counts in the lag phase, *J. Bone Joint Surg.*, 50A, 547, 1968.

Northup, S.J., Mammalian cell culture methods, in *Handbook of Biomaterials Evaluation.*, von Recum, A.F. (Ed.), Macmillan, New York, 1986, 209.

Pappas, A.M. and Cohen, J., Toxicity of metal particles in tissue culture. Part I: a new assay method using cell counts in the phase of replication, *J. Bone Joint Surg.*, 50A, 535, 1968.

Purchase, I.F.H. et al., An evaluation of six short-term tests for detecting organic chemical carcinogens, *Br. J. Cancer*, 37, 873, 1978.

Rae, T., A review of tissue culture techniques suitable for testing biocompatibility of implant materials, in *Advances in Biomaterials*, Vol. 1: *Evaluation of Biomaterials*, Winter, G.D., Leray, J.L. and de Groot, K. (Eds.), John Wiley & Sons, Chichester, U.K., 1980, 289.

Schmalz, G., Concepts in biocompatibility testing of dental restorative materials, *Clin. Oral Invest.*, 1(4), 154, 1997.

Shanbhag, A.H. et al., Macrophage/particle interactions: effect of size, composition, and surface area, *J. Biomed. Mater. Res.*, 28, 81, 1994.

Skarja, G.A. et al., A cone-and-plate device for the investigation of platelet biomaterial interactions, *J. Biomed. Mater. Res.*, 34, 427, 1997.

Wieslander, A., Magnusson, Å. and Kjellstrand, P., Use of cell culture to predict toxicity of solid materials in blood contact, *Biomater. Artif. Cells Artif. Org.*, 18(3), 367, 1990.

Wilsnack, R.E., Quantitative cell culture biocompatibility testing of medical devices and correlation to animal tests, *Biomater. Med. Dev. Artif. Org.*, 4(3–4), 235, 1976.

Bibliography

Anderson, D., An appraisal of the current state of mutagenicity testing, *J. Soc. Cosmet. Chem.*, 29, 207, 1978.

Autian, J., The new field of plastics toxicology — methods and results, *CRC Crit. Rev. Toxicol.*, 2, 1, 1973.

Brown, S.A. (Ed.), *Cell-Culture Test Methods, ASTM STP 810*, American Society for Testing and Materials, Philadelphia, 1983.

Douglas, J.F., *Carcinogenesis and Mutagenesis Testing*, Humana Press, Totowa, NJ, 1984.

Grandjean–Laquerriere, A. et al., Importance of surface area ratio on cytokines production by human monocytes *in vitro* induced by various hydroxyapatite particles, *Biomaterials*, 26, 2361, 2005.

Hanson, S.R., Blood–material interactions, in *Handbook of Biomaterial Properties*, Black, J. and Hastings, G. (Eds.), Chapman & Hall, London, 1998, 545.

Helgason, C.D. and Miller, C.L., *Basic Cell Culture Protocols*, 3rd ed., Humana Press, Totowa, NJ, 2004.

Kitchin, K.T., *Carcinogenicity: Testing, Predicting, and Interpreting Chemical Effects*, Marcel Dekker, New York, 1999.

Kleinschmidt, J.C. and Hollinger, J.O., in *Bone Grafts & Bone Substitutes*, Habal, M.B. and Reddi, A.H. (Eds.), W.B. Saunders, Philadelphia, 1992, 133.

Moroff, G., Methods for evaluating alterations in platelet and red cell properties, in von Recum, A.F. (Ed.), *Handbook of Biomaterials Evaluation*, 1st ed., Macmillan, New York, 1986, 233.

Rice, R.M. et al., Biocompatibility testing of polymers: *in vitro* studies with *in vivo* correlations, *J. Biomed. Mater. Res.*, 12, 43, 1978.

Venitt, S., Crofton–Sleigh, C. and Forster, R., Bacterial mutation assays using reverse mutation, in Venitt, S. and Perry, J.M. (Eds.), *Mutagenicity Testing: A Practical Approach*, IRL Press, Oxford, 1984, 45.

Venitt, S. and Perry, J.M. (Eds.), *Mutagenicity Testing: A Practical Approach*, IRL Press, Oxford, 1984.

von Recum, A.F. (Ed.), *Handbook of Biomaterials Evaluation*, 1st ed., Macmillan, New York, 1986; 2nd ed., Taylor & Francis, Boca Raton, FL, 2004.

Waters, R., DNA repair tests in cultured mammalian cells, in Venitt, S. and Perry, J.M. (Eds.), *Mutagenicity Testing: A Practical Approach*, IRL Press, Oxford, 1984, 99.

Wennberg, A. et al., A method for toxicity screening of biomaterials using cells cultured on millipore filters, *J. Biomed. Mater. Res.*, 13, 109, 1979.

Wilson, R.S. et al., Blood–material interactions: assessment of *in vitro* and *in vivo* test methods, in *Techniques of Biocompatibility Testing*, Vol. II, Williams, D.F. (Ed.), CRC Press, Boca Raton, FL, 1986, 151.

Yuspa, S.H., Tumor promotion in epidermal cells in culture, in *Mechanisms of Tumor Promotion*, Vol. III: *Tumor Promotion and Carcinogenesis in Vitro*, Slaga, T.J. (Ed.), CRC Press, Boca Raton, FL, 1984, 1.

18

In Vivo Implant Models

18.1 Introduction

18.1.1 Approaches to *In Vivo* Tests

After acute screening by physical or biological *in vitro* techniques, it is the practice to test new implant materials, or old materials in significantly different applications, in extended-time, whole-animal tests. Although the use of nonhuman species involves many limitations and compromises, it is the common judgment that such tests involving the exposure of materials to systemic physiological processes are a necessary practical and ethical precedent to human clinical testing.

With the exception of materials for application in the cardiovascular system, the site chosen for initial nonfunctional (see Section 18.2.1) testing is usually in soft tissue. This decision is based on the assumption that cytotoxic effects have a generality of action and because soft tissue sites can be approached in animals with relatively minor surgery. For these reasons, the peritoneal cavity (Wortman et al. 1983) and subcutaneous "air pouch" (Willoughby et al. 1986) have been widely used as sites for acute *in vivo* screening studies. For joint replacement or fracture fixation applications, initial implantation is in cortical and, occasionally, cortico-cancellous bone. Specialized sites such as the cornea and the cerebral cortex are used for materials intended for specific, limited applications.

Chick embryo and fetal rodent models have been used; however, most testing now uses mature, higher animals. Although still used in multispecies tests, rodents are rarely used alone since the experience of the Oppenheimers (see Chapter 13). A variety of sites have been used for chronic testing; the most popular ones are:

- Subcutaneous
- Intramuscular (e.g., supraspinatus)
- Intraperitoneal

- Transcortical (e.g., femur, tibia, and cranium)
- Intramedullary (e.g., femur and tibia)

Functional testing (see Section 18.2.2) requires a wider range of species due to the specific requirements of the material or device configuration selected. No single species presents an ideal general model for the human species, and some human structural functions, such as patellar motion, are not attainable in animal models. Anderson and Hughes (1986) provide a still relevant overview to the problems of selection of appropriate animal models.

18.1.2   Animal Welfare

In recent years, the use of animals in medical research has come under strong criticism from a number of organizations, particularly People for the Ethical Use of Animals (PETA).* This criticism, strident at times, tends to ignore two key features of animal use:

- Investigators are generally sensitive individuals concerned about the well-being of their test subjects.
- Sound research applicable to problems of human disability and disease requires that the test subjects, of whatever species, generally be healthy and not subject to avoidable stress (unrelated to the experimental design).

Nevertheless, there is now a well-developed system for monitoring and controlling animal research in the U.S. The enabling legislation is the Animal Welfare Act (7 USC 2131, December 23, 1985) and a final regulation issued by the U.S. Department of Agriculture regarding inspection and compliance (Dept. of Agriculture 1991). The requirements of the Animal Welfare Act are summarized in an NRC publication (National Research Council, 1996) that should be on the desk** of any investigator involved in research using animals. The central points of this system of regulation and inspection are:

- Research involving animals may be performed only under a prospective protocol that describes the purpose and significance of the experiment; the species, source, and number of animals to be studied; the procedures to be performed; and the general care and housing conditions of the experimental animals and identifies the personnel involved in animal experimentation and animal care and the qualifications of these personnel.

---

* http://www.peta.org.
** Also available online: http://oacu.od.nih.gov/regs/guide/guidex.htm.

- The protocol must be reviewed and approved before initiation by an institutional animal care committee, although this review applies only to the animal welfare aspects of the protocol and not the scientific content or objectives of the study.
- The facilities in which surgical and experimental procedures are performed and animals are housed must meet specific minimum requirements.
- The personnel, including students, who conduct the procedures, must be adequately trained and prepared.
- The animal housing facilities and all procedures involving animals must be under the supervision of a veterinarian.

Additionally, standards are set forth concerning specific housing requirements (cage type, size, etc.) for each species and for the provision of veterinary care to minimize pain and treat conditions unrelated to the experiment.

The vast majority of U.S. fund-granting agencies and organizations now require that research proposals be reviewed before submission to determine that they meet the requirements of the Animal Welfare Act. This is a worthwhile and humane system that may at times seem burdensome to the investigator, particularly because some institutional review committees have experienced confusion when trying (in many cases mistakenly) to balance concerns about animal welfare against the scientific and technological requirements of the proposed studies. This occasionally produces the unusual result of withholding permission to perform procedures on animals that are routine in human clinical practice, such as multiple procedures on the same individual. However, such reviews are necessary because of societal requirements and ethical considerations, and their conduct emphasizes the investigator's professional and ethical responsibilities for experimental animals.

If the *in vivo* testing is intended to support future claims of safety in the clinical use of the material used in fabricating the animal implants, additional requirements are imposed by the Good Laboratory Practices (GLPs) regulation of the U.S. Food and Drug Administration.* Although these practices generally describe good procedures for conducting research, three sections explicitly relate to animal care facilities and the provisions made for care within them. Although these generally duplicate the provisions of the Animal Welfare Act, the overall requirements imposed by the GLPs make safety studies difficult to perform in university or other educational settings. Such studies are often more easily carried out by one of the commercial enterprises that have sprung up in recent years.

Three additional ethical responsibilities must be emphasized at this point:

- The general obligation is to avoid unnecessary use of animals as experimental subjects. Part of the decision to use an animal model

---

* http://www.access.gpo.gov/nara/cfr/waisidx_01/21cfr58_01.html. 2001 CFR Title 21, Vol. 1, Part 58.

should involve careful *a priori* investigation (and rejection) of alternative approaches (cell culture; mechanical, electronic, or computational simulations; etc.).

- A determination should be made that the experiment has not been done before or that reliable data are not available from other sources.
- Once a determination has been made to use animals and a surgical model has been selected, the experiment should be designed to use the minimum but sufficient number to provide a reasonable assurance of a statistically valid result. Failure to provide adequate prospective statistical design in an animal experiment can lead to the need to replicate the experiment and, in some cases, to use a significantly larger total number of animals than would have been required by a better thought out approach. In this regard, sequential designs that use a few animals to work out experimental design and procedure uncertainties before larger statistically valid main experiments are done are strongly recommended.

The National Institutes of Health (U.S.) now provide an extramural competitive grant program for development of alternatives to the use of animals in drug and biomaterials evaluation. In some areas, this has resulted in significant progress, as in the development of a number of cell and tissue culture screening techniques as candidates to replace the Draize rabbit ocular irritation test (Curren and Harbell 1998). However, more complex clinical applications, especially those involving blood contact and/or chronic implantation, will probably always require the use of animal testing before there is sufficient confidence in safety to conduct initial human studies.

18.2   Test Types

18.2.1   Nonfunctional Tests

Tests divide globally into two types: functional and nonfunctional. In the nonfunctional type, the implant is of an arbitrary shape, perhaps in a form required for later mechanical tests of material response, and "floats" passively in the tissue site. Ferguson et al. (1960) popularized the prototype for such tests. This is a supraspinatus implantation in the rabbit in a cavity produced by blunt dissection, followed by a 16-week observation period. This test series formed the basis for a peer-reviewed, national-consensus protocol now in use, the F 981 method of the American Society for Testing and Materials (ASTM, 2004b) (see Chapter 18, Appendix 1).

Nonfunctional tests focus on the direct interactions between the substance of the material and the chemical and biological species of the implant environment. The absence of mechanical loads and other elements of function

limits the usefulness of such tests. Thus, they tend to be of short to intermediate duration, usually a few weeks to 24 months in length. For these results
and those of later functional tests to be useful predictors of biological performance in patients, the implants must be in a condition as close as possible
to the physical and chemical condition proposed to be used in the final
clinical application. Care must be taken, especially in cleaning and sterilization, because surface contaminants may affect the host response (Greenfield
et al. 2005).

A typical short-term study of this type is described in the British Standards
Institute Method BS 5736, part 2 (1981). This test protocol utilizes 1- × 10-
mm strips of material, with positive and negative controls, implanted by
blunt stylet in the paravertebral (supraspinatus) muscle of the rabbit and
recovered by sacrifice after 7 days. Thus, although it is an *in vivo* method, it
evaluates only acute soft-tissue response. Turner et al. (1973) have shown
that such a 7-day model, although capable of producing false negatives,
produces no false positives (when compared with local host response to 12
weeks), thus justifying the use of this model for acute *in vivo* screening. A
similar updated procedure for 7-, 30-, and 90-day studies is F 763 (ASTM,
2004a). To examine more fully the effects of systemic physiology on material
and host response, a longer term study of materials that pass such a short-
term *in vivo* screen is needed.

F 981 (Chapter 18, Appendix 1) illustrates the typical course of such a
longer term study. Standard-sized implants fabricated from the material in
question, as well as one or more well-characterized comparative control
materials, are used. They are selected so as to come close to SA/BW ratios
for major implantation in humans (see Section 15.4.4), at least for soft-tissue
sites. The method uses muscle sites in the rat, rabbits, and larger animals,
as well as femoral transcortical sites, if indicated by the proposed application.
Rats are maintained and sacrificed at 12, 26, and 52 weeks postimplantation.*
Evaluation consists primarily of inspection of the test and control implants
and the sites of implantation.

At present, no control materials for the F 981 protocol are universally
available. The method specifies the use of a number of metals and one
ceramic and one polymer that have a long history of experimental evaluation
and human clinical use as reference or control materials. However, individual variations in composition, surface properties, etc. in these materials make
intertest comparisons difficult. There is considerable continuing interest in
developing positive and negative metallic and polymeric controls that might
be made available through a national program such as the Standard Reference Material program administered by the National Institute of Standards
and Testing (NIST). No reference standards for studies of porous implants
are currently recognized.

---

* Previous practice had been to use dogs when larger species were needed and to utilize a 2-year
implantation period in addition. Improved understanding of host response has permitted the
routine use of alternative large animal species such as sheep and goats and eliminated the 104-
week sacrifice period as redundant in most cases. See SectionX1.9, Appendix 1 (Chapter 18).

Major defects in the design and practice of F 981 have been recognized. Notwithstanding its strong position as a consensus test method providing standardized results that can be compared with others (Escalas et al. 1975)* even when variants from the method are used, these shortcomings must be recognized. In its concentration on study of the implant site, F 981 overlooks systemic or remote site effects unless they are extreme enough to produce visible morbidity or mortality. Thus, remote site neoplastic transformation will not be seen in this test even if adequate implantation time has elapsed. Additionally, implantation times are probably too short in the rabbit or dog, or even the rat, to overcome latency effects (see Section 13.2.5). Furthermore, for practical reasons, the numbers of test animals used are so small that even observation of a tumor at the implant site or at a remote site cannot be evaluated statistically with any acceptable level of certainty. Thus, the method is unsuited for yielding information beyond the magnitude of the acute and chronic inflammatory processes and subsequent fibrotic responses.

A question can be raised about the quantitative significance of the fibrotic response. Measurement of capsule thickness in muscle-site implant studies tends to show large variances. In most studies, differences must exceed 25 µm to be statistically significant. This result is usually ascribed to "biological" variation. A study (Kupp et al. 1982) suggests a different explanation. In this study, sites were identified in the rat hind quarter that produced considerable motion between implant and muscle (intermuscular) when the leg was moved passively from full extension to full flexion and that produced negligible relative motion (intramuscular). The relative degrees of motion in the two sites were verified radiologically. Spherical capped cylindrical implants of a polyester (PE) and a polyacetal (PA) were placed in each of these two sites, and capsule mean thicknesses were studied at 21 days. The results are given in Table 18.1.

A one-way analysis of variance (ANOVA) was performed, using the method of contrasts. A near significant effect of motion may be seen in the response to PA (25.1 vs. 14.1 µm) (H_2). However, the greater intrinsic reactivity of PE masks this effect (H_1). This greater reactivity may be seen by comparison of the minimal motion sites, a more usual place for implant evaluation (24.3 vs. 14.1 µm) (H_3). An apparent additive effect of motion in the maximal motion implant site masks this difference (H_4). Thus, capsule thickness seems to reflect the additive response to two factors: an intrinsic (chemical) activity and an extrinsic (mechanical) activity.

It is clear from this study that relative tissue-implant motion may have a large influence on the observed capsule thickness. It may be that specimen geometries should be changed in this type of test or the specimen secured to the surrounding tissue to minimize such motion variables. Experiments of this sort are called two-factor experiments because they examine effects related to chemical and mechanical factors. For more complete evaluations,

* Escalas et al. (1975) used a precursor method, ASTM F 361. See Rationale (X1), Appendix 1 (Chapter 18) for a more complete discussion.

TABLE 18.1

Interaction of Intrinsic Reactivity and Motion in Implant Capsule
Thickness

	Motion	
	Minimal[a]	Maximal[b]
Material	Thickness of Capsule (mean ± S.E.M.)	
PE	24.3 ± 2.9 μm	31.4 ± 2.7 μm
PA	14.1 ± 2.8 μm	25.1 ± 3.5 μm

	ANOVA Contrasts	
Hypothesis	F	Significance
H_1: $T_{pe,min} = T_{pe,max}$	2.05	$p > 0.2$
H_2: $T_{pa,min} = T_{pa, max}$	3.07	$p = 0.125$
H_3: $T_{pe,min} = T_{pa, min}$	3.01	$p = 0.125$
H_4: $T_{pe,max} = T_{pa,max}$	0.60	$p > 0.5$

[a] 0.00 ± 0.07 cm.
[b] 0.18 ± 0.07 cm.

Source: Kupp, T. et al., in *Advances in Biomaterials, Vol. 3: Biomaterials 1980*, Winter, G.D., Gibbons, D.F. and Plenk, H., Jr. (Eds.), John Wiley & Sons, Chichester, 1982, 787.

one must move to three-factor experiments that include (or control for) electrical effects. Thus, in this study, it may have been the case that differing electrical charge densities at the polymer–tissue interfaces could account in part for the observed effects.

The findings of Kupp and colleagues (1982) are particularly important when one is considering host response to the implant's degradation products, such as wear debris or precipitated corrosion products, rather than to the implant. Several models utilizing deliberate imposed motion at the implant–tissue interface demonstrate effects on materials response (Overgaard et al. 1996) and host response (Howie et al. 1988).

In any case, implant shape must be carefully selected and standardized for each test protocol to avoid effects on capsule thickness associated with surface features of the biomaterial. It has long been recognized that sharp edges on an implant produce a locally increased capsule thickness. Thus, when a flat-ended cylinder is used (Wood et al. 1970), the familiar dog-bone shaped capsule results from a local thickening over the circular edges of the rod ends. This effect has been more generally studied by Matlaga et al. (1976), and it has been shown that tissue response is inversely related to the included angle at the edge of the implant. Finally, all soft-tissue sites, in any given species, are probably not equivalent in terms of the fibrous response evoked by an implant (Bakker et al. 1988).

One might further point out that observation of capsule thickness is an indirect measure of cellular response. Dillingham (1983) has shown a good correlation between capsular response and *in vitro* cytotoxicity; however, a useful addition to this type of test might be to evaluate the concentration and spatial distribution of cellular enzymes directly (Salthouse and Willigan 1972; Salthouse and Matlaga 1975).

Even if a refined histochemical evaluation system is not used, it might be a good idea to evaluate tissue around animal implants in a more detailed way than simply by measuring capsule thickness. Salthouse (1980) has suggested using a scheme that incorporates a number of observations into an overall index, analogous to the CTI approach of Autian (1977) in his level 1 test scheme. The scheme suggested by Salthouse is a modification of one proposed by Gourlay et al. (1978), which is based upon the earlier work of Sewell et al. (1955). An outline of the method is given in Chapter 18, Appendix 2. The advent of modern image analysis systems now permits the use of quantitative measures of tissue response (Hunt and Williams 1995); however, earlier semiquantitative grading scales still remain in use.

In the long run, the most severe criticism of F 981 is its nonfunctional aspect. Even when this drawback is offset by selecting tissue sites more typical of the application — for instance, in the rabbit cornea for intraocular applications — the results remain inferior in providing confidence in prediction of human clinical experiences to those obtained from functional tests.

An alternate approach is to isolate the material from the tissue so as to remove the mechanical features and examine the chemical (and presumably electrical) effects on cellular aspects of local host response directly. Perhaps the best known example of this approach is the cage implant system developed by James Anderson and his students (Marchant 1989; Kao and Anderson 1998). In this case, the implanted material is placed within a wire or mesh enclosure and, after appropriate sterilization, implanted. This "cage" will rapidly fill with a mixture of extracellular exudate and inflammatory cells. The fluid may be sampled from time to time by transdermal puncture and analyzed for enzymatic and cellular content, and a chronological picture can be built of the local response to the implant. Although elegant in conception and widely applied by its originators, the major criticism of this approach is that the local host response to the implanted material is that of cells already exposed to the cage material, which is usually different in composition and surface condition. Although it is possible to overcome this problem by fabricating the enclosure from the same material as that of the test specimen; in the general case this is difficult and costly.

18.2.2   Functional Tests

18.2.2.1   *General Requirements and Problems*

Functional tests require that, in addition to being implanted, the material, at least in some degree, be placed in the functional mode that it would experience in human implant service. This is required to study, for instance, tissue ingrowth into porous materials for fixation purposes, formation of neointima in vascular processes, and production of wear particles in load-bearing devices (and possible clinically relevant tissue response to them).

Functional tests are obviously of much greater complexity and cost than nonfunctional ones. Simple devices have been designed to exert dynamic loads typical of the desired application on the material. An example of this approach is the dynamic aortic patch (von Recum et al. 1978) for evaluating materials for cardiac assist devices in the canine aorta.

Tests of materials for partial or total joint replacements present different problems. In some cases, small human implants may be used directly, as in the case of insertion of a phalangeal interphalangeal (PIP) joint in the fore leg of a cat (Woodman et al. 1983). On the other hand, the design of a completely functional animal version of the proposed device is frequently required. Design, fabrication, mechanical testing, and implantation of these devices may be more difficult than the final production of the device for human use. In both cases, problems arise from the small size of economically priced animals, differences in animal anatomy, and the inability of the animal "patients" to cooperate actively with the experiment.

Despite these difficulties, total hip joint replacement designs, for example, have been made and tested in rats, cats, dogs, sheep, and goats. Figure 18.1 illustrates the evaluation of a fibrous material for fixation by bony ingrowth. Initial tests utilized nonfunctional, cylindrical transcortical plugs. This was followed by implantation of a proximal medullary device that permitted mechanical "pull-out" testing to evaluate the shear strength of the interface, albeit under essentially unloaded conditions. Finally, the material was incorporated into a custom designed tibial component for a fully functional canine total knee replacement (Berzins et al. 1994; Rivero et al. 1988).

In some cases, veterinary models of implants exist that can be used as material test devices. Figure 18.2 is a radiograph of a total hip implanted in a cat. The femoral component is a modified small size of a canine femoral (Gorman) prosthesis; the UHMWPE cup was custom designed and is held in a metallic retainer attached to the iliac crest with bone screws.

In other cases, a human clinical design can simply be scaled down to a suitable size for an animal. Figure 18.3 illustrates a metallic femoral component designed for cemented total hip replacement in 450-g rats, maintained at constant skeletal dimensions by dietary control (Powers et al. 1995). The head diameter is 2 mm; advantage was taken of rodentine anatomy to implant the devices functionally (head placed medially) and nonfunctionally (head placed laterally). One of the advantages of such small implants and test animals is that full histological sections may be made with the components in place.

Fracture fixation designs have been tested in all of the species mentioned earlier, as well as in larger ones such as cows and horses. For such relatively small devices in larger species, it is often possible to use actual human dimension prototype models rather than having to produce modified designs.

Particular problems arise in each of these test methods. Some difficulties, however, are common to all of them. Considerable interspecies variation is found in the histological appearance of tissue. Additionally, local tissue conditions that are abnormal in some species may be chronic in others.

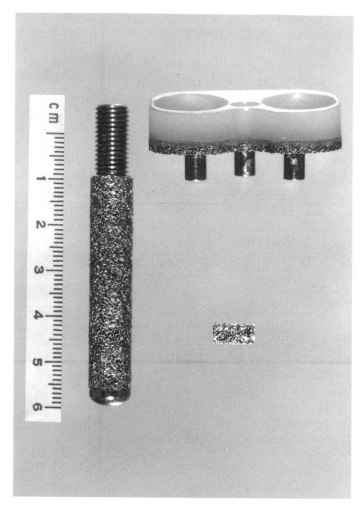

FIGURE 18.1

Specimens for canine evaluation of fiber metal (titanium) as an ingrowth material. Clockwise from bottom: transcortical plug, medullary pullout specimen (Ti6Al4V substrate), tibial component for total knee replacement (Ti6Al4V substrate and pins, ultra high molecular weight polyethylene articular surface). (From Berzins, A. et al., *J. Appl. Biomater.*, 5(4), 349, 1994; Rivero, D.P. et al., *J. Biomed. Mater. Res.*, 22, 191, 1988; previously unpublished, used by permission.)

Misinterpretations of test results, insofar as local tissue response and remote organ condition are concerned, have arisen from the involvement of clinical (rather than veterinary) pathologists in evaluation of histology from implant studies. Satisfactory and reliable evaluation of tissue from multispecies tests can only be achieved by an individual specifically trained in comparative histology and animal pathology.

The inability of animals to cooperate with treatment has already been mentioned. Specifically, it is not possible to return an animal to full activity

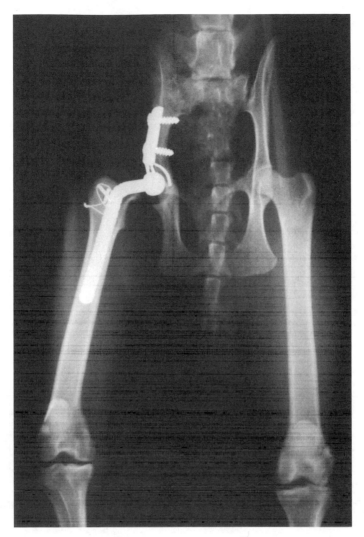

FIGURE 18.2
Radiography of feline THR. (From author's research in collaboration with D. Nunamaker. Implants provided by Richards Manufacturing, now Smith+Nephew Richards, Memphis, TN.)

on a planned schedule. The animal will move as it sees fit and set its own schedule. Similarly, an animal cannot indicate or describe internal problems of discomfort or pain. Experienced animal handlers may be able to detect early signs of pain accompanying infection or tissue reaction. More commonly, these problems are not detected until the animal is systemically ill or loses function in a limb, or, incidentally, at autopsy. The presence of culturable infection of any origin at an implant site invalidates any observations on that animal (unless an infectious agent was deliberately introduced as part of the experimental plan). Systemic infection imposes a

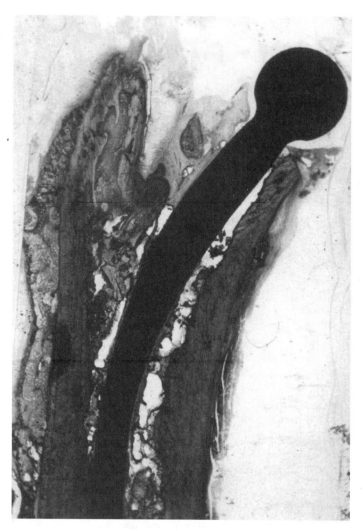

FIGURE 18.3
Section of femoral component of a rodentine total hip replacement (~25× magnification). Material: stem/head F-75 type cast CoCr alloy; cement: F 451 acrylic bone cement. (Component fabricated by DePuy, Inc., Warsaw, IN; section by L. Smith, Clemson University.)

significant stress on experimental animals, may cause weight loss, and casts doubts on the validity of observations.

Test animals such as cats, dogs, rats, etc. have shorter life spans and higher metabolic rates than humans (Brody 1945). Over and above particular variations in physiology, these factors introduce other problems of unknown magnitude. For instance, what is the appropriate factor by which to scale down an implant for an animal to experience the same apparent body load of foreign material as man does (see Section 15.4.4)? Because lifetime as well as neoplastic transformation induction times are shorter in these animals than in humans, how can these be scaled up to expected human experience? The importance of this latter point is underlined by occasionally finding implant site sarcomas in dogs in conjunction with high corrosion rate stainless steel implants in clinical veterinary practice (see Section 13.5). In dogs, these have occurred after an average implantation time of 5.8 years. What is the comparable period in man after which one should expect to see this type of tumor, if the assumption is that the transformation mechanisms are the same in both species?

Questions of this type are unresolved and are the subject of continuing research. A final question related to these interspecies differences is how long to test before true chronic conditions are realized. Although current practice is to limit chronic implant models to 1-year duration, this question remains unresolved on a universal basis. The initial expense of animals and an annual holding cost for dogs frequently exceeding $2000 per animal make this last question one of vital importance.

18.2.3 Cardiovascular Functional Tests

18.2.3.1 Material Tests

The previous comments have applied primarily to implants in locations other than in the cardiovascular system. The nature of such implants is largely functional and, as in the case of *in vitro* testing, must be discussed separately.

In vivo testing in the cardiovascular system is an extension of the *ex vivo* or dynamic type of testing previously discussed in Section 17.4.3. The simpler form of such testing is the use of an implant of an idealized geometry rather than a full-scale working device. Instead of reproducing the exact functional design of the implant, a standard design of simple geometry is used to introduce the material into a vascular process. Patches or daggers may be attached to the vascular wall in various locations — in some cases with provision for mechanical loading (von Recum et al. 1978). Sections of blood vessels may be replaced, often with devices with deliberate flow-disturbing defects in them such as in the Gott and Kusserow tests.

The Gott or canine vena cava test (Gott and Furuse 1971) is the better known of these two methods. In this technique, rings 9 mm long by 8 mm (OD), with a 7-mm-diameter lumen, are surgically inserted to replace a portion of the inferior vena cava in the dog. The rings may have a small internal constriction or web to increase blood turbulence. Groups of five animals are used with implantation periods of 2 hours and, if the initial group remains patent, 2 weeks. Evaluation is by examining patency of the rings and degree of coverage by thrombosis on removal.

The Kusserow or renal embolus test (Kusserow et al. 1970) involves replacing a portion of the suprarenal aorta with a similar ring. An infrarenal constriction is produced by partial ligation to force a large portion of the aortic circulation (an estimated 90%) through the renal arteries into the kidneys. Groups of five to eight animals are used, with implantation times of 3 days to 2 weeks. Evaluation is by examination of the rings and histological quantization of kidney infarcts secondary to emboli "shed" by the implants.

The Gott test appears more severe with respect to adherent thrombi due to lower flow rates in the canine vena cava than in the aorta, even after partial ligation. However, the Kusserow test provides better overall evaluation because it permits examination of adherent thrombus and remote emboli (in the kidney primarily), thus more closely modeling human clinical exposure.

18.2.3.2   Transitional Tests

A transitional form of this sort of testing may involve the use of a portion of a clinical design implanted in a different location in an animal. Sawyer et al. (1976) described an early example. In this study, sections of cardiac catheters intended for human clinical use were implanted as segmental replacements in jugular and femoral veins of dogs as well as being placed in the more usual location in the right atrium through right jugular insertion.

This study illustrates a feature common to most cardiovascular tests of the idealized type; that is, the response at 2 hours after implantation mirrors and closely predicts that seen at 2 weeks. It is this acute response of the cardiovascular system to foreign materials that makes functional testing so difficult. The early events are complicated by the establishment of equilibrium between material and host and by the events of trauma associated with implantation, and they are difficult to study due to the requirements to support the test animal clinically. However, from the point of view of the test and of the eventual clinical response, the acute response may be the most important. Thus, it is often said of materials tested *in vivo* for cardiovascular applications: "If they will last 2 hours, they will last 2 weeks; if they will last 2 weeks, they will last 2 years."

18.2.3.3   Device Tests

The more complex form of functional testing for cardiovascular application is the evaluation of a material fabricated into a final device design. The costs and difficulties associated with such tests can be easily appreciated. A major problem is the same as that which faces evaluation of any human clinical device: the animal implant site is not the same as the human site, so problems of comparison and scaling arise. These scaling problems are particularly acute in the case of blood contact materials because of the relative interspecies constancy of the viscosity of mammalian blood. Calves are often used for such studies; however, their continuing growth usually limits such tests to 9 months' duration. In the final analysis, materials for cardiovascular applications can only achieve qualification by tests in actual clinical applications. On the face of it, this may seem to be an insupportable position;

however, it must be recognized that such testing is always based upon two prerequisites:

- The material must first perform sufficiently well *in vitro* and in animal tests in which likelihood of success is good and chance of failure is small.
- There must be a real potential benefit to the specific patients involved in this study. (Chapter 19 deals with this point at greater length.)

Functional device tests using typical clinical geometries and methods of construction and implantation are essential to examine the effects of the details of construction on response to materials. For instance, for a new design, it is difficult to predict the rate of hemolysis that will result from relative movements of parts in a heart valve and the portion of this that can be ascribable to materials selection. In this respect, full clinical testing is highly desirable despite its risks and inherent ethical problems.

18.2.4 Human Tests

In the final analysis, clinical testing is the only technique by which the true biological performance of implantable biomaterials can be determined. In short, the only completely valid subject for study is the human being. When necessary preconditions are met (Chapter 19), human implantation will begin; the challenge is to obtain data from this experience.

The second consideration cited in the previous section — that is, that any human clinical experiment must provide a potential benefit to the patients involved — essentially prevents the use of humans as test subjects for biomaterials per se. There are very rare exceptions to this rule, as in the study of Hofmann and colleagues (1990) involving patients who were to receive staged bilateral total knee replacement arthroplasties (TKAs). During the first surgery, a TKA was performed on one side and plugs of porous implant materials were inserted in the medial femoral condyle of the opposite knee. At the second surgery 9 weeks later, the plugs were retrieved and the second TKA performed without deviation from the technique that would have been employed in the absence of the experimental implants. This study, which was approved by a local review committee (see Section 19.2.1) and for which each patient gave informed consent, probably represents the extreme limit to which the "potential benefit" principle can be stretched. The need for such tests is underlined by the observation of the investigators that their results (ingrowth of bone into porous cobalt- and titanium-base alloy plugs) did not replicate the responses seen earlier in a canine model (Hofmann 1993).

Although there is a marked lack of study of device function (and biological performance of the materials involved) in patients (as noted in Interpart 2), opportunities exist for examination of these issues during device retrieval subsequent to clinical failure or at autopsy. References to a number of such studies are provided in Interpart 2; Chapter 22 discusses them in further detail. Although engineering tests on the device to ascertain, among other data, the material response are routine, examination of the local host response is somewhat more difficult. Efforts have been made to develop comparative overall scores for local host response in parallel to those used in animal studies. The "Mirra scale" (Mirra et al. 1976) (Chapter 18, Appendix 3) or modifications of it are still in general use to describe the largely materials-mediated response of patient tissues to partial and total hip and knee replacement devices. Although it is highly desirable that this scale continue to be used (so that historical comparisons can be made), more sophisticated ones are needed, especially as materials and material configurations used in implanted clinical devices continue to change.

18.3   A Final Comment

As consensus emerges concerning qualification of new materials, better judgments about the role that each of the generic test methods will play can be made. However, animal tests of the functional and nonfunctional type play a vital part in determining material and host response in the application of biomaterials. Despite their expense, complexity, and difficulty of interpretation, they will continue to be used for the foreseeable future.

Nevertheless, it is necessary to recognize that the limitations of animal testing are becoming an increasing problem as clinical experience with established biomaterials extends. It may be that their use in development and selection of materials for novel devices and applications should be emphasized, rather than depending upon them for preclinical qualification for older materials in established or new devices. For the latter situations, an increased dependence on studying the actual clinical experience seems preferable.

References

American Society for Testing and Materials, Standard practice for short-term screening of implant materials, F 763-04, in, *2004 Annual Book of ASTM Standards, Vol. 13.01: Medical Devices; Emergency Medical Services*, ASTM International, West Conshohocken, 2004a.

American Society for Testing and Materials, Standard practice for assessment of compatibility of biomaterials for surgical implants with respect to effect of materials on muscle and bone, F 981-04, in, *2004 Annual Book of ASTM Standards, Vol. 13.01: Medical Devices; Emergency Medical Services*, ASTM International, West Conshohocken, pp. 290ff, 2004b.

Anderson, L.C. and Hughes, H.C., Experimental animal selection, in, *Handbook of Biomaterials Evaluation*, 1st ed., von Recum, A.F. (Ed.), Macmillan, New York, 1986, 255.

Autian, J., Toxicological evaluation of biomaterials: primary acute toxicity screening program, *Artif. Organs*, 1(1), 53, 1977.

Bakker, D. et al., Effect of implantation site on phagocyte/polymer interaction and fibrous capsule formation, *Biomaterials*, 9, 14, 1988.

Berzins, A. et al., Effects of fixation technique on displacement incompatibilities at the bone-implant interface in cementless total knee replacement in a canine model, *J. Appl. Biomater.*, 5(4), 349, 1994.

British Standards Institute, Evaluation of medical devices for biological hazards, BS 5736, Part 2: method of testing for tissue implantation, BSI, London, 1981.

Brody, S., Basal energy and protein metabolism in relation to body weight in mature animals of different species, in *Bioenergetics and Growth, with Special Reference to the Efficiency Complex in Domestic Animals*, Reinhold, New York, 1945, 352.

Curren, R.D. and Harbell, J.W., In vitro alternatives for ocular irritation, *Environ. Health Perspect.*, 106 (Suppl 2), 485, 1988.

Department of Agriculture, Animal welfare; standards; final rule, 9 CFR Part 3, *Fed. Reg.* 56(Feb. 15), 6426, 1991.

Department of Health and Human Services, *Guide for the Care and Use of Laboratory Animals*, NIH Publication 85-23, U.S. Government Printing Office, Washington, D.C., 1985.

Dillingham, E.O., Primary acute toxicity screen for biomaterials: rationale, in vitro/ in vivo relationship and interlaboratory performance, in *Cell-Culture Test Methods*, ASTM STP 810, Brown, S.A. (Ed.), American Society for Testing and Materials, Philadelphia, 1983, 51.

Escalas, F. et al., $MP_{35}N$: a corrosion resistant, high strength alloy for orthopedic surgical implants: bioassay results, *J. Biomed. Mater. Res.*, 9, 303, 1975.

Ferguson, A.B., Jr. et al., The ionization of metal implants in living tissues, *J. Bone Joint Surg.*, 42A, 77, 1960.

Gott, V.L. and Furuse, A., Antithrombogenic surfaces, classification, and in vivo evaluation, *Fed. Proc.*, 30(5), 1679, 1971.

Gourlay, S.J. et al., Biocompatibility testing of polymers: in vivo implantation studies, *J. Biomed. Mater. Res.*, 12, 219, 1978.

Greenfield, E.M. et al., Does endotoxin contribute to aseptic loosening of orthopedic implants? *J. Biomed. Mater. Res., Appl. Biomater.*, 72B, 179, 2005.

Hofmann, A.A, Bachus, K.N. and Bloebaum, R.D., In vivo implantation of identically structured and sized titanium and cobalt alloy porous coated cylinders into human cancellous bone, *Trans. Soc. Biomater.*, 13, 80, 1990.

Hoffman, A.A., Response of human cancellous bone to identically structured commercially pure titanium and cobalt chromium alloy porous-coated cylinders, *Clin. Mater.*, 14, 101, 1993.

Howie, D.W. et al., A rat model of resorption of bone at the cement-bone interface in the presence of polyethylene wear particles, *J. Bone Joint Surg.*, 70A, 257, 1988.

Hunt, J.A. and Williams, D.F., Quantifying the soft tissue response to implanted materials, *Biomaterials*, 16, 167, 1995.

Kao, W.J. and Anderson, J.M., The cage implant system, in *Handbook of Biomaterials Evaluation*, 2nd ed, von Recm, A.F. (Ed.), Taylor & Francis, Philadelphia, 1998, 659.

Kupp, T. et al., Effect of motion on polymer implant capsule formation in muscle, in *Advances in Biomaterials, Vol. 3: Biomaterials 1980*, Winter, G.D. Gibbons, D.F. and Plenk, H., Jr. (Eds.), John Wiley & Sons, Chichester, U.K.,1982, 787.

Kusserow, B. et al., Observations concerning prosthesis-induced thromboembolic phenomena made with an *in vivo* embolus shunt test system, *Trans. Am. Soc. Artif. Intern. Organs*, XVI, 58, 1970.

Marchant, R.E., The cage implant system for determining *in vivo* biocompatibility of medical device materials, *Fund. Appl. Toxicol.*, 13, 218, 1989.

Matlaga, B.F. et al., Tissue response to implanted polymers: the significance of sample shape, *J. Biomed. Mater. Res.*, 10, 391, 1976.

Mirra, J.M. et al., The pathology of the joint tissues and its clinical relevance in prosthesis failure, *Clin. Orthop. Rel. Res.*, 117, 221, 1976.

National Research Council, *Guide for the Care and Use of Laboratory Animals*, National Academy Press, Washington, D.C. 1996.

Nunamaker, D.M. and Black, J., Tissue response associated with ingrowth into porous stainless steel, *Trans. Orthop. Res. Soc.*, 3, 160, 1978.

Overgaard, S. et al., Role of different loading conditions on resorption of hydroxya-patite coating evaluated by histomorphometric and stereological methods, *J. Orthop. Res.*, 14, 888, 1996.

Powers, D.L. et al., The rat as an animal model for total hip replacement arthroplasty, *J. Invest. Surg.*, 8, 249, 1995.

Rivero, D.P. et al., Calcium phosphate-coated porous titanium implants for enhanced skeletal fixation, *J. Biomed. Mater. Res.*, 22, 191, 1988.

Salthouse, T.N., Personal communication, 1980.

Salthouse, T.N. and Matlaga, B.F., An approach to the numerical quantitation of acute tissue response to biomaterials, *Biomater. Med. Dev. Artif. Org.*, 3(1), 47, 1975.

Salthouse, T.N. and Willigan, D.A., An enzyme histochemical approach to the eval-uation of polymers for tissue compatibility, *J. Biomed. Mater. Res.*, 6, 105, 1972.

Sawyer, P.N. et al., Experimental and clinical evaluation of a new catheter material, *Trans. Am. Soc. Artif. Intern. Organs*, XXII, 527, 1976.

Sewell, W.R., Wiland, J. and Craver, B.N., A new method of comparing sutures of ovine catgut with sutures of bovine catgut in three species, *Surg. Gynecol. Obstet.*, 100, 483, 1955.

Turner, J.E., Lawrence, W.H. and Autian, J., Subacute toxicity testing of biomaterials using histopathologic evauation of rabbit muscle tissue, *J. Biomed. Mater. Res.*, 7, 39, 1973.

von Recum, A.F. et al., Biocompatibility tests of components of an implantable cardiac assist device, *J. Biomed. Mater. Res.*, 12, 743, 1978.

Willoughby, D.A. et al., The use of the air pouch to study experimental synovitis and cartilage breakdown, *Biomed. Pharmacother.*, 40(2), 45, 1986.

Wood, N.K., Kaminski, E.J. and Oglesby, R.J., The significance of implant shape in experimental testing of biological materials: disc vs. rod, *J. Biomed. Mater. Res.*, 4, 1, 1970.

Woodman, J.L., Black, J. and Nunamaker, D.N., Release of cobalt and nickel from a new total finger joint prosthesis made of vitallium, *J. Biomed. Mater. Res.*, 17, 655, 1983.

Wortman, R.S., Merritt, K. and Brown, S.A., The use of the mouse peritoneal cavity for screening for biocompatibility of polymers, *Biomater. Med. Dev. Artif. Org.*, 11(1), 103, 1983.

Bibliography

Anderson, J.M., Biological response to materials, *Annu. Rev. Mater. Sci.*, 31, 81, 2001.

Berry, C.L. (Ed.), *The Pathology of Devices*, Springer–Verlag, Berlin, 1994.

Department of Health and Human Services, *Guidelines for Blood–Material Interactions*, NIH Pub. 85-2185, U.S. Government Printing Office, Washington, D.C., 1985.

Gad, S.C., *Safety Evaluation of Medical Devices*, 2nd ed., Marcel Dekker, New York, 2001.

Greco, R.S. (Ed.), *Implantation Biology: The Host Response and Biomedical Devices*, CRC Press, Boca Raton, FL, 1994.

Homsy, C.A. et al., Surgical suture–canine tissue interaction for six common suture types, *J. Biomed. Mater. Res.*, 2, 215, 1968.

Horowitz, E. and Torgesen, J.L. (Eds.), *Biomaterials*, NBS Special Pub. 415, Washington, D.C., 1975.

Leininger, R.L., Polymers as surgical implants, *CRC Crit. Rev. Bioeng.*, 1, 333, 1972.

Loomis, T.A. and Hayes, A.W., *Loomis's Essentials of Toxicology*, 4th ed., Academic Press, New York, 1996.

von Recum, A.F. (Ed.), *Handbook of Biomaterials Evaluation*, 2nd ed., Macmillan, New York, 1998.

Revell, P.A., *Pathology of Bone*, Springer–Verlag, Berlin, 1986, 215.

Schmidt–Nielsen, K., *Scaling: Why Is Animal Size so Important?* Cambridge University Press, Cambridge, U.K., 1985.

Skurla, C.P. and James, S.P., Assessing the dog as a model for human total hip replacement: analysis of 38 postmortem-retrieved canine cemented acetabular components, *J. Biomed. Mater. Res., Part B. Appl. Biomater.*, 73B, 260, 2005.

Williams, D. (Ed.), *Biocompatibility of Implant Materials*, Sector Publishing, London, 1976.

Williams, D.F. (Ed.), *Techniques of Biocompatibility Testing*, Vols. I and II, CRC Press, Boca Raton, FL, 1986.

Appendix 1*

Designation: F 981 – 04

Standard Practice for

Assessment of Compatibility of Biomaterials for Surgical Implants with Respect to Effect of Materials on Muscle and Bone[1]

This standard is issued under the fixed designation F 981; the number immediately following the designation indicates the year of original adoption or, in the case of revision, the year of last revision. A number in parentheses indicates the year of last reapproval. A superscript epsilon (ε) indicates an editorial change since the last revision or reapproval.

1. Scope

1.1 This practice provides a series of experimental protocols for biological assays of tissue reaction to nonabsorbable biomaterials for surgical implants. It assesses the effects of the material on animal tissue in which it is implanted. The experimental protocol is not designed to provide a comprehensive assessment of the systemic toxicity, immune response, carcinogenicity, teratogenicity, or mutagenicity of the material since other standards deal with these issues. It applies only to materials with projected applications in humans where the materials will reside in bone or soft tissue in excess of 30 days and will remain unabsorbed. It is recommended that short-term assays, according to Practice F 763, first be performed. Applications in other organ systems or tissues may be inappropriate and are therefore excluded. Control materials will consist of any one of the metal alloys in Specifications F 67, F 75, F 90, F 136, F 138, or F 562, high purity dense aluminum oxide as described in Specification F 603, ultra high molecular weight polyethylene as stated in Specification F 648 or USP polyethylene negative control.

1.2 This practice is a combination of Practice F 361 – 80 and Practice F 469 – 78. The purpose, basic procedure, and method of evaluation of each type of material are similar; therefore, they have been combined.

1.3 *This standard does not purport to address all of the safety concerns, if any, associated with its use. It is the responsibility of the user of this standard to establish appropriate safety and health practices and determine the applicability of regulatory limitations prior to use.*

2. Referenced Documents

2.1 *ASTM STANDARDS:*[2]
F 67 Specification for Unalloyed Titanium for Surgical

Implant Applications (UNS R50250, UNS R50400, UNS R50550, UNS R50700)
F 75 Specification for Cobalt-28Chromium-6Molybdenum Alloy Castings and Casting Alloy for Surgical Implants (UNS R30075)
F 86 Practice for Surface Preparation and Marking of Metallic Surgical Implants
F 90 Specification for Wrought Cobalt20-Chromium15-Tungsten10-Nickel Alloy for Surgical Implant Applications (UNS R30605)
F 136 Specification for Wrought Titanium-6Aluminum-4Vanadium ELI (Extra Low Interstitial) Alloy for Surgical Implant Applications (UNS R56401)
F 138 Specification for Wrought-18Chromium-14Nickel-2.5Molybdenum Stainless Steel Bar and Wire for Surgical Implants (UNS S31673)
F 361 Practice for Assessment of Compatibility of Metallic Materials for Surgical Implants with Respect to Effect of Materials on Tissue[3]
F 469 Practice for Assessment of Compatibility of Nonporous Polymeric Materials for Surgical Implants with Regard to Effect of Materials on Tissue[3]
F 562 Specification for Wrought Cobalt-35Nickel-20Chromium-10Molybdenum Alloy for Surgical Implant Applications (UNS R30035)
F 603 Specification for High-Purity Dense Aluminum Oxide for Surgical Implant Application
F 648 Specification for Ultra-High-Molecular-Weight Polyethylene Powder and Fabricated Form for Surgical Implants
F 763 Practice for Short-Term Screening of Implant Materials

3. Summary of Practice

3.1 This practice describes the preparation of implants, the number of implants and test hosts, test sites, exposure schedule, implant sterilization techniques, and methods of implant retrieval and tissue examination of each test site. Histological criteria for evaluating tissue reaction are provided.

---

[1] This practice is under the jurisdiction of ASTM Committee F04 on Medical and Surgical Materials and Devices and is the direct responsibility of Subcommittee F04.16 on Biocompatibility Test Methods.
Current edition approved May 1, 2004. Published June 2004. Originally approved in 1986. Last previous edition approved in 2003 as F 981 – 99 (2003).
[2] For referenced ASTM standards, visit the ASTM website, www.astm.org, or contact ASTM Customer Service at service@astm.org. For *Annual Book of ASTM Standards* volume information, refer to the standard's Document Summary page on the ASTM website.

[3] Withdrawn.

---

4. Significance and Use

4.1 This practice covers a test protocol for comparing the local tissue response evoked by biomaterials, from which medical implantable devices might ultimately be fabricated, with the local tissue response elicited by control materials currently accepted for the fabrication of surgical devices. The materials may include metals (and metal alloys), dense aluminum oxide, and polyethylene that are standardized on the basis of acceptable long-term well-characterized long-term response. The controls consistently produce cellular reaction and wound healing to a degree that has been found to be acceptable to the host.

5. Test Hosts and Sites

5.1 Rats (acceptable strains such as Fischer 344), New Zealand White rabbits, and other small laboratory animals may be used as test hosts for soft tissue implant response. It is suggested that the rats be age and sex matched. Rabbits or larger animals may be used as test hosts for bone implants. When larger animals such as dogs, goats, or sheep are used, the decision should be based upon special considerations of the particular implant material or study.

5.2 The sacro-spinalis, paralumbar, gluteal muscles, and the femur or tibia can serve as the test site for implants. However, the same site must be used for test and material implants in all the animal species.

5.3 There shall be a minimum of four animals at each sacrifice interval for a total of twelve animals per study. If larger animals are used, in which a greater number of implants can be placed, there shall be at least two animals sacrificed at each time period.

6. Implant Specimens

6.1 *Fabrication*—Each implant shall be made in a cylindrical shape with hemispherical ends (see 6.3 and 6.4 for sizes). If the ends are not hemispherical, this shall be reported. Each implant shall be fabricated, finished, and its surface cleaned in a manner appropriate for its projected application in human subjects in accordance with Practice F 86. If the specimens are porous, the method of preparation of the porous specimens shall be representative of the contemplated human implant applicationan shall yield a specimen with characteristic pore size, pore volume, and pore interconnection diameter. The choice between using solid core specimens with porous coatings and specimens that are porous throughout shall be a decision of the investigator and shall be reported.

6.2 Reference metallic specimens shall be fabricated in accordance with 6.1 from materials such as the metal alloys in Specifications F 67, F 75, F 90, F 138, or F 562, ceramic in Specification F 603, or polymers such as in Specification F 648 polyethylene or USP Negative Control Plastic. If the test materials are porous, consideration should be given to using porous specimens for reference specimens. Alternatively, nonporous reference specimens may be used.

6.3 *Suggested Sizes and Shapes of Implants for Insertion in Muscle*:

6.3.1 The implants shall be cylindrical in shape and may range from 1 mm to 6 mm in diameter and from 10 mm to 20 mm in length depending upon the relative size of the species under study.

6.3.2 The dimensions used shall be reported in accordance with 8.1.

6.3.3 Depending upon the particular device application, other sample shapes may be used. For instance, an investigator might wish to test the biocompatibility of a new material for screws in the form of a screw. If an alternative specimen shape is used, this should be reported in accordance with 8.1.

6.4 *Sizes and Shapes of Implants for Insertion in Bone*:

6.4.1 Implant diameters for use in bone shall be approximately equal to the cortex thickness. Implant lengths shall allow them to reside in one cortex and the medulla without excessive protrusion beyond the periosteum.

6.4.2 The dimensions used shall be reported in accordance with 8.1.

6.5 *Number of Test and Control Implants*:

6.5.1 In each rat, due to size, there may be two implants; one each test and control material implant.

6.5.2 In each rabbit, due to size, there may be six implants; four test materials and two control material implants.

6.5.3 In larger animals, there may be twelve implants; eight test materials and four control material implants.

6.5.4 In rabbits or larger animals, there shall be tested at least sixteen test material implants and eight control material implants at each time period.

6.6 *Conditioning*:

6.6.1 Remove all surface contaminants with appropriate solvents and rinse all test and control implants in distilled water prior to sterilization. It is recommended that the implant materials be processed and cleaned in the same way the final product will be.

6.6.2 Clean, package, and sterilize all implants in the same way as used for human implantation.

6.6.3 After final preparation and sterilization, handle the test and control implants with great care to ensure that they are not scratched, damaged, or contaminated in any way prior to insertion.

6.6.4 Report all details of conditioning in accordance with

6.7 *Implantation Period*—Insert all implants into each animal at the same surgical session for implantation periods of 12, 26, and 52 weeks.

7. Procedure

7.1 *Implantation (Muscle)*:

7.1.1 Place material implants in the paravertebral muscles in such a manner that they are directly in contact with muscle tissue.

7.1.2 Introduce material implants in larger animals by the technique of making an implantation site in the muscle by using a hemostat to separate the muscle fibers. Then insert the implant using plastic-tipped forceps or any tool that is nonabrasive to avoid damage to the implant.

7.1.3 Introduce material implants using sterile technique. Sterile disposable needles or hypodermic tubing and trochar may be used to implant the material implants into the paravertebral muscles along the spine. In rats, insert a negative control implant on one side of the spine and a test material implant on the other side. In rabbits, implant one negative control material on each side of the spine and implant two test materials on each side of the spine. If larger diameter specimens are used, an alternative implantation technique is that described in 7.1.2.

7.2 *Implantation (Femur)*—Expose the lateral cortex of each rabbit femur and drill undersized pilot holes through the lateral cortex using the technique and instrument appropriate for the procedure. Final reaming of the holes should be performed by hand to yield holes which are smaller than the implant specimens by 0.1 mm or less. Into each one of these holes, insert one of the implants by finger pressure. Then close the wound.

Note 1—Caution should be taken to minimize the motion of the implant in the tissue to prevent the effects of motion on the desired result.

7.3 Postoperative Care:

7.3.1 All animal studies must be done in a facility approved by a nationally recognized organization and in accordance with all appropriate regulations.

7.3.2 Carefully observe each animal during the period of assay and report any abnormal findings.

7.3.3 Infection or injury of the test implant site may invalidate the results. The decision to replace the animal so that the total number of retrieved implants will be as represented in the schedule shall be dependent upon the design of the study.

7.3.4 If an animal dies prior to the expected date of sacrifice, perform a necropsy in accordance with the procedure in 7.4 to determine the cause of death. Replacement of the animal to the study shall be dependent upon the design of the study. Include the animal in the assay of data if the cause of death is related to the procedure or test material.

7.4 *Sacrifice and Implant Retrieval*:

7.4.1 Euthanize animals by a humane method at the intervals specified in 6.7.

NOTE 2—The necropsy periods start at 12 weeks because it is assumed that acceptable implant data has been received for earlier periods from short term implant testing according to Practice F 763. If the 90-day sacrifice period has been utilized under Practice F 763, that group need not be repeated under this protocol, and thus, the 12-week group may be eliminated.

7.4.2 At necropsy, record any gross abnormalities of color or consistency observed in the tissue surrounding the implant. Remove each implant with an intact envelope of surrounding tissue. Include in the tissue sample a minimum of a 4-mm thick layer of tissue surrounding the implant. If less than a 4-mm thick layer of tissue is removed, report in accordance with 8.1.

7.5 *Postmortem Observations*—In accordance with standard laboratory practice, perform a necropsy on all animals that are sacrificed for the purposes of the assay or die during the assay period. Establish the status of the health of the experimental animal during the period of the assay. Report as described in Section 8.

7.6 *Histological Procedure*:

7.6.1 *Tissue Sample Preparation*—Prepare appropriate blocks from each implantation site and indicate the orientation of the axis of the femur relative to the axis of the implant (for bone implants). Also indicate the orientation of the implant relative to the axis of rotation of the femoral condyles.

1 .   7.6.1.1 Process the excised tissue block containing either a test implant or control implant for histopathological examination and such other studies as are appropriate. Cut the sample midway from end to end into appropriate size and in the appropriate orientation for each study. Transfer, or record, or both, the orientational details noted in 7.6.1 to each part of the sample. Record the gross appearance of the implant and the tissue. If the sample is porous, it is imperative that sectioning procedures be used that maintain the implant within its tissue envelope to allow the evaluation of tissue within the pores. Such procedures may include ground section preparation.

2 .   7.6.1.2 If special stains are deemed necessary, prepare additional sections and make appropriate observations.

3 .   7.7 *Histopathological Observations*—Compare the amount of tissue reaction adjacent to the test implant to that adjacent to a similar location and orientation on the control implant with respect to thickness of scar, presence of inflammatory or other cell types, presence of particles, and such other indications of interaction of tissue and material as might occur with the actual material under test. A suggested method for the evaluation of tissue response after implantation is Turner, et al. (**1**) .Ifa porous sample is being tested, the evaluation of the tissue reaction must include areas within the pores of the test and control samples at similar locations.

7.7.1 *Suggested Method for Tissue Response Evaluation*:

7.7.1.1 A suggested format with tissue response and cell accumulation to be evaluated and a scoring range of 0 to 3 is shown in Table 1.

7.7.1.2 The scoring system of 0 to 3 is based upon the observation of high power fields (400-500X) and an average of five fields.

⁴

    The boldface numbers in parentheses refer to the list of references at the end of this standard.

TABLE 1 Suggested Evaluation Format and Scoring Range

Animal Number						
Duration of Implant (weeks)						
Sample Description						
Gross Response						
Histopath-Number						
Score		0	0.5	1	2	3
Necrosis						
Degeneration						
Inflammation						
	Polymorphonuclear Leukocytes					
	Lymphocytes					
	Eosinophils					
	Plasma Cells					
	Macrophages					
Fibrosis						
Giant Cells						
Foreign Body Debris						
Fatty Infiltration						

Relative Size of Involved Area in mm				
Histopathologic Toxicity Rating				

Tissue Response/Cell Score Accumulation

0	0
1–5	0.5
6–15	1
16–25	2
26 or more	3

7.7.1.3 The necrosis and/or degeneration score is determined using the same range of 0 to 3, as follows:

Degree	Score
No reaction	0
Very slight reaction	0.5
Mild reaction	1
Moderate reaction	2
Marked reaction	3

7.7.1.4 An overall rating of test samples may be given using a rating range of 0 to 4, as follows:

Rating	Score
No reaction	0
Very slight reaction	1
Mild reaction	2
Moderate reaction	3
Marked reaction	4

7.7.1.4.1 Pathologists may choose to use the scoring system of comparing the negative control to the test material as an aid in their evaluation. The overall reaction to the test material as compared to the negative control is to be evaluated independently for all time periods.

7.7.2 *Suggested Criteria for Comparing Responses to Test and Control Specimens*—In discussing and reporting the results of this testing, a test article may be reported as

having satisfied the requirements of this test if the response of tissues surrounding the test article is not significantly greater than that for the control specimen.

8. Report

8.1 Report the following information:

8.1.1 All details of implant characterization, fabrication, conditioning (including cleaning, handling, and sterilization techniques employed). For porous implants, a measure of the porosity and pore interconnection diameters shall have been measured and reported.

8.1.2 Procedures for implantation and implant retrieval.

8.1.3 Details of any special procedure (such as unusual or unique diet fed to test animals).

8.1.4 The observations of each control and test implant as well as the gross appearance of the surrounding tissue in which the implants were implanted.

8.1.5 The observation of each histopathological examination including a descriptive pathology narration and the pathologist's evaluation as to the reaction to the test material provided.

9. Keywords

9.1 biocompatibility; bone implant materials; cellular reaction; histology/histopathology; implants muscle; New Zealand rabbits; orthopaedic medical devices—bone; plastic surgical devices/applications; polyethylene (PE)—surgical implant applications; rabbits; rats; scar; test animals; tissue compatibility; tissue response evaluation

APPENDIX

(Nonmandatory Information)

X1. RATIONALE FOR PRACTICE F981

X1.1 This practice is based on the research techniques utilized by Cohen (2), and by Laing, Ferguson, and Hodge (3, 4) in the early 1960's. These studies involved the implantation of metal cylinders in paravertebral muscle of rabbits. The biological reaction to the cylinders was described as the thickness of the fibrous membrane or capsule formed adjacent to the implant. The thickness of the capsule and the presence of inflammatory cells was used as a measure of the degree of adverse reaction to the test material.

X1.2 As first published in 1972, Practice F 361 was a test for the biological response to metallic materials. The scope had been expanded beyond that of the published reports to include bone as well as muscle as an implant test site. To avoid species specific reactions, the method called for the use of rats and dogs as well as rabbits. Cylindrical test specimens with rounded ends were used to avoid biological reactions associated with sharp corners or other variations in specimen shape.

X1.3 In 1978, Practice F 469 was published as a parallel document for the test of polymeric materials. In that the methods were essentially the same, the scope of Practice F 361 has been expanded to include the testing of specimens made of metallic, polymeric or ceramic materials, thereby including and superseding Practice F 469.

X1.4 Stainless steel, cobalt chromium, and titanium alloys are used as reference materials since the biological response to these materials has been well characterized by their extensive use in research. The response to these materials is not defined as compatible, but rather the response is used as a reference against which reactions to other materials are compared.

X1.5 This practice is a modification of the original Practice F 361 in that it only involves long term test periods. The short term response to materials is to be evaluated using Practice F 763.

X1.6 This practice was revised in 1987 to allow for

alternative specimen dimensions for rats and rabbits for muscle implantation. The original specimen dimensions were intended to be implanted through a needle, which was a change from Practice F 361 and Practice F 469. The alternate dimensions restore those specified since 1972, which some members felt were more appropriate for some material types.

experience in the use of these techniques for the evaluation of the response of tissue to implant materials. In revision, there

X1.7 This practice was revised in 1990 to add a ceramic was discussion of the appropriate length of a long term study. material (Specification F 603) as a reference material when testing ceramics.

X1.8 In 1991, this practice was revised to add the testing of year interval for larger animals could be removed. porous materials to the scope of the practice. Previously, the committee had been unable to achieve consensus on the appropriate modifications to the technique to allow the

testing of porous materials.

X1.9 This practice is based upon over 30 years of published experience in the use of these techniques for the evaluation of the response of tissue to implant ,materials. In revision, there was discussion of the appropriate length of a long term study. Comments received suggested that one or two year studies were excessive. It was the decision of the task force that the one year interval would be maintained but that the two year interval for larger animals could be removed.

X1.10 The revision of this document in 1992 removed all reference to the use of the canine for these studies to encourage the use of rats and rabbits when practical. Larger animals such as dogs, goats, and sheep may be utilized when found to be appropriate by the investigator.

REFERENCES

(1) Turner, J. E., Lawrence, W. H., and Autian, J., "Subacute Toxicity Testing of Biomaterials using Histopathologic Evaluation of Rabbit Muscle Tissue," *Journal Biomedical Material Research*, Vol. 7, No. 39, 1973.
(2) Cohen, J., "Assay of Foreign-Body Reaction," *Journal of Bone and Joint Surgery*, No. 41A, 1959, pp. 152–166.
(3) Ferguson, A. B., Jr., Laing, P. G., and Hodge, E. S.," The Ionization of Metal Implants in Living Tissues," *Journal of Bone and Joint Surgery*, No. 42A, 1960, pp. 77–90.
(4) Laing, P. G., Ferguson, A. B., Jr., and Hodge, E. S.," Tissue Reaction in Rabbit Muscle Exposed to Metallic Implants," *Journal Biomedical Materials Research*, No. 1, 1967, pp. 135–149.

Appendix 2: Rating System for Tissue at Animal Implant Sites*

This system, based upon earlier studies (Gourlay et al. 1978, Sewell et al. 1955) involves measuring the capsule thickness, evaluating the local cellular response, and then assigning weighting factors to arrive at an overall rating. Specific values (of weighting factors) are given for implants in the form of 2-0 sutures; modification for standard implants in other configurations might be advisable.

Capsular Thickness:

Grade	Thickness range (μm)
1	0 - 25
2	26 - 50
3	51 - 250
4	251 - 500
5	501 - 750

Cellular Response:
> Grade from 0 to 5 depending upon the concentration of cells observed in the capsule and adjacent tissue per high power (500x) field..

Weighting Factors:
> Capsular thickness: x 5
> Cellular response: x 3
> Cells present:
>> Neutrophils: x 5
>> FB Giant Cells: x 2
>> Lymphocytes: x 1
>> Macrophages: x 1
>> Fibroblasts: x 1

A final score might appear as follows:
> Capsule thickness: grade 3 x factor 5 = 15
> Cellular response: grade 2 x factor 3 = 6
> Cell types:
>> Neutrophils: 5 x factor 5 = 25
>>   Total: 46

The numerical ratings might be verbally expressed by descriptors:
0: no reaction; 1-10: minimal; 11-25: slight; 26-40: moderate; 41-60: marked; >60: excessive.

The example given above would then be in the marked tissue reaction range. Note that this rating system is intended as a model system. Specific rating scales should be developed for specific applications.

---

* source: adapted from Salthouse (1980)

Appendix 3:
System for Evaluation of Human Local Host Response to Implants in the Musculoskeletal System (synovial and capsular tissues)[*]

Tissues fixed in 10% buffered formalin, routinely processed (paraffin mounted), stained with hematoxylin and eosin and viewed by ordinary light and polarized microscopy. Tissues are to be examined without any prior knowledge of clinical or radiographic status of patient. The maximum concentrations are counted, averaged and graded from at least five different microscopic fields per section using the following eight categories:

1. Acute inflammatory cells (polymorphonuclear leukocytes) and mononuclear histiocytes
    0 = absent
    1+ = 1 - 5 cells/(500x) field
    2+ = 6 - 49 cells/(500x) field
    3+ = 50 or more cells/(500x) field

2. Chronic inflammatory cells (lymphocytes, plasma cells, lymphoid follicles)
    1+ = 1 - 9 cells/(500x) field and/or one lymphoid follicle/(100x) field
    2+ = 10 - 49 cells/(500x) field and/or 2 - 3 lymphoid follicles/(100x) field
    3+ = 50 or more cells/(500x) field and/or 4 or more lymphoid follicle/(100x) field

3. Giant cells (multinucleated histiocytes)
    1+ = 1 - 2 cells/(250x) field
    2+ = 3 - 8 cells/(250x) field
    3+ = 9 or more cells/(250x) field

4. Metal particles
    1+ = 1 - 19 particles/(500x) field
    2+ = 20 - 499 particles/(500x) field
    3+ = 500 or more particles/(500x) field

5. Polyethylene** fibers, small type (less than 100mm in length)
    1+ = 1 - 9 fibers lying extracellularly and/or 1 - 9 histiocytes containing one or more fibers per (500x) field
    2+ = 10 - 19 fibers lying extracellularly and/or 10 - 19 histiocytes containing one or more fibers per (500x) field
    3+ = 20 or more fibers lying extracellularly and/or 20 or more histiocytes containing one or more fibers per (500x) field

6. Polyethylene** fibers, (greater than 100mm and less than 500mm in length)
    1+ = 1 - 3 fibers/(45x) field
    2+ = 4 - 9 fibers/(45x) field
    3+ = 10 or more fibers/(45x) field

_____

[*] source: adapted from Mirra et al. 1976

7. Polyethylene flakes** (greater than 500mm in length)
    1+ = 1 - 2/tissue section
    2+ = 2 - 5/tissue section
    3+ = 6 or more/tissue section

8. Methyl methacrylate globules***
    1+ = 1 - 3/tissue section
    2+ = 4 - 6/tissue section
    3+ = 7 or more/tissue section

** identified by birefringence in polarized light
*** may be seen as void spaces, with possible $BaSO_4$ granules, due to dissolution by section
    clearing solvent

19

Clinical Testing of Implant Materials

19.1 Goal of Clinical Trials

After material selection, device design, *in vitro* tests, and implantation in animals, a material must eventually be tested in humans. Such tests are necessary because the goal of implant materials development, selection, and testing is the alleviation of human disability and disease and because knowledge about biological performance of materials is insufficient to predict clinical success with confidence on the basis of only laboratory and animal testing. In this chapter, some aspects of the design and conduct of clinical trials will be briefly considered.

Before considering a clinical trial, it is well to consider the goal of such evaluation. Unless an implant is designed for acute use, trials cannot extend beyond a short fraction of intended device life. Furthermore, testing a new or novel biomaterial in a particular device cannot result in qualification of the material. Therefore, clinical trials must be regarded as serving primarily as detectors of bad news; in much the same way that canaries in coal mines warned of impending life-threatening gas concentrations, a clinical trial represents a limited, controlled, well-observed introduction of a new material and/or design. The use of the term *introduction* is deliberate because, unlike in the case of animal trials, the experimental subjects will continue to be exposed to the device and its material components even after the period of observation. The longer the time elapsed is and the greater the number of patients studied during such limited introduction is, without detection of adverse results, one is entitled to have greater confidence in acceptable biological performance following general introduction.

19.2   Design of Clinical Trials

19.2.1   General Requirements

Burdette and Gehan (1970) identify four types or sequential phases of clinical trials:

- Phase I — early trial: selecting a new treatment from among several options for further study
- Phase IIA — preliminary trial: if the new treatment is not effective in the early trial, this phase examines whether further studies should be performed or the treatment abandoned
- Phase IIB — follow-up trial: estimating the effectiveness of a new treatment that appears promising based upon phase I or phase IIA trials
- Phase III: comparison of the effectiveness of the new treatment with a standard method of management or some other treatment

In the human testing of materials within devices, phases I, IIA, and IIB are rarely planned in a formal sense. Their function is usually fulfilled by the use of individual custom devices for selected patients under the direct care or supervision of the surgeon member of the research group. Only when the new material/device (usually in comparison to other material/device arrangements) is perceived to have relative benefit does formal clinical testing begin with a phase III trial. This phase in implant development may be further subdivided into two subphases (Burdette and Gehan 1970):

- Phase IIIA: examination of clinical outcome of a defined new treatment for a group of patients with defined indications
- Phase IIIB: following success in a subphase IIIA trial, examination of the clinical outcome for a defined (refined) new treatment for a group of patients with defined (refined) indications, usually involving multiple investigators and institutions*

It is standard practice in new drug trials to employ the double-blind method; that is, a drug and a harmless inactive material (placebo) are used in a treatment plan for a defined group of patients with a common set of symptoms. Which patients receive the drug and which the placebo is predetermined at random. Neither the patients (single blind) nor the treating physician (double blind) knows whether they are receiving the active drug. When the experimental trial is complete, an identifying code assigned to the drug and placebo doses is deciphered and an analysis of effectiveness of the

---

* A very useful source for up-to-date information on clinical trials in the U.S. can be found at http://www.clinicaltrials.gov.

treatment is made. A further sophistication is employed in some designs: the treatments for the two groups are "crossed over" or interchanged half-way through the trial. Thus, each subject has a near equal chance of benefit from the drug and of adverse effects from the drug or the placebo (because administering the placebo prevents the use of other [previous] drugs known to have beneficial effects on the patient's condition).

When an implant is surgically inserted, whatever the phase of the trial, it is not possible to pair the implanted patient with a placebo-treated patient. The case of no insertion is clearly not blind to patient or doctor, and it would not be ethically or practically acceptable in longer term trials. A study comparing identical devices made of different materials is at best blind to the patient. Differences in appearance, weight, shape, etc. between devices made of different materials usually render them easily distinguishable to the physician and the patient. Furthermore, as is noted in Chapter 21, the interrelationship between materials selection and device design is such that it would be unlikely that the two devices would differ only in respect to materials of construction. It is more usual that several factors, including surgical technique, are changed. Although this still permits comparison between the old and new treatments, the effect of materials change is statistically confounded and thus cannot be observed with any certainty.

Therefore, clinical trials of implant materials must be based upon different experimental designs. Comparisons may be made as follows:

- Between the condition of the patient before and after implant surgery. This is useful to detect acute changes that may take place in an individual with underlying disease (for which the implant is indicated) that may be associated with response to the implant material.
- Among patients with similar implants made of different materials. When possible, this is useful to investigate acute and chronic differences in material and host responses.
- Between patients with implants and nondiseased (control) individuals of the same age and sex, and with a similar home/workplace environment. This may be useful for detection of subtle chronic effects of materials (host response). Spousal or partner controls are used in many such studies.

A number of efforts have been made to set standards for selection and treatment of patients in clinical trials. Some of the general rules that have emerged are:

- Medical care must be under the direction of a medical professional.
- The patients must give informed consent to any experimental procedure. This consent can only be obtained after a full explanation of

possible benefits and risks of the proposed procedure in comparison to alternatives, including no treatment.

- The identity of the patients must be protected and the confidentiality of their medical records must be preserved.

- Perhaps the most important point is that, for the trial to be justified, whatever the phase, there must be a reasonable possibility of specific benefit to the patients in the trial combined with reasonable assurance of the absence of unusual risk.

The governing ethical considerations of which these are a part are the 12 basic principles of the Declaration of Helsinki II, revised and extended by the 29th World Medical Assembly (Silverman 1985).

It is clear that clinical trial protocols for drugs or devices are difficult to design and implement. As an aid in such efforts, virtually all medical research and treatment facilities involved with patients maintain Human Subjects Committees (also known as Internal Review Boards [IRBs]). These committees are available to help in preparing protocols and generally must review the procedures and safeguards in any experimental program involving human subjects before the clinical trial is started. Federal agencies now make such reviews by IRBs a prerequisite to public funding of clinical research. In addition, many of the Device Classification Panels of the Center for Medical Devices and Radiological Health (CDRH) of the Food and Drug Administration (FDA) have developed guidelines for design of clinical trials and for statistical treatment and format for reporting results. If relevant guidelines exist in the area under consideration, they should be consulted at an early point of protocol development.

Although these detailed guidelines are of use, they have now generally been supplanted by an FDA control document. This arises from the need to obtain an exemption from certain provisions of the Medical Device Amendments (1976) (see Section 20.2) in order to manufacture, ship interstate, and implant the quantities of implants required for phase III clinical trials.* The necessary authorization is obtained through a successful (approved) application for an investigational device exemption (IDE).** The referenced portions of the Code of Federal Regulations describe the procedure for application for an IDE and the responsibilities of the sponsor, investigators, and Human Subjects Committees (here called IRBs), as well as set standards for informed consent, protection of patient confidentiality, and reporting of study results.

It should be further noted that an IDE would not be granted unless the supporting tests of the type to be discussed later in this chapter, as well as others, meet the requirements of the regulations on good laboratory practice

---

* Devices required for earlier phases are manufactured individually at the surgeon's or physician's prescription and are permitted to be used under the custom devices provisions of the Medical Device Amendments (1976).

** *Federal Register* 45(13):3732, 1980. See also Dobelle et al. (1980).

(GLP).* These regulations set forth standards concerning design and documentation of preclinical trials, qualification of personnel, and preservation and presentation of experimental results. Although the GLP regulations apply only to aspects of testing to support claims of safety at this time, it is not improbable that they will eventually be extended to apply to all aspects of preclinical testing, as well as to a wide variety of biomedical research efforts not directly associated with direct material and device development.

Before clinical trials of a new material (in a device configuration) can be countenanced, at least two preliminary types of nonclinical tests of the material seem imperative. These are in addition to tests that may be required to demonstrate the safety and effectiveness of the material and the device design before phase III clinical trials may begin. However, if GLPs are observed, these preliminary test results may be used as part of a later IDE application submission.

19.2.2   Preclinical Tests

The first of these two preliminary tests is acute screening based upon *in vitro* and tissue culture techniques as outlined in Chapter 17. This area has no general standards and many different protocols are in use. Completion of these acute screening trials should lead to a second type of preliminary test, the chronic animal demonstration test. The ASTM F 981 protocol (Chapter 18) is such a test. Chronic animal tests should essentially meet or exceed the requirements of F 981. Equivalency to F 981 involves, as a minimum, the use of:

* Multiple species
* The same control (reference) materials used in acute testing
* Group sizes and sacrifice schedules substantially equal to or greater than those required by F 981
* Operative sites similar to those of the intended human application

If a material demonstrates that it is equal or superior to materials in present use in both of these types of tests and no extraordinary hazards specifically associated with it arise, the planning and execution of phases I and II clinical trials seems warranted. The requirements for such clinical trials are probably more stringent than those needed to demonstrate performance of new device designs. This is the case due to the subtlety of many materials' problems and the general "endorsement" that a new material may achieve inferentially after successfully completing its first clinical trial series.

The question of what tests are necessary and sufficient before phase III clinical trials of new materials are warranted is extremely controversial in all aspects. It would be very inviting to develop a consensus viewpoint or

---

* *Federal Register* 43(247):59986, 1978.

matrix into which all new materials, material combinations, and material applications could be classified, thus settling the generic problem once and for all. A number of groups, including working groups within various U.S. and foreign national governmental agencies and national standards-making organizations, are examining this approach to the question. Progress has been slow, and the end product is clearly a long way away.

The first step was the development of ASTM F 748: Practice for Selecting Generic Biological Test Methods for Materials and Devices. The standard contains a recommended test matrix that distinguishes among external devices, external communicating devices, and implants, and between tissue types and contact periods (Figure 19.1). When originally written, generic host response tests, including an F 981 type chronic implantation test, were recommended for each exposure class. Although the tests were defined generically, the ASTM F-4 committee has gone on to recommend specific test procedures in each area that are now incorporated by reference (Table 19.1).

The success of this voluntary practice, originally adopted in 1982, led to the so-called Tripartite Biocompatibility Guidance (TBG) (Kammula 1991), which was ratified on April 24, 1987. This document was developed by a joint U.S., Canada, and U.K. working group and was intended to assist manufacturers and government health agencies in the three countries in anticipating the information necessary for preclinical evaluation of new materials. The TBG retained the matrix approach of F 748, deleted the distinction between contact periods (intraoperative, short term, or chronic) and added several additional possible tests, including determination of the pharmacokinetics of released material ("biological fate") and of reproductive and developmental toxicity. Unlike F 748, the TBG does not refer to specific recommended test methods but simply puts forward recommended aspects of such tests.

The formation of the European Economic Union (EU), effective at the end of 1992, led to interest within the International Standards Organization (ISO) in producing a systematic approach to selection of tests for biological evaluation of materials. This standard (ISO 10993-1, 1991) was drafted by Technical Committee 194 and draws very strongly on the TBG, which it has effectively superseded. In fact, it uses a similar matrix and recommended tests but restores the exposure classes of F 748 by distinguishing among three conditions:

- Limited exposure ($\leq$24 hours; includes intraoperative)
- Prolonged or repeated exposure (>24 hours but <30 days) (= short term)
- Permanent contact (>30 days) (= chronic)

In addition, the ISO guidance document is somewhat subtler in its approach in that it distinguishes among nine initial and four supplementary evaluation tests. This approach recognizes the criticality of nine initial tests,

Recommended Applicable Tests

Classification of Material or Device and Application	Cell Culture Cytotoxicity	Sensitization	Skin Irritation/Intracutaneous	Mucus Membrane Irritation	Sys. Toxicity — Acute/Subchronic	Blood Compatibility	Hemolysis	Pyrogenicity	Implantation — Short-Term	Implantation — Long-Term	Immunogenicity	Genotoxicity	Carcinogenicity
External devices													
Intact surfaces (all time periods)	X	X	X										
Breached surfaces													
Intraoperative	X	X	X										
Short term	X	X	X		X								
Chronic	X	X	X		X							X	
External devices communicating with													
Intact natural channels													
Intraoperative	X	X	X	X									
Short term	X	X	X	X	X				X				
Chronic	X	X	X	X	X				X		X	X	X
Body tissues and fluids													
Intraoperative	X	X	X		X			A					
Short term	X	X	X		X			A	X		X		
Chronic	X	X	X		X			A	X		X	X	X
Blood path, indirect													
Intraoperative	X	X	X		X	X	X	X					
Short term	X	X	X		X	X	X	X					
Chronic	X	X	X		X	X	X	X			X	X	
Blood path, direct													
Intraoperative	X	X	X		X	X	X	X					
Short term	X	X	X		X	X	X	X	X		X		
Chronic	X	X	X		X	X	X	X	X		X	X	X
Implanted devices principally contacting													
Bone/tissue/tissue fluid													
Intraoperative	X	X	X		X								
Short term	X	X	X		X			X	X				
Chronic	X	X	X		X			X	X	X	X	X	X
Blood													
Intraoperative	X	X	X		X	X	X	X					
Short term	X	X	X		X	X	X	X	X			X	X
Chronic	X	X	X		X	X	X	X	X	X	X	X	X

Notes: X: recommended; A: may be considered (especially for central nervous system); intraoperative: < 24 hours; short term: up to and including 30 days; chronic: >30-days. Consult standard for definitions of tissue types.

FIGURE 19.1
Selection of preclinical tests (ASTM F 748 Recommended Practice) (Adapted from ASTM F 748-04, *ASTM Annual Book of Standards,* Vol. 13.01, ASTM International, West Conshohocken, PA, 2004 (see Table 20.3).

TABLE 19.1

Test Methods Referred to in F 748-04

Test Type (per F 748-04)	Recommended Test Protocol
Cell culture cytoxicity	F 813, F 895, F 1027, F1903
Sensitization	F 720 F 2147, F 2148
Skin irritation or intracutaneous	F 719
Mucus membrane irritation	F 749[a]
Systemic toxicity, acute or subchronic	USP, F 750
Blood compatibility	F 2151[b]
Hemolysis	F 756
Pyrogenicity	USP, LAL
Short-term implantation	F 736, F 1408, F 1904
Long-term implantation	F 981, F 1983
Immunogenicity	F 1905, F 1906
Genotoxicity	[c]
Carcinogenicity	F 1439

Notes: For USP, see Section 20.2.1, for F XXX, see Table 20.3. LAL: limulus amebocyte lysate test.

[a] In suitable animal/tssue.
[b] See also tests for complement activation (F 1984, F 2065).
[c] No single test agreed.

Sources: Ross, V.C. and Twohy, C.W., *Prog. Clin. Biol. Res.*, 189, 267, 1985; Munson, T.E., *Prog. Clin. Biol. Res.*, 231, 143, 1987.

excluding chronic toxicity and carcinogenicity, for the majority of short- and intermediate-term applications; it makes no recommendations concerning testing for reproductive and developmental toxicity and the biological fate of degradation products, except for an application-by-application consideration.

Comparing ISO 10993-1 and ASTM F 748, one observes that the former emphasizes cytotoxicity, sensitization, and intracutaneous irritation more than the latter. In addition, ISO 10993-1 is less tailored to differences in exposure class. This probably reflects the overall EU regulatory outlook that, in comparison to the U.S. approach, depends less on preintroduction testing and more on clinical observation of outcomes of materials (and device) use. Finally, ISO is following the example of F 748 and developing specific test methods for many of the 13 generic test categories used in its selection matrix (published as additional parts of standard ISO 10993).*

Although the matrix approaches taken to date in ISO 10993 and ASTM F 748 are extremely beneficial, the ideal generic test selection matrix should incorporate the following criteria:

1. Separation of test requirements by the following technical aspects:

   a. Type of tissue that the implant will contact (muscle, blood, etc.)

---

* Subsequent revisions over the years suggest that eventually no useful distinctions will be possible between F 748 and IS 10993-1.

    b. Duration of implant, by classes of time intervals (short-term, intermediate-term, etc.)

    c. Relative exposure of materials to the patient's body (SA/BW ratio, etc.)

2. Selection of tests by generic description (with minimum requirements) rather than by detailed specification of procedures

3. Specification of levels of certainty ("confidence levels") rather than setting specific sample or group sizes in individual tests

The ISO standard addresses some but not all of these concerns. In particular, it fails to deal with 1c and 3. Great care must be taken in defining specific test methods for host response in this context. Although the intent is clear to set minimum requirements, the high cost of testing often converts these minima into maxima. In the case of new classes of materials, this may permit subtle but deleterious aspects of host response to be overlooked.

In practice, it appears that F 748, the TBG, and ISO 10993 have not been strictly adhered to; that is, they appear to serve a useful role as benchmarks by defining the consensus minimum preclinical testing required. Industrial sponsors tend to develop their own test matrices, involving additional testing, based upon these views (Stark 1991).

19.2.3   Clinical Trials

Finally, the time will arrive when confidence in a new material has risen sufficiently that clinical trials can be begun with caution. Clinical trials must be performed under the control of a defined (written) prospective protocol that includes the following provisions:

- Description of the implant device (note that the implant site must be that of the proposed application)
- Outline of indications for the surgical procedure
- Outline of the uniform surgical procedure used
- Outline of postoperative treatment
- Outline of follow-up schedule and postoperative evaluation techniques

The following information is needed for adequate consideration and evaluation of clinical testing results (with respect to biological performance of materials):

- Protocol as listed previously

- Identification of 200 patients, by code number, who constitute consecutive individuals seen by the treating physician and meet item 2 of the protocol
- Results of follow-up of these patients for a minimum of 5 years and average of 7 to 10 years for those not lost to follow-up at an earlier date (minimum of 100)*
- Summary of all adverse results (note that a statistical summary is desirable; individual results with code should not be reported)

The last point should be dwelt upon. Presumably, at the time at which the trial protocol was being developed, consideration was given to each of the questions to be asked and the statistical measures to be used in answering them. At the end of the trial, it is thus appropriate to suggest that statistical measures be employed. Therefore, reports of clinical trials should take care to:

- Discuss accuracy and precision of all measurements, where possible.
- Define a minimum confidence level for all statistical measures of the data, usually $p < 0.05$.
- Report confidence intervals or other measures of significance associated with all derived parameters.
- Indicate the significance of any conclusion arrived at by analysis of the trial.

19.3 Conclusions from Clinical Trials

19.3.1 Introduction

As pointed out in Interpart 2, no clinical trial can approach the numbers and period of exposure that will be experienced when a material enters into general use. Thus, in a sense, it is imperative that clinical testing never end. The treating physician and his consultants should distinguish between new and old materials and should continue to be sensitive to possible biological performance problems associated with the use of either kind.

A well-designed and conducted clinical trial does not serve to qualify a material. In addition to design studies, physical measurements, and acute and animal tests, it provides data that are required for a decision to release a product for general use. The decisions made along the path to release

---

* In practice, it is difficult to distinguish material trials from device trials. Unfortunately the *de facto* standard for device trials is only 2 years' minimum follow-up, and no additional follow-up is generally recommended in the case of new materials. This is grossly inadequate for the evaluation of new materials.

should all be based on appropriate statistical tests at a minimum confidence level of 95%. Such release, when it occurs with the approval of the appropriate regulating agencies, is necessarily a risk. That is, the benefits attendant to the use of the device incorporating the material in question are felt at the moment of decision to outweigh the risks involved.

Throughout this book, aspects of biological performance, including material and host response, have been considered. The latter sections of this work have begun to examine the details of test methods for examining biological performance leading to clinical use. Two factors are common to all of these methods:

- Large investments of time and money are required to produce results with reasonable levels of reliability and statistical significance due to the variability of the biological systems involved.
- Large quantities of inductive reasoning must be used to apply the results of *in vitro* and animal testing to the prediction of clinical performance.

These two general conclusions overshadow all considerations of clinical testing and introduction into routine clinical use of new materials or old materials in new designs or applications.

19.3.2 Complication Incidence Rates

In discussions of clinical evidence for materials incompatibility (failure to exhibit adequate levels of biological performance), time and again, incidence rates of complications are small. For instance, the "variant poppet" problem in early heart valve designs probably did not affect more than 3% of patients receiving the prosthesis. The more adverse experience with an early design of an anterior cruciate ligament replacement prosthesis (Chen and Black 1980) resulted in failure in a larger percentage of cases, but still probably less than 20%. In many high-use applications, such as total hip and knee joint replacement, device-related failures for all causes, including failure of biological performance, are now appreciably less than 1% per year after surgery.

Why then is the concern expressed here for examining biological performance? A manufacturer could fairly argue that modern implant materials have proven beneficial for 95 to 99%+ of patients receiving them. Similarly, a study by the Carnegie–Mellon Institute of costs and benefits associated with research to improve then current orthopaedic prosthetic devices concluded that failure/complication rates, even in the 1970s, were acceptably small and that the investment required to reduce these rates significantly would be costly out of proportion to the resulting benefits (Piehler 1978). This remains clearly the case today, with an additional problem: in some cases, such as total hip replacement, present technology is so successful that, even if they are actually superior to current choices, newer developments, such as changes in the materials of the articulating wear pair, cannot reasonably be expected to demonstrate statistical superior clinical outcomes due to practical limitations on size and duration of clinical trials (Black 1996)

Thus, one is faced with the problem that one cannot define a failure or complication rate during clinical trials and that such a rate, *a priori*, could not be judged to be acceptable except in extreme cases. How then is one to decide when a material has proven itself sufficiently, with respect to biological performance, to move into general use?

19.4   Aspects of the Decision for General Clinical Use

19.4.1   Current Concerns

I believe that it is necessary to address this question in two frames of reference. The first is the current medical/legal environment. The general arguments cited earlier concerning cost of additional testing and the "acceptable" level of performance of current devices were raised time and again during the hearings on the Kennedy (U.S. Senate) and Rogers (House of Representatives) bills that resulted in the Medical Device Amendments of 1976 (see Section 20.2). However, they were more than offset by the force of individual testimony concerning the human and financial costs to individuals as a result of device malfunction and failure. Thus, although statistical failure rates are low, the failure rate in a given individual with a defective device is perceived as 100%. Despite the implementation of the 1976 legislation, continuing concerns about the impact of individual device malfunction and failure led to two subsequent safe medical devices acts (1990, 1992) (see Section 20.2).

This humane view of individuals rather than average statistics has resulted in a dramatic rise in medical malpractice and damage suits associated with device failure. A typical early report* summarizes five suits concerning "defective" heart valves. Only one of the five alleged defects was connected with the death of a patient; the damage claimed in the other four cases was disability and the need for additional surgery. Total damages sought in the five cases were $55 million. Although the final outcome of such cases will not be known for some time, malpractice/device failure awards have already exceeded $1 million in individual nonfatal cases and, by 1990, new cases were being filed at a rate of 900/day, with average final awards of $300,000 (Kiplinger 1991).

As reflected in congressional testimony and in the results of malpractice suits, public opinion contributed in no small part to the formula adopted in the Medical Device Amendments (1976). The test of adequate performance laid out in this law is that the device be "safe and effective" and expose the

---

* *The New York Times*, Dec. 4, 1977.

patient to no "unreasonable" risk or hazard. Thus, decisions on what will be acceptable failure rates remain subjective and depend on the continued interaction of public opinion, expert advice, and administrative action.

Individuals are torn between two views. The heart says that no failure is acceptable, especially if it were to happen to oneself or to one dear to one. The head says that such a goal may be unattainable and approachable only at prohibitive cost.

19.4.2   Response to Current Concerns

The search for a defect-free materials technology for medical and surgical implants and devices has a precedent. Early in the development of intercontinental ballistic missiles, it was recognized that, in the normal course of events, the complexity of the electronic control systems required would lead to nonfunctioning systems. That is, the level of reliability of individual electronic components, then exceeding 99.9%, was insufficient to permit systems with 10^6 to 10^8 components to have any real level of satisfactory performance.

Two approaches were taken to deal with this problem. The first was the idea of redundancy. Each section of a control system was to have one or more "backup" sections that operated in support or in parallel and could take over if the primary system failed. This led to the practice in the present space shuttle program of having three (and in some cases four) parallel systems serving each critical function.

The second approach was to adopt the position that no absolute level of performance for an individual component was definitively acceptable. This latter view led to a highly successful initiative, first instituted by the Martin–Marietta Company (Denver) and later by the U.S. Air Force and NASA, called the Zero Defects Program. The basic concept is to test devices continually, even after they pass into active service, and feed the results back into product improvement with a view to eventual "100%" satisfactory performance through evolutionary change. The combination of these two approaches contributed to the success of the Apollo Lunar Program and the continued high level of performance of civilian and military aerospace hardware.

I suggest that both of these concepts and an additional idea of a fail-safe product can be applied to considerations of biological performance in the current environment. The idea of redundancy is hard to apply directly toward the design of devices for a number of reasons. It is applicable to active devices, such as heart pacers, but far less so to joint replacements, sutures, etc. However, redundancy can be incorporated into materials and device testing. The F 981 protocol already does this to a degree in its use of multiple animal species. Despite efforts to the contrary, multiple, parallel, and overlapping tests should be continued, driven in part by financial considerations and in part by greater, perhaps misplaced, confidence in short-term test results.

The concept of zero defects can be incorporated into clinical evaluation and experience by refusing to accept any given level of performance as permanently satisfactory. Thus, one can insist that performance equal to or better than that of materials in use today be demonstrated before new materials can go into clinical trials and routine use. However, this should not blind one to the need to examine the performance of current (old) and future (new) materials constantly with a view toward continual evolutionary improvements where and when possible — thus the emphasis in Interpart 2 on increased attention to the human epidemiology of biomaterials.

The third idea of a fail-safe product can also be adopted. This is the concept that the ill effects of the failure of a device to function in its intended mode may be minimized by design* provisions. An example of fail-safe design in everyday life is the Westinghouse type AB air brake used on railroad cars. If the train separates at a coupling or the brake control system fails, the system is designed to apply the brakes automatically in the individual cars and to maintain braking until each system is manually released and reset. In fracture fixation applications, such a concept might lead to the choice of a material with lower strength and higher ductility, such as a stainless steel, over alloys with higher strength but limited ductility. Here the fail-safe feature is that the observation of permanent deformation of an internal fixation device can lead to a change in external support prescribed by the physician. Even though it may result in an angulation in the healed fracture, the "failed" situation for a device fabricated from a ductile material (that is, angulation) is far more acceptable to patient and physician than the "failed" situation for the less deformable device — acute device fracture — that may lead to additional disability, surgery, and, possibly, legal action.

19.4.3 Future Concerns

The second frame of reference that should be briefly examined with respect to cost/risk/benefit aspects of material introduction is that of the future. How can one judge when a new material or device is ready to enter use and perhaps supplant present, apparently less effective products?

I think the answer is rather simple. If the ideas of safe failure modes in design, redundancy in testing, and, especially, continual evolutionary performance improvement are adopted, a real distinction between old and new materials will no longer be present. No one would knowingly substitute an inferior new product for a current product unless driven by inhumane motives. With this in mind, I hope that progressive attitudes on the parts of researchers, manufacturers, surgeons, and regulatory authorities will lead to a continual upgrading of the performance of current materials and the gradual introduction of new materials when subjective levels of safety and efficacy, most probably defined by then-current experience, are reached.

---

* See Chapter 21 for a discussion of the materials' design process.

Critics would suggest the need for some absolute (minimum) level of safety that must be obtained before introduction of a new material. With respect to devices, it has been proposed that the following definition be used: "A device is safe enough to use when it is no worse than others in use and presents no greater hazard than the condition it is to be used to treat." This appears clear enough in instances in which large improvements in devices (and materials) can be demonstrated and the conditions treated are life threatening. In situations in which a new material represents an evolutionary change in composition and/or processing and in subsequent behavior and the aim is to improve the quality of life of the patient by alleviating a condition of low mortality and morbidity, such a statement is a poor guide. Hazards may be of a new and noncomparable type. Meaningful comparison of hazards, in any case, is possible only when potential outcomes differ greatly. Thus, I suggest that decisions on device and materials introductions must be made on the individual merits and demerits of each situation and not shackled by a set of rigid rules.

Except at an early point in this discussion, I have said nothing about the costs associated with this approach to materials application in the medical and surgical field. This was deliberate. I suggest that the analyses of the type made by Piehler (1978) and others fail in the face of the human and emotional aspects of this field. As long as the financial costs of devices remain a relatively small component of the true cost of disease and disability, including the cost of health care (as they currently are in the U.S.), money should not be an important factor in these considerations. In individual cases, it is clear that the increased cost of research, development, and testing of materials and devices that is the legacy of the Medical Device Amendments and the Safe Medical Devices Acts, the increased number and size of malpractice and product liability suits, and increased public attention will act to stifle innovation. A situation parallel to that in the drug field has developed: an improvement in the nature of products newly introduced and a tendency to move research and development activities "offshore." It is hard to pass judgment on this continuing development. Whether it is good or bad, it is coming about in response to a clear public demand for safe and effective materials for medical and surgical implants and devices.

One can pass judgment, however, on the increasing trend towards market-driven rather than technology-driven introduction of new devices and materials. Clinical experience with many existing materials now exceeds three decades; thus, it is very difficult to argue that short-term (2- to 5-year) testing of new materials is capable of revealing subtle or long-term defects in them or, more directly, of providing the information needed to determine whether the new material is equal to or exceeds the performance of the older material that it may replace simply on a novelty basis. A Gresham's law appears to be operating in the development of medical and surgical devices and their materials through which novelty has a market value. The drive to use new materials is depriving patients of the proven performance of older ones. In a free market system that provides many benefits and maximizes individual freedom, it is hard to see how such a situation can be corrected. Physician and patient education, more sophisticated regulatory approaches, and economic restrictions imposed by widespread recognition of the need to curtail the growth of medical expenses may help. However, one can expect to avoid future problems associated with inadequate biological performance of materials in patients only through the bioengineer's endorsement of the Hippocratic injunction to, in the first place, do no harm.

19.5 Final Comments

One of the chronic problems that the materials scientist or engineer encounters in the medical device clinical literature is an inability to determine from what materials devices were made and, even if that is possible, the details of composition, processing, etc. selected within the generic material. For this reason, I suggest that a radical change is needed in how the clinical use of materials is viewed. The clinical introduction of a material should be viewed more as the beginning of the qualification process rather than the end of it. Studies of retrieved devices have helped to provide information concerning biological performance in actual clinical settings. In the last two decades, such studies have slowly been extended from examination of clinically retrieved failed devices to study of successful devices obtained at autopsy or, in some cases, still in use. However, lacking reliable incidence and prevalence data, such studies tend to be isolated examples of numerators for which reliable denominators are, as yet, unavailable. Therefore, it seems advisable to be at least as serious about durable medical devices, especially chronic (>30-day) implants as one is about motor vehicles and devise some form of internationally acceptable registration and tracking system. Chapter 22 discusses early efforts towards this goal in the U.S.

To further illuminate this need, consider two situations: the first use of an adapted or new material as a biomaterial and the subsequent use of that material in a second design or application. In the first case, the device designer, surgical developer, IRB, and regulatory agency are all tempted to ask, "Is the material biocompatible?" The main thrust of this work is to suggest that the more appropriate question is, "What is the predicted biological performance of the material in the intended application?" The answer to this question is then approached through theoretical and practical considerations, laboratory testing, and a progression of *in vitro* and *in vivo* biological testing before clinical evaluation, as described in this chapter, begins. However, the second case is different. The material has been in clinical use now for some years and the questions that need to be asked and answered are different. Now actual experience can be drawn upon — unfortunately not with the material but with devices fabricated in part or in whole from it.

Each component of an implant has three elements: a functional element, a connectional element, and a structural element. That is, each component has a desired function in relation to its site of implantation, a method of connecting it to the surrounding tissues so that it remains in the intended site and orientation, and a structural aspect to preserve the spatial relationship between the sites of connection and of function. In some cases, components may consist of a single material that can constitute all three elements, such as a monofilament surgical suture. In other cases, different materials may be joined in a single component, with each contributing one or more of these elements. For instance, a femoral component of a hip replacement may have an articulating ceramic head and a metal intramedullary stem with a porous ingrowth fixation coating to attach it to bone.

Now suppose that a material has been in use as an articulating (functional) element in the hip, but using it as an articulating element in the shoulder is desired. The temptation is to revert to the initial question of biological performance. However, this is not logical because there is (or should be) information on the actual, rather than conjectural, performance of the material in the biological environment of a human joint — in this case, one fairly similar to that of the new application (hip vs. shoulder). Then the appropriate initial question becomes, "What data and clinical experience support the assertion that the material in question will prove safe and effective in the proposed (new) clinical application?"

A study leading to answering this question now should have the following charge:

> Considering the material in question (a ceramic used for femoral heads in the hip), in the proposed design in the proposed application (prosthetic replacement of the humeral head), find and analyze the laboratory and clinical predicates that support the assertion that its use will meet appropriate regulatory standards for safety and effectiveness.*

The analysis then proceeds through the following secondary questions:

- For each component of the proposed design fabricated in whole or in part from the material in question, the question is "What are the laboratory and clinical predicates for friction and wear, structural integrity, and fixation (including possible adverse local and systemic reactions to wear debris and other degradation products) that would

---

* *Safe* and *effective* are foundational descriptors in medical device regulation. However, as is the case for biocompatibility, they cannot be defined or determined on absolute bases. Therefore, satisfaction of locally prevailing regulatory definitions and standards provides the usual test, rather than any intrinsic *de novo* considerations. Note, however, that in U.S. experience, no legal connection exists between a regulatory decision that a device is safe and effective for a given set of indications and the actual observed clinical performance. This issue has been extensively litigated, pro and con. However, this complex topic is beyond the scope of this work. For general regulatory considerations, see Chapter 20.

lead one to conclude that this design in the proposed clinical application will be safe and effective?"*

- For interfaces between such components and other components of the proposed design, the question is "What are the predicates to support the assertion that the use of the material in question will not produce clinical outcomes inferior to those experienced with materials now in general clinical use in the proposed market?"

It should be clear that the ability to answer this progression of questions depends acutely on the quality and quantity of data that exist concerning the actual material in question, its material and host responses in patients, and the overall clinical outcomes as a function of time. In this situation, it should be remembered and taken to heart that data are not the plural of anecdote.

References

F 748-04 Standard Practice for Selecting Generic Biological Test Methods for Materials and Devices, *ASTM Annual Book of Standards,* Vol. 13.01, ASTM International, West Conshohocken, PA, 2004.

F 981-04 Standard practice for assessment of compatibility of biomaterials for surgical implants with respect to effect of materials on muscle and bone, *ASTM Annual Book of Standards,* Vol. 13.01, ASTM International, West Conshohocken, PA, 2004.

Black, J., Metal on metal bearings: a practical alternative to metal on polyethylene bearings? *Clin. Orthop. Rel. Res.,* 329S, S244, 1996.

Burdette, W.J. and Gehan, E.A., *Planning and Analysis of Clinical Studies,* Charles C Thomas, Springfield, IL, 1970.

Chen, E.H. and Black, J., Materials design analysis of the prosthetic anterior cruciate ligament, *J. Biomed. Mater. Res.,* 14, 567, 1980.

Dobelle, W.H. et al., How to comply with the Food and Drug Administration's new "investigational device exemption (IDE)" regulations, including an application form, *Artif. Organs,* 4(4), 1, 1980.

International Standards Organization, Biological testing of medical and dental materials and devices, Part 1: guidance on selection of tests. ISO/DIS 10993-1:1994. ISO, Switzerland.

Kammula, R.G., Tripartite biocompatibility guidance for medical devices, in *Biocompatibility Workshop Notebook,* Duncan, P.E. and Wallin, R.F. (Eds.), Society for Biomaterials, San Antonio, TX, 1991.

Kiplinger, A., *The Kiplinger Washington Letter,* 68(20), 4, 1991.

Munson, T.E., FDA LAL guideline — update, *Prog. Clin. Biol. Res.,* 231, 143, 1987.

---

* Note that the question has been specialized for the application: friction and wear reflect the functional element of this application; structural integrity the structural element, and fixation the connectional element; the listing of possible adverse observations reflects a general understanding of clinical performance of joint replacements.

Piehler, H.R., Regulating orthopedic surgical implants, *Orthopaedic Rev.*, 7(1), 75, 1978; effect of FDA Medical Device Amendments on the benefit and cost of implants, (2), 65; better data acquisition and analysis are needed to pinpoint device failure sources, (3), 97; orthopedic implant retrieval studies document a part of failure story, (4), 79; orthopedic surgeon and patient play important roles in success of implant, (5), 99; FDA Medical Device Amendments regulation of orthopedic implants is misdirected, (7),103, 1978.

Ross, V.C. and Twohy, C.W., Endotoxins and medical devices, *Prog. Clin. Biol. Res.*, 189, 267, 1985.

Silverman, W.A., *Human Experimentation: A Guided Step into the Unknown*, Oxford University Press, Oxford, 1985.

Stark, N.J., How to organize a biocompatibility testing program: a case study, *Med. Dev. Diag. Ind.*, 13(6), 68, 1991.

Bibliography

Fleiss, J.L., *The Design and Analysis of Clinical Experiments*, John Wiley & Sons, New York, 1986.

Friedman, L.M. et al., *Fundamentals of Clinical Trials*, 3rd ed., Springer, New York, 1999.

Plantadosi, S., *Clinical Trials: A Methodological Approach*, Wiley-InterScience, New York, 1997.

Peto, R. et al., Design and analysis of randomized clinical trials requiring prolonged observation of each patient. I. Design, *Brit. J. Cancer*, 34, 585, 1976; Part II. Analysis and examples, *Brit. J. Cancer*, 35, 1, 1976.

Rozovsky, F.A. and Adams, R.K., *Clinical Trials and Human Research: A Practical Guide to Regulatory Compliance*, Jossey–Bass (John Wiley), New York, 2003.

Whitehead, J., *The Design and Analysis of Sequential Clinical Trials*, John Wiley & Sons, New York, 1997.

20

Standardization and Regulation of Implant Materials

20.1 Historical Perspective

The manufacture and sale of drugs in the U.S. has been under gradually increasing federal regulation since passage of the Wiley Act in 1897 and the first Pure Food and Drug Act of 1906. These acts, as well as subsequent ones, were adopted against a background of the sale of patent medicines with exaggerated claims and the production of food with extensive and deliberate contamination. There are many horror stories about the effects of patent medicines from the pre-Wiley Act era and the later period of weak legislation up to the 1930s (see Lamb 1936; Mintz 1965). Perhaps the strongest single factor in the initiation of federal regulation of food additives and purity was the publication of *The Jungle* by Upton Sinclair (1906). This novel describes the conditions in the processed meat industry in Chicago at the time in horrifying detail and caused widespread revulsion to and rejection of processed meats such as sausage, ham paste, etc.

Various legislative acts directed towards regulation of content and safety of food, drugs, and cosmetics brought the U.S. Food and Drug Administration (FDA) into being. Although legislative authority probably existed from 1923 to regulate implants, practical regulation did not begin until the 1970s. A series of amendments to the Food, Drug, and Cosmetic Act (1976), collectively termed The Medical Device Amendments, was adopted and signed into law on May 28, 1976. These amendments gave the then recently organized Bureau of Medical Devices and Diagnostic Aids* of the FDA broad powers to regulate implants, surgical instruments, and medical devices as articles of commerce. These powers generally parallel the powers afforded in the regulation of drugs; differences in the law and the regulatory arrangements reflect some of the differences between devices and drugs. These amendments have been supplemented and modified to minor degrees by

---

* Now called the Center for Devices and Radiological Health.

legislative action; however, they underwent significant recent extension beginning in 1990 by adoption of the Safe Medical Devices Act.

Numerous efforts at standardization and thus control of medical and surgical devices and materials predate these legislative efforts and continue in a supplementary and parallel fashion today.

20.2   Drug Standardization Activities

20.2.1   The *U.S. Pharmacopeia*

The idea of standardization of drugs and, more recently, of medical and surgical devices and materials is quite an old one. The motives involved are usually the related desires to assure reproducible effect (efficacy) while protecting the patient against hazards associated with adulteration, mislabeling, misuse, etc. (safety).

The first concrete effort in this area in the U.S. was the proposal by Dr. Lyman Spalding in January 1817 to establish a national pharmacopeia. The pharmacopeia was seen as a widely agreed upon and accepted document that would set out the composition, identity, properties, and, to some extent, clinical behavior of drugs and other medical substances shown to be useful — that is, beneficial in action. In response to Dr. Spalding's proposal, the First United States Pharmacopeial Convention (USPC) assembled in Washington, D.C., on January 1, 1820. The *First U.S. Pharmacopeia* was published on December 15, 1820, in Latin and English. Its 272 pages listed some 217 drugs considered worthy of recognition. At that time, provisions were made to hold subsequent meetings of the convention and to issue a revised pharmacopeia every 10 years.

The first USPC and the First Revision Committee were composed exclusively of physicians. By 1830, pharmacists had been invited to join the convention and numbers of them have continued to join over the years. The present bylaws of the United States Pharmacopeia require, however, that at least one-third of the members of the Board of Trustees and the Committee of Revision continue to represent the medical profession.

The initial policy of the USPC was to select the most fully established and best understood substances from among those that possess medicinal power. Over the years and through its various revisions, this principle had been adhered to. The last independent version, *The Pharmacopeia of the United States of America* (USP XIX 1975), was the 19th revision, published subsequent to the USPC of April, 1970. It contains 1284 articles describing a somewhat lower number of drugs and other medical agents. Implants and other medical devices are not discussed in USP XIX, with two exceptions. The first and more important of these exceptions is that provision is made for the definition and testing of glass and plastic containers for drugs. The methods of test for containers outlined in USP XIX are:*

- Light transmission
- Chemical resistance (glass containers)
- Biological tests (plastic containers): injection of extracts and examination of 72-hour implants in rabbits and mice
- Physiochemical tests (plastic containers): extraction, residue identification, residue ignition, heavy metal content, and buffering capacity

The other medical device described is the absorbable surgical suture. This is the so-called "catgut" suture, although the basic material is now derived from other sources. USP XIX sets out methods of test and standards for length, diameter, tensile strength, content of soluble chromium compounds, and color of extracts, as well as describing methods of needle attachment for these sutures.

Although neither of these device areas is directly applicable to implant materials, many of the methods, particularly those used to qualify container materials, have been used extensively by biomaterials investigators. Of interest is the provision for the use of a standard implant reference material for evaluation of the 72-hour animal tests. The material is a low-molecular-weight polyethylene fiber that can be inserted through a hypodermic needle. It is stocked in a supply maintained by the USPC.

In 1974, the USP and the *National Formulary* (NF) (see next section) were combined. The current edition (USP 28 2005) continues the USP series as the 28th revision and includes the 23rd revision of the NF. Although they are now published together, an internal distinction is maintained, with the USP articles addressing drug composition and dosage (as well as general issues of testing and packaging) and NF articles dealing with pharmaceutical ingredients other than drugs. The combined USP/NF has been published every 5 years since 1975 and is enlarged by annual supplements and by a bimonthly magazine, *Pharmacopeial Forum*; with the 2002 edition, it will now be published annually. The rate of growth can be appreciated by noting the addition of 112 chapters and monographs as well as 637 revisions of previous ones in the 28th edition.

The current revision, USP 28 (2005), in addition to continuing the nonbiological tests of previous revisions, now lists a total of six host response tests (Table 20.1). It is of great interest that the *in vitro* test methods now cite ASTM standards as references.

---

* USP XIX, p. 642.

TABLE 20.1

Host Response Test Methods in USP 28

General article <82>: biological reactivity tests, *in vitro*
Agar diffusion
Direct contact
Elution
General article <83>: biological reactivity tests, *in vivo*
Systemic injection
Intracutaneous injection
Implantation

Source: USP 28, *The Pharmacopeia of the United States of America*, *28th revision*, incorporating *The National Formulary*, *23rd revision*, The United States Pharmacopeial Convention, Inc., Washington, D.C., 2005.

20.2.2   The National Formulary

As mentioned earlier, another compilation of drugs and their properties is the *National Formulary*, which first appeared in 1888. This is prepared and published by the American Pharmaceutical Association, which was organized in 1852. The stated goals of the NF are similar to those of the USP, with the exception that not only the drugs of the greatest therapeutic merit are to be included, but also drugs of any demonstrated merit. This factor and the domination of the NF by the manufacturers rather than the users of drugs, leads to a somewhat different format and emphasis. The NF was originally published at 10-year intervals, more recently in 5-year intervals and, since 2002, annually. The last independent edition (see previous section) was the 14th edition (NF 14 1975) and includes 1009 articles defining and describing a somewhat greater number of drugs and medical materials.

NF 14 describes materials, in the nondrug sense, in only two areas. It makes provisions for examination and qualification of glass containers for drug packaging that are similar to and depend upon USP 19 provisions. In addition, special provisions are made for qualification of containers for ophthalmic preparations. These provisions include a previously mentioned eye-irritation test using saline and cottonseed oil extracts in the eye of the albino rabbit.

20.3   Biomaterials Standardization Activities

20.3.1   The American Dental Association

A number of efforts have been made in the standardization of biomaterials (in the sense of materials without primary pharmacological effects). Beginning in 1926, the American Dental Association (ADA) has sponsored and conducted a program to define the physical and chemical properties of materials used in restorative dentistry. Over the years a large number of specifications have been developed for various metal alloys, cements, impression materials, casting and investment waxes, plaster, resin, and elastomeric products, as well as cutting instruments and equipment for radiation diagnosis and therapy.

In addition to these specifications, the ADA maintains a program to certify specific dental material products and manufacturers of these certified products. The results of this program, carried out through a cooperative effort with the National Bureau of Standards (now the National Institute for Standards and Technology [NIST]), was a periodic publication entitled *Guide to Dental Materials and Devices* most recently published in a seventh edition (ADA 1974).* This contains a great deal of technical information as well as some 25 materials specifications. Today there are about 67 standards; however, they may be obtained only individually from the ADA or from the American National Standards Institute, Washington, D.C. Table 20.2 lists dental materials and materials test standards currently in use.

20.3.2   The American Society for Testing and Materials**

An effort of greater generality is that on the part of the American Society for Testing and Materials (ASTM). This organization was founded in 1898 and is the principal scientific and technical organization for the voluntary development of standards on characteristics and performance of materials, products, systems, and services in the U.S. It performs its work through 130 main technical committees with more than 20,000 active members.*** These committees function in prescribed fields under regulations that ensure balanced representation by producers, users, and general interest participants.

In 1962, the Committee F4 on Medical Devices was organized (Brown and Cook 1982). More recently, this committee was reorganized and renamed the Committee F4 on Medical and Surgical Materials and Devices. It includes within its organization a resources subcommittee with individual sections devoted to specific materials classes such as polymeric materials, metallurgical materials, etc., as well as biocompatibility, and a series of subcommittees in various surgical specialties such as orthopaedics, cardiovascular surgery, neurosurgery, etc. The division of areas addressed by these latter medical subcommittees approximately parallels that of the Device Classification Panels established by the Food and Drug Administration subsequent to the passage of the Medical Device Amendments (1976).

---

* The reason for discontinuation of this publication is unclear; however, the subsequent approval of these standards by the American National Standards Institute (ANSI) and their joint publication renders the decision moot.
** Since 2004, called ASTM International; however, I have preserved the older name here because it is more familiar to readers.
*** http://www.astm.org.

TABLE 20.2

ANSI/ADA Dental Biomaterials Standards and Test Methods

Biomaterials

1	Alloy for dental amalgam
5	Dental casting alloys
6	Dental mercury
11	Agar impression materials
12	Denture base polymers
13	Denture cold-curing repair resins
14	Dental base metal casting alloys
15	Synthetic polymer teeth
16	Dental impression paste — zinc oxide-eugenol type
17	Denture base temporary relining resins
18	Alginate impression materials
19	Dental elastomeric impression material
20	Dental duplicating material
22	Intraoral dental radiographic film
24	Dental baseplate wax
27	Resin-based filling materials
30	Dental zinc oxide–eugenol and zinc oxide–noneugenol cements
32	Orthodontic wires
37	Dental abrasive powders
38	Metal-ceramic dental restorative systems
39	Pit and fissure sealants
42	Polymer-based crowns and bridges
57	Endodontic sealing material
69	Dental ceramic
75	Resilient lining materials for removable dentures — part 1: short-term materials
82	Dental reversible/irreversible hydrocolloid impression material systems
87	Dental impression trays
88	Dental impression alloys
96	Dental water-based cements

Test Methods

41	Biological evaluation of dental materials
82	Dental materials — determination of color stability
97	Corrosion test methods

Source: American Dental Association (ADA) http://www.ada.org.

The scope of this committee is the development of definitions of terms and nomenclature, methods of test, specifications, and performance requirements for medical and surgical materials and devices. By 2004, the committee had adopted and approved through society vote more than 75 biomaterials specifications and 50 methods of test for biological response (Table 20.3), as well as device standards and other methods of test. The biomaterials specifications are consensus documents that describe the results of present practice in the fabrication of these materials. In that they are adhered to and the incorporated standardized materials are used as reference materials, the methods of test can be considered as standard tests, within the meaning of

TABLE 20.3

ASTM Biomaterials Standards and Methods of Testing for Host and Material Response[a]

Biomaterials

F0067-00 Specification for Unalloyed Titanium, for Surgical Implant Applications (UNS R50250, UNS R50400, UNSR50550, UNS R50700)

F0075-01 Specification for Cobalt-28 Chromium-6 Molybdenum Alloy Castings and Casting Alloy for Surgical Implants (UNS R30075)

F0086-04 Practice for Surface Preparation and Marking of Metallic Surgical Implants

F0090-01 Specification for Wrought Cobalt-20Chromium-15Tungsten-10Nickel Alloy for Surgical Implant Applications (UNS R30605)

F0136-02A Specification for Wrought Titanium-6Aluminum-4Vanadium ELI (Extra Low Interstitial) Alloy for Surgical Implant Applications (UNS R56401)

F0138-03 Specification for Wrought 18Chromium-14Nickel-2.5Molybdenum Stainless Steel Bar and Wire for Surgical Implants (UNS S31673)

F0139-03 Specification for Wrought 18Chromium-14Nickel-2.5Molybdenum Stainless Steel Sheet and Strip for Surgical Implants (UNS S31673)

F0451-99AE01 Specification for Acrylic Bone Cement

F0560-05 Specification for Unalloyed Tantalum for Surgical Implant Applications (UNS R05200, UNS R05400)

F0562-02 Specification for Wrought 35Cobalt-35Nickel-20Chromium-10Molybdenum Alloy for Surgical Implant Applications (UNS R30035)

F0563-00 Specification for Wrought Cobalt-20Nickel-20Chromium-3.5Molybdenum-3.5Tungsten-5Iron Alloy for Surgical Implant Applications (UNS R30563)

F0602-98AR03 Criteria for Implantable Thermoset Epoxy Plastics

F0603-00 Specification for High-Purity Dense Aluminum Oxide for Medical Application

F0604 Specification for Silicone Elastomers Used in Medical Applications

F0620-00 Specification for Alpha plus Beta Titanium Alloy Forgings for Surgical Implants

F0621-02 Specification for Stainless Steel Forgings for Surgical Implants

F0639-98AR03 Specification for Polyethylene Plastics for Medical Applications

F0641-04 Specification for Implantable Epoxy Electronic Encapsulants

F0648-00E01 Specification for Ultra-High-Molecular-Weight Polyethylene Powder and Fabricated Form for Surgical Implants

F0665-98R03 Classification for Vinyl Chloride Plastics Used in Biomedical Application

F0688-05 Specification for Wrought Cobalt-35 Nickel-20 Chromium-10 Molybdenum Alloy Plate, Sheet, and Foil for Surgical Implants (UNS R30035)

F0702-98AR03 Specification for Polysulfone Resin for Medical Applications

F0745-00 Specification for 18Chromium-12.5Nickel-2.5Molybdenum Stainless Steel for Cast and Solution-Annealed Surgical Implant Applications

F0754-00 Specification for Implantable Polytetrafluoroethylene (PTFE) Polymer Fabricated in Sheet, Tube, and Rod Shapes

F0755-99R05 Specification for Selection of Porous Polyethylene for Use in Surgical Implants

F0799-02 Specification for Cobalt-28Chromium-6Molybdenum Alloy Forgings for Surgical Implants (UNS R31537, R31538, R31539)

F0899-02 Specification for Stainless Steels for Surgical Instruments

F0961-03 Specification for 35Cobalt-35Nickel-20Chromium-10Molybdenum Alloy Forgings for Surgical Implants (UNS R30035)

F0983-86R05 Practice for Permanent Marking of Orthopedic Implant Components

F0997-98AR03 Specification for Polycarbonate Resin for Medical Applications

(continued)

TABLE 20.3 (CONTINUED)

ASTM Biomaterials Standards and Methods of Testing for Host and Material Response[a]

Biomaterials (continued)

F1058-02 Specification for Wrought 40Cobalt-20Chromium-16Iron-15Nickel-7Molybdenum Alloy Wire and Strip for Surgical Implant Applications (UNS R30003 and UNS R30008)

F1088-04A Specification for Beta-Tricalcium Phosphate for Surgical Implantation

F1091-02 Specification for Wrought Cobalt-20Chromium-15Tungsten-10Nickel Alloy Surgical Fixation Wire [UNS R30605]

F1108-04 Specification for Titanium-6Aluminum-4Vanadium Alloy Castings for Surgical Implants (UNS R56406)

F1185-03 Specification for Composition of Hydroxylapatite for Surgical Implants

F1251-89R03 Terminology Relating to Polymeric Biomaterials in Medical and Surgical Devices

F1295-05 Specification for Wrought Titanium-6 Aluminum-7 Niobium Alloy for Surgical Implant Applications (UNS R567000)

F1314-01 Specification for Wrought Nitrogen Strengthened 22 Chromium/N 13 Nickel/N 5 Manganese/N 2.5 Molybdenum Stainless Steel Alloy Bar and Wire for Surgical Implants (UNS S20910)

F1341-99 Specification for Unalloyed Titanium Wire UNS R50250, UNS R50400, UNS R50550, UNS R50700, for Surgical Implant Applications

F1350-02 Specification for Wrought 18Chromium-14Nickel-2.5Molybdenum Stainless Steel Surgical Fixation Wire (UNS S31673)

F1377-04 Specification for Cobalt-28 Chromium-6 Molybdenum Powder for Coating of Orthopedic Implants (UNS-R30075)

F1472-02A Specification for Wrought Titanium-6Aluminum-4Vanadium Alloy for Surgical Implant Applications (UNS R56400)

F1537-00 Specification for Wrought Cobalt-28 Chromium-6 Molybdenum Alloy for Surgical Implants

F1538-03 Specification for Glass and Glass Ceramic Biomaterials for Implantation

F1579-02E01 Specification for Polyaryletherketone (PAEK) Polymers for Surgical Implant Applications

F1580-01 Specification for Titanium and Titanium-6 Aluminum-4/tVanadium Alloy Powders for Coatings of Surgical Implants

F1581-99 Specification for Composition of Anorganic Bone for Surgical Implants

F1586-02 Specification for Wrought Nitrogen Strengthened 21 Chromium/M10 Nickel/M3 Manganese/M2.5 Molybdenum Stainless Steel Alloy Bar for Surgical Implants (UNS S31675)

F1609-03 Specification for Calcium Phosphate Coatings for Implantable Materials

F1713-03 Specification for Wrought Titanium-13Niobium-13Zirconium Alloy for Surgical Implant Applications (UNS R58130)

F1813-01 Specification for Wrought Titanium/N 12 Molybdenum /N 6 Zirconium/N 2 Iron Alloy for Surgical Implant (UNS R58120)

F1839-01 Specification for Rigid Polyurethane Foam for Use as a Standard Material for Testing Orthopedic Devices and Instruments

F1855-00R05 Specification for Polyoxymethylene (Acetal) for Medical Applications

F1873-98 Specification for High-Purity Dense Yttria Tetragonal Zirconium Oxide Polycrystal (Y-TZP) for Surgical Implant Applications

F1876-98R03E01 Specification for Polyetherketoneetherketoneketone (PEKEKK) Resins for Surgical Implant Applications

(continued)

TABLE 20.3 (CONTINUED)

ASTM Biomaterials Standards and Methods of Testing for Host and Material Response[a]

Biomaterials (continued)

F1925-99R05 Specification for Virgin Poly(L-Lactic Acid) Resin for Surgical Implants

F2005-00 Terminology for Nickel-Titanium Shape Memory Alloys

F2026-02 Specification for Polyetheretherketone (PEEK) Polymers for Surgical Implant Applications

F2038-00R05 Guide for Silicone Elastomers, Gels and Foams Used in Medical Applications Part I/M Formulations and Uncured Materials

F2042-00R05 Guide for Silicone Elastomers, Gels, and Foams Used in Medical Applications Part II/M Crosslinking and Fabrication

F2063-00 Specification for Wrought Nickel-Titanium Shape Memory Alloys for Medical Devices and Surgical Implants

F2066-01 Specification for Wrought Titanium-15 Molybdenum Alloy for Surgical Implant Applications (UNS R58150)

F2146-01 Specification for Wrought Titanium-3Aluminum-2.5Vanadium Alloy Seamless Tubing for Surgical Implant Applications (UNS R56320)

F2210-02 Guide for Processing Cells, Tissues, and Organs for Use in Tissue Engineered Medical Products

F2211-02 Classification for Tissue-Engineered Medical Products (TEMPs)

F2224-03 Specification for High-Purity Calcium Sulfate Hemihydrate or Dihydrate for Surgical Implants

F2229-02 Specification for Wrought, Nitrogen-Strengthened 23Manganese-21Chromium-1Molybdenum Low-Nickel Stainless Steel Alloy Bar and Wire for Surgical Implants (UNS S29108)

F2257-03 Specification for Wrought Seamless or Welded and Drawn 18 Chromium-14Nickel-2.5Molybdenum Stainless Steel Small Diameter Tubing for Surgical Implants (UNS S31673)

F2311-03 Guide for Classification of Therapeutic Skin Substitutes

F2312-04 Terminology Relating to Tissue-Engineered Medical Products

F2313-03 Specification for Virgin Poly(glycolide) and Poly(glycolide-co-lactide) Resins for Surgical Implants with Mole Fractions Greater than or Equal to 70% Glycolide

F2315-03 Guide for Immobilization or Encapsulation of Living Cells or Tissue in Alginate Gels

F2386-04 Guide for Preservation of Tissue-Engineered Medical Products (TEMPs)

F2393-04 Specification for High-Purity Dense Magnesia Partially Stabilized Zirconia (Mg-PSZ) for Surgical Implant Applications

Methods of Test for Host and Material Response

F0561-05 Practice for Retrieval and Analysis of Implanted Medical Devices and Associated Tissues

F0619-03 Practice for Extraction of Medical Plastics

F0624-98AR03 Guide for Evaluation of Thermoplastic Polyurethane Solids and Solutions for Biomedical Applications

F0719-81R02E01 Practice for Testing Biomaterials in Rabbits for Primary Skin Irritation

F0720-81R02E01 Practice for Testing Guinea Pigs for Contact Allergens: Guinea Pig Maximization Test

F0732-00 Test Method for Wear Testing of Polymeric Materials Used in Total Joint Prostheses

(continued)

TABLE 20.3 (CONTINUED)

ASTM Biomaterials Standards and Methods of Testing for Host and Material Response[a]

Methods of Test for Host and Material Response (continued)

F0746-04 Test Method for Pitting or Crevice Corrosion of Metallic Surgical Implant Materials

F0748-04 Practice for Selecting Generic Biological Test Methods for Materials and Devices

F0749-98R02E02 Practice for Evaluating Material Extracts by Intracutaneous Injection in the Rabbit

F0750-87R02E01 Practice for Evaluating Material Extracts by Systemic Injection in the Mouse

F0756-00 Practice for Assessment of Hemolytic Properties of Materials

F0763-04 Practice for Short-Term Screening of Implant Materials

F0813-01 Practice for Direct Contact Cell Culture Evaluation of Materials for Medical Devices

F0895-84R01E01 Test Method for Agar Diffusion Cell Culture Screening for Cytotoxicity

F0897-02 Test Method for Measuring Fretting Corrosion of Osteosynthesis Plates and Screws

F0981-04 Practice for Assessment of Compatibility of Biomaterials for Surgical Implants with Respect to Effect of Materials on Muscle and Bone[*]

F1027-86R02 Practice for Assessment of Tissue and Cell Compatibility of Orofacial Prosthetic Materials and Devices

F1408-97R02E01 Practice for Subcutaneous Screening Test for Implant Materials

F1439-03 Guide for Performance of Lifetime Bioassay for the Tumorigenic Potential of Implant Materials

F1635-04 Test Method for *in Vitro* Degradation Testing of Hydrolytically Degradable Polymer Resins and Fabricated Forms for Surgical Implants

F1801-97 Practice for Corrosion Fatigue Testing of Metallic Implant Materials

F1830-97 Practice for Selection of Blood for *in Vitro* Evaluation of Blood Pumps

F1841-97 Practice for Assessment of Hemolysis in Continuous Flow Blood Pumps

F1877-98R03E01 Practice for Characterization of Particles

F1903-98R03 Practice for Testing for Biological Responses to Particles *in vitro*

F1904-98R03 Practice for Testing the Biological Responses to Particles *in vivo*

F1905-98R03 Practice for Selecting Tests for Determining the Propensity of Materials to Cause Immunotoxicity

F1906-98R03 Practice for Evaluation of Immune Responses in Biocompatibility Testing Using ELISA Tests, Lymphocyte Proliferation, and Cell Migration

F1926-03 Test Method for Evaluation of the Environmental Stability of Calcium Phosphate Coatings

F1983-99R03 Practice for Assessment of Compatibility of Absorbable/Resorbable Biomaterials for Implant Applications

F1984-99R03 Practice for Testing for Whole Complement Activation in Serum by Solid Materials

F2003-02 Practice for Accelerated Aging of Ultra-High Molecular Weight Polyethylene after Gamma Irradiation in Air

F2025-00 Practice for Gravimetric Measurement of Polymeric Components for Wear Assessment

F2027-00E01 Guide for Characterization and Testing of Substrate Materials for Tissue-Engineered Medical Products

F2064-00 Guide for Characterization and Testing of Alginates as Starting Materials Intended for Use in Biomedical and Tissue/Engineered Medical Products Application

F2065-00E01 Practice for Testing for Alternative Pathway Complement Activation in Serum by Solid Materials

---

[*] See Appendix 1 in Chapter 18.

(continued)

TABLE 20.3 (CONTINUED)

ASTM Biomaterials Standards and Methods of Testing for Host and Material Response[a]

Methods of Test for Host and Material Response (continued)

F2102-01E01 Guide for Evaluating the Extent of Oxidation in Ultra-High-Molecular-Weight Polyethylene Fabricated Forms Intended for Surgical Implants

F2103-01 Guide for Characterization and Testing of Chitosan Salts as Starting Materials Intended for Use in Biomedical and Tissue-Engineered Medical Product Applications

F2129-04 Test Method for Conducting Cyclic Potentiodynamic Polarization Measurements to Determine the Corrosion Susceptibility of Small Implant Devices

F2131-02 Test Method for *in Vitro* Biological Activity of Recombinant Human Bone Morphogenetic Protein-2 (rhBMP-2) Using the W-20 Mouse Stromal Cell Line

F2147-01 Practice for Guinea Pig: Split Adjuvant and Closed Patch Testing for Contact Allergens

F2148-01 Practice for Evaluation of Delayed Contact Hypersensitivity Using the Murine Local Lymph Node Assay (LLNA)

F2149-01 Test Method for Automated Analyses of Cells/The Electrical Sensing Zone Method of Enumerating and Sizing Single Cell Suspensions

F2150-02E01 Guide for Characterization and Testing of Biomaterial Scaffolds Used in Tissue-Engineered Medical Products

F2151-01 Practice for Assessment of White Blood Cell Morphology after Contact with Materials

F2183-02 Test Method for Small Punch Testing of Ultra-High Molecular Weight Polyethylene Used in Surgical Implants

F2212-02 Guide for Characterization of Type I Collagen as Starting Material for Surgical Implants and Substrates for Tissue Engineered Medical Products (TEMPs)

F2255-05 Test Method for Strength Properties of Tissue Adhesives in Lap-Shear by Tension Loading

F2256-05 Test Method for Strength Properties of Tissue Adhesives in T-Peel by Tension Loading

F2258-05 Test Method for Strength Properties of Tissue Adhesives in Tension

F2259-03 Test Method for Determining the Chemical Composition and Sequence in Alginate by Proton Nuclear Magnetic Resonance (1H NMR) Spectroscopy

F2260-03 Test Method for Determining Degree of Deacetylation in Chitosan Salts by Proton Nuclear Magnetic Resonance (1H NMR) Spectroscopy

F2347-03 Guide for Characterization and Testing of Hyaluronan as Starting Materials Intended for Use in Biomedical and Tissue-Engineered Medical Product Applications

F2382-04E01 Test Method for Assessment of Intravascular Medical Device Materials on Partial Thromboplastin Time (PTT)

F2392-04 Test Method for Burst Strength of Surgical Sealants

Note: F-999-02R03E02 means standard F999, adopted 2002, revised 2003, two editorial changes (to 2003 version).

[a] ASTM standards are routinely revised on a 5-year cycle. A number of those listed here have been reprinted more recently with minor or editorial changes only. Please refer to most recent editions of ASTM annual standards books for current texts and explanatory notes.

Source: 2005 Annual Book of ASTM Standards, Vol. 13.01. ASTM International, West Conshohocken, PA, 2004, xi–xv.

Section 1.2. Individual standards are available from ASTM, as well as annual collections. Most technical libraries maintain recent full sets of ASTM standards in their reference collections; biomaterials standards are in annual volume 13.01.

It is worth noting that, although ASTM F-4 standards for test methods are consensus documents and have wide support in government, academia, and industry, they are rarely used. That is, most investigators derive variations of these procedures; however, when care is taken to meet the requirements of the parent procedure, the revised and extended procedure is properly said to adhere to the ASTM standard or recommended method of test.

20.3.3   Other Efforts

A number of other organizations have entered into the specification and standardization of medical materials and devices. However, none are as advanced in their efforts as the ADA and the ASTM. Perhaps the best known of the remainder of these organizations is the Association for Advancement of Medical Instrumentation (AAMI). This organization has been involved for a number of years in developing specifications for active medical devices such as heart pacers and neurostimulators. A number of these specifications are coming into general use.

Outside the U.S., other countries have made progress in this field. Some, like Canada, have decided to follow the progress of American groups such as the ASTM and ADA. As standards have been adopted as American National Standards (by the American National Standards Institute [designation: ANSI]), they are also being adopted after review as Canadian standards. For instance, all of the ADA standards listed in Table 20.2 are now ANSI standards, as are many ASTM standards. Some countries, such as Germany, France, and England, have developed, relatively independently, their own national standards for implant materials and devices. An international standards-making group, the International Standards Organization (ISO),* has organized two committees with broad international representation:

- ISO TC 150 is evaluating national device and material standards and attempting to adopt common international versions. This effort is under way in the fields of orthopaedic, cardiovascular, and neurosurgery and will eventually spread to encompass all medical disciplines.
- ISO TC 194 is conducting similar activities in the area of measurement of biological response.

Subject to approval by the European Commission, ISO standards began to supplant or override national standards with the formation of the Euro-

---

* http//www.iso.org.

pean Common Market in 1992 and, as a result, are becoming *de facto* standards for firms involved in international trade in medical and surgical materials and devices.* Table 20.4 lists the ISO standards currently in force for biomaterials and methods of test for host response. Individual AAMI and ISO standards are available from the Association for Advancement of Medical Instrumentation.**

Trade associations such as the Orthopedic Surgical Manufacturers Association (OSMA) and the Health Industry Manufacturers Association (HIMA) have taken active roles in developing standards on their own or through activity of their representatives in standards-writing organizations such as ASTM, ISO, etc. Traditional professional organizations in the health and engineering professions also have standards committees that act as focal points for technical input into standards preparation by standards-making organizations.

20.4 U.S. Federal Regulation of Medical Devices and Biomaterials

20.4.1 Medical Device Amendments (1976)

Although the various standardization efforts described in previous sections continue through today, they were not generally perceived to be sufficient to provide safe and effective medical and surgical materials and devices for the public and to control unsafe and ineffective materials and devices. The result in the U.S. was a legislative mandate for the executive branch of government to control and regulate medical device manufacturing in the public interest. The initial chosen legislative tool was the Medical Device Amendments (1976) whose overall goal is to assure the safety and efficacy of devices. This legislation provides for classification of devices, which will be considered later in this chapter. They also lay out a scheme of general controls including provisions for dealing with adulterated and misbranded devices, for registering device types and device manufacturers, for premarket notification of the introduction of new devices, and for dealing with banned devices. Details of manufacturers' obligations to repair, replace, or refund in the case of defective devices are also included. The amendments also permit the establishment of regulations to define "good manufacturing practices" and of performance standards as well as premarket product development protocols for new materials and devices.

---

* For a detailed idea of how these various standards and specifications interact generically with the process of federal regulation of medical materials and devices, the reader is referred to *Everything You Always Wanted to Know about the Medical Device Amendments...and Weren't Afraid to Ask*, HHS, FDA, Rockville, MD, FDA 92-4173.
** http://www.aami.org.

TABLE 20.4

ISO Biomaterials Standards and Methods of Testing for Host Response[a]

General Biomaterials

ISO 5832-1:1997 Implants for surgery — metallic materials — part 1: wrought stainless steel
ISO 5832-2:1999 Implants for surgery — metallic materials — part 2: unalloyed titanium
ISO 5832-3:1996 Implants for surgery — metallic materials — part 3: wrought titanium 6–aluminum 4–vanadium alloy
ISO 5832-4:1996 Implants for surgery — metallic materials — part 4: cobalt–chromium–molybdenum casting alloy
ISO 5832-5:1993 Implants for surgery — metallic materials — part 5: wrought cobalt–chromium–tungsten–nickel alloy
ISO 5832-6:1997 Implants for surgery — metallic materials — part 6: wrought cobalt–nickel–chromium–molybdenum alloy
ISO 5832-7:1994 Implants for surgery — metallic materials — part 7: forgeable and cold-formed cobalt–chromium–nickel–molybdenum–iron alloy
ISO 5832-8:1997 Implants for surgery — metallic materials — part 8: wrought cobalt–nickel–chromium–molybdenum–tungsten–iron alloy
ISO 5832-9:1992 Implants for surgery — metallic materials — part 9: wrought high-nitrogen stainless steel
ISO 5832-10:1996 Implants for surgery — metallic materials — part 10: wrought titanium 5–aluminum 2,5–iron alloy
ISO 5832-11:1994 Implants for surgery — metallic materials — part 11: wrought titanium 6–aluminum 7–niobium alloy
ISO 5832-12:1996 Implants for surgery — metallic materials — part 12: wrought cobalt–chromium–molybdenum alloy
ISO 5833:2002 Implants for surgery — acrylic resin cements
ISO 5834-1:1998 Implants for surgery — Ultrahigh molecular weight polyethylene — part 1: powder form
ISO 5834-2:1998 Implants for surgery — ultrahigh molecular weight polyethylene — part 2: molded forms
ISO 10334:1994 Implants for surgery — malleable wires for use as sutures and other surgical applications
ISO 13356:1997 Implants for surgery — ceramic materials based on yttria-stabilized tetragonal zirconia (Y-TZP)
ISO 13779-1:2000 Implants for surgery – part 1 — ceramic hydroxyapatite
ISO 13781:1997 Poly (L-lactide) resins and fabricated forms for surgical implants — *in vitro* degradation testing
ISO 13782:1996 Implants for surgery — metallic materials — unalloyed tantalum for surgical implant applications

Dental Materials

ISO 1561:1995 Dental casting wax
ISO 1563:1990 Dental alginate impression material
ISO 1564:1995 Dental aqueous impression materials based on agar
ISO 1567:1988 Dentistry — denture base polymers
ISO 6871-1:1994 Dental base metal casting alloys — part 1: cobalt-based alloys
ISO 6871-2:1994 Dental base metal casting alloys — part 2: nickel-based alloys
ISO 6872:1995 Dental ceramic
ISO 6874:1988 Dental resin-based pit and fissure sealants
ISO 6876:2001 Dental root canal sealing materials

(continued)

TABLE 20.4 (CONTINUED)

ISO Biomaterials Standards and Methods of Testing for Host Response[a]

Dental Materials (continued)

ISO 6877:1995 Dental root-canal obturating points
ISO 7491:2000 Dental materials — determination of color stability of dental polymeric
materials
ISO 8891:1998 Dental casting alloys with noble metal content of 25% up to but not including 75%
ISO 9333:1990 Dental brazing materials
ISO 9693:1997 Metal-ceramic dental restoration systems
ISO 9694:1996 Dental phosphate-bonded casting investments
ISO 9917:1991 Dental water-based cements
ISO 9917-2:1998 Dental water-based cements — part 2: light-activated cements
ISO 10139-1:1991 Dentistry — resilient lining materials for removable dentures — part 1:
short-term materials
ISO 10139-2 Dentistry — resilient lining materials for removable dentures — part 2: long-
term materials
ISO 11244:1998 Dental brazing investments
ISO 11245: 1999 Dental restorations — phosphate-bonded refractory die material
ISO 11246:1996 Dental ethyl silicate-bonded casting investments
ISO 12163:1999 Dental baseplate modeling waxes
ISO 16744:2003 Dentistry — base metal materials for dental restorations
ISO 24234:2004 Dentistry — mercury and alloys for dental amalgam

Methods of Test for Host Response

ISO 7405:1997 Dentistry — preclinical evaluation of biocompatibility of medical devices used
in dentistry — test methods for dental materials
ISO 10993–1:2003 Biological evaluation of medical devices — part 1: evaluation and testing
ISO 10993-2:1992 Biological evaluation of medical devices — part 2: animal welfare
requirements
ISO 10993-3:2003 Biological evaluation of medical devices — part 3: tests for genotoxicity,
carcinogenicity and reproductive toxicity
ISO 10993-4:2002 Biological evaluation of medical devices — part 4: selection of tests for
interactions with blood
ISO 10993-5:1999 Biological evaluation of medical devices — part 5: tests for *in vitro*
cytotoxicity
ISO 10993-6:1994 Biological evaluation of medical devices — part 6: tests for local effects after
implantation
ISO 10993-10:2002 Biological evaluation of medical devices — part 10: tests for irritation and
delayed-type hypersensitivity
ISO 10993-11:1993 Biological evaluation of medical devices — part 11: tests for systemic toxicity
ISO 10993-12:2002 Biological evaluation of medical devices — part 12: sample preparation
and reference materials
ISO 10993-16:1997 Biological evaluation of medical devices — part 16: toxicokinetic study
design for degradation products and leachables
ISO 10993-17:2002 Biological evaluation of medical devices — part 17: establishment of
allowable limits for leachable substances
ISO 11979-5:1999 Opthalmic Implants — intraocular lenses — part 5: biocompatibility
ISO 12891-1-4:1998, 2000 Retrieval and analysis of surgical implants

[a] In some cases, ISO standards have multiple designations, reflecting texts identical with
national standards (such as ANSI); however, only ISO designations are listed here.

Source: International Standards Organization (ISO) http://www.iso.org.

If the Medical Device Amendments can be said to have a central theme, it is one that closely parallels the ideas of the safety and effectiveness of drugs, cosmetics, and food additives. That is, the legislation foresaw a pattern in which materials and devices would be developed, tested, and demonstrated to be safe and efficacious before being offered for sale. Once this point was reached, their future safety and effectiveness would then be controlled by the institution of general standards and controls or by the provisions of specific performance standards.

20.4.2   Safe Medical Devices Act (1990)

The Safe Medical Devices Act (1990) was the first major revision of the Medical Device Amendments and occurred largely as a result of public dissatisfaction with the implementation (rather than the content) of medical and surgical device regulations envisioned at the time of passage of the 1976 legislation. The many provisions of the act (Kahan et al. 1991) are intended largely to strengthen, streamline, better define, and speed up regulatory activities. Thus, the provisions primarily enlarge on and modify rather than replace those of the earlier Medical Device Amendments. However, several new provisions are introduced, including lifetime tracking of permanently implanted life-supporting or life-sustaining devices, more and improved reports of life-threatening device malfunction, regulatory authority to order mandatory recalls and allow seizure of defective devices, rules for postmarket introduction surveillance of experience with permanent implants, and creation of a humanitarian device exemption, similar to an "orphan" drug provision within drug regulation, to simplify and reduce the cost of development of devices for diseases or conditions affecting fewer than 4000 individuals in the U.S.

20.4.3   FDA Modernization Act (1997)

At the time of the adoption of the Medical Device Amendments (1976), no one could predict the vast increase in number and complexity of medical and surgical devices that would occur in the 1980s and 1990s. The result was a gradual slowdown of FDA review and approval activities and a growing frustration on the part of manufacturers and the public. Various small changes were made to FDA procedures, including a second Safe Medical Devices (1992) act; however, the major change came about in 1997 with the adoption of a widely heralded and long awaited "modernization" act. This act (Kahan et al. 1998a, b) is complex and its effects are still just beginning to be felt. Perhaps the most important aspects of its intentions are:

- To reduce the arbitrary and unpredictable nature of FDA device regulatory activities by clarifying previsions of the 1976 amendments and spelling out procedures previously left to administrative definition

- To make the FDA a partner with industry and physicians during the device design, development, and qualification process, rather than merely a judge of the end product performance, thus improving chances of a new device's release for use after an initial application; this is to be brought about by development and approval of a product design protocol early in the design process
- To require a higher level of professional achievement within the FDA regulatory staff by providing for better training, liaison, and reporting

Review times, which had in some cases stretched out to years, are apparently shortening significantly and the FDA's role in medical device development seems less threatening to manufacturers as a consequence of this act. More recently, subsequent to yet another effort to provide legislative relief,* various efforts have been made to speed up the review process further, in some cases by raising fees or imposing special charges on the manufacturers. However, these have come under significant criticism from industry because they appear to embody the old political principle of "pay to play." The longer term consequences of these many changes and the continuing influence of the political leadership of the FDA remains to be seen.

20.5 Regulation of Materials for Implants

20.5.1 Requirements of the Medical Device Amendments

The need for regulatory standards arises from the requirements of the Medical Device Amendments (1976) and the Safe Medical Devices Act (1990). These are embodied in a classification system that attempts to distinguish among various generic types of devices on the basis of risk to the patient. The general pattern of device classification is as follows. Devices are classified into three categories by one of 14 specialty-oriented Device Classification Panels:

- Class I, general controls: a device for which controls other than standards and premarket approval are sufficient to assure safety and effectiveness
- Class II, performance standards: a device for which general controls are insufficient to assure safety and effectiveness but for which information is sufficient for the establishment of a performance standard to provide such assurance

---

* Medical Device User Fee and Modernization Act, PL 107-250.

- Class III, premarket approval: a device for which insufficient information exists to assure that general controls and performance standards would provide reasonable assurance of safety and effectiveness and that is represented to be life sustaining, life supporting, or implanted in the body or that presents a potential unreasonable risk of illness or injury

Devices classified as class III and any new device that comes on the market after May 28, 1976 must pass through some form of scientific premarket review before market introduction. At the point at which these products are judged to be reasonably safe, effective, and controllable by a performance standard, they may be reclassified into class II. Thus, the existence of standards can be seen to be critical to the introduction of new materials and devices into general use. It is hoped that many of the voluntary standards developed by the various organizations mentioned here, as well as others, can be adapted to be regulatory standards.

To date, very few regulatory standards have been approved for devices and none for materials. However, many permanent implants have been reclassified from class III to class II on the basis of long pre- and postenactment experience. The need for regulatory standards, particularly for materials of construction, will become more acute as more devices achieve such reclassification.

As a consequence and in line with similar changes throughout the U.S. government, the effort to substitute voluntary standards (see Section 20.5.2) for regulatory standards is continuing. This effort is driven by a directive of the Office of Management and Budget (OMB-119*) (Kono 1998). The basic provision of OMB 119 is permission (and encouragement) to substitute a consensus standard, such as those developed by ASTM or ISO, for a specially drawn regulatory standard if the provisions of the voluntary standard are appropriate to meet the needs of the regulatory agency, in this case the FDA. This directive was recognized in a provision of the FDA Modernization Act (1997) (section 204) to make conformance with an appropriate (preaccepted) standard the basis for approval for the sale and use of certain devices.

20.5.2   Voluntary vs. Regulatory Standards

It should be clear to the reader that a voluntary standard and a regulatory standard are not necessarily the same thing. Voluntary standards, whether consensus derived or otherwise, are designed to describe the content, design, construction, and performance of existing devices, as well as to set forth methods of verifying compliance with these aspects of the standard. By their nature, regulatory standards are designed to regulate — that is, to assure specific attributes of products. In the case of the (regulatory) performance

---

* OMB 119: Federal Participation in Development and Use of Voluntary Consensus Standards and in Conformity Assessment Activities. *Fed. Reg.* 61:8548, 1998.

standards required by the Medical Device Amendments (1976), the specific attributes to be regulated are safety and efficacy. It is not clear at this time what combination of standards on content, design, and construction, as well as simulation tests *in vitro* and *in vivo*, are necessary and sufficient to meet such a general requirement for (*in vivo*) patient performance. Thus, although it is possible to prepare a voluntary standard for an existing device or for its materials of construction, the relationship of this standard to a future generic regulatory standard is tenuous, at best.

It seems safe to presume that as genuinely new materials come under consideration as candidate biomaterials, they will be qualified in a similar way to that envisaged specifically for devices. In the course of selection and development, they pass through series of tests along the lines of those discussed in Section 19.2. As their behavior becomes better understood and devices incorporating them pass into clinical trials, the process of voluntary standards preparation begins. The results of these tests and the proposed form of the standard then constitute the body of material, with supporting clinical reports, that can be submitted for initial review by a regulating agency such as the FDA.

In that case, the use of the words "performance standard" in the 1976 enabling legislation harmonizes well with the ideas of biological performance laid out here in earlier chapters. Thus, a performance standard for an implant material is one that describes the chemical, physical, and processing requirements for a material that are needed to assure a reproducible level of biological performance, as well as to meet the engineering requirements, of a proposed application. As soon as it is possible to prepare such a document, the material becomes in an important sense a known material. Its biological performance can be examined objectively and its suitability (and admissibility) for specific applications can be determined. At this point, as embodied in devices, it should pass easily into class II and be a natural competitor for use in future specific medical and surgical device applications. Perhaps the recent revision of OMB 119 (Kono 1998) will encourage this evolution and lead to materials "generally recognized as safe" for specific groups of applications.

As an initial step in responding to OMB-119, the FDA maintains an online registry of standards that it recognizes in regulatory submissions.* In large part, these standards remain consensus standards that reflect current industrial practice and carry with them no assurance of safety and efficacy of the devices designed and constructed utilizing them.**

---

* http://www.accessdata.fda.gov/scripts/cdrh/cfdocs/cfStandards/search.cfm.

** For completeness, it is worth noting also that product liability litigation has failed to establish that FDA approval for sale and use implies a guarantee of safety and efficacy; such regulatory action only establishes that the then current FDA requirements for such approval have been met. The converse is also true: lack of FDA approval for a specific indication does not *de facto* render a medical device and its materials of construction unsafe and/or ineffective.

Safety will continue to be a relative rather than an absolute attribute because it will always be related, as I have pointed out, to a balance between risk and benefit (Black 1995).

20.6   The Biomaterials Supply "Crisis"

Largely as a consequence of litigation associated with the use of silicone gel in breast augmentation implants and polytetrafluoroethylene in tempero-mandibular joint (TMJ) replacements, concern about future availability of many biomaterials rose during the 1990s (Hallab et al. 1997). The problem was apparently that materials suppliers, whose products contribute only a few cents or dollars to the cost of medical devices selling for thousands of dollars, have repeatedly been named by plaintiffs in actions alleging injury through malperformance of the device or merely maloutcome of the overall procedure. For some materials producers, the result has been legal defense costs — even in the absence of adverse judgments against them — that far exceed any reasonable profit. As a consequence, some manufacturers have ceased to provide materials to medical device manufacturers. The end effect is unclear; in the case of medical-grade silicones, the withdrawal of Dow Corning from the marketplace led to the entry of several new small companies that now provide a wider range of well characterized materials, albeit at significantly higher prices, than were previously available (Hallab et al. 1997).

This situation, still regarded by some as an impending "crisis," seems unfortunate on two grounds. In the first place, because the device manufacturer makes the selection of the material and then tests it as a material and indirectly during preclinical and clinical device evaluation, the so-called "learned intermediary" principle seems sufficient to protect the material manufacturer as long as the materials supplied are made to identified standards (Harper 1996). That is, the responsibility of the material manufacturer is to assure that the material is what it is represented to be and that of the device manufacturer (the "learned intermediary" between the material supplier and the patient) is to make the judgment that the material selected has suitable biological performance in the intended application.

Although this concept is clear in U.S. litigation experience, it does not overcome the problem of paying for legal defense before and until the material manufacturer is discharged from the plaintiff's action. Numerous attempts have been made, led by then Rep. Lieberman (D-Conn), to embody this principle in a federal statute. Despite widespread resistance to product liability reform, the Biomaterials Access Assurance Act (1998)* was finally

---

* PL 105-230. See http://www.advamed.org/publicdocs/legal021599.htm for an extensive legal analysis.

passed and signed into law. The provisions of this legislation parallel the arguments of Harper (1996) and provide for summary (immediate) discharge from medical product liability litigation for any materials supplier that meets appropriate standards and conditions of general salability for its medical grades of materials.

In the second place, the idea that withdrawal of medical grades of materials will make those materials unavailable is, to a degree, naive. Although some biomaterials are specifically manufactured for medial and surgical applications, many, such as ultrahigh molecular weight polyethylene and many titanium- and cobalt-base alloys, are simply selected batches or modest variants of very large quantity production commercial materials. Thus, because the FDA does not explicitly regulate biomaterials manufacture or manufacturers, it is quite possible that intermediaries or the device manufacturers could continue to procure suitable materials from commercial sources and qualify them (i.e., determine their conformance with relevant standards) for use in medical devices and implants.

An unforeseen negative result of the 1998 act has begun to emerge. Recently, biomaterials and process suppliers named with device manufactures as plaintiffs in cases in which failure modes appear to center on materials' properties rather than device design have begun to assert the defense that the device manufacturer is, *de facto*, a learned intermediary and, as a result, they share no possible liability for clinical maloutcome as long as their product meets the representations (specifications, etc.) for which they make it. This defense theory is novel enough that it has not yet been definitively tested in U.S. courts.

At this time, the situation remains very unclear. However, more than a decade after the specter of future biomaterials unavailability was seriously raised, the U.S does not appear to have any important shortages. Suppliers have changed and materials substitutions have been made, albeit at increased cost, but device availability to patients appears not to have been adversely affected so far.

References

American Dental Association, *Guide to Dental Materials and Devices*, 7th ed. ADA, Chicago, 1974.

American Society for Testing and Materials, *2005 Annual Book of ASTM Standards*, Vol. 13.01: *Medical Devices and Services*, ASTM International, West Conshohocken, PA, 2005.

Black, J., "Safe" biomaterials (editorial), *J. Biomed. Mater. Res.*, 29, 791, 1995.

Brown, P. and Cook, A.G., The background, formation, and maturation of committee F-4, *ASTM Standardization News*, October, 10, 1982.

Department of Health and Human Services, *Everything You Always Wanted to Know about the Medical Device Amendments…and Weren't Afraid to Ask*, HHS, FDA, Rockville, MD, FDA 92-4173, 1992.

Hallab, N.J. et al., Biomaterials crisis looms, *AAOS Bull.*, 45(1), 13, 1997.

Harper, G.L., An analysis of the potential liabilities and defenses of bulk suppliers of titanium biomaterials, *Gonzaga Law Rev.*, 32(1), 195, 1996.

Kahan, J.S., The Safe Medical Devices Act of 1990, *Med. Dev. Diag. Ind.*, 13(1), 66, 1991.

Kahan, J.S. and Holstein, H.M., The FDA Modernization Act of 1997: part 1, *Med. Dev. Diag. Ind.*, 20(3), 105, 1998a.

Kahan, J.S. and Holstein, H.M., The FDA Modernization Act of 1997: part 2, *Med. Dev. Diag. Ind.*, 20(4), 77, 1998b.

Kahan, J.S. et al., The implications of the Safe Medical Devices Act of 1990, *Med. Dev. Diag. Ind.*, 13(2), 44, 1991.

Kono, K., OMB A-119 revised, *ASTM Stand. News*, June, 1998, 19.

Lamb, R. DeF., *American Chamber of Horrors: The Truth about Food and Drugs*, Farrar & Rinehart, New York, 1936.

Mintz, M., *The Therapeutic Nightmare*, Houghton–Mifflin Co., Boston, 1965.

NF XIV, *The National Formulary*, 14th ed., American Pharmaceutical Association, Washington, D.C., 1975.

Sinclair, U., *The Jungle*, New American Library, New York, 1906.

USP XIX, *The Pharmacopeia of the United States of America, 19th revision*, The United States Pharmacopeial Convention, Inc., Washington, D.C., 1975.

USP 28, *The Pharmacopeia of the United States of America, 28th revision*, incorporating *The National Formulary, 23rd revision*, The United States Pharmacopeial Convention, Inc., Washington, D.C., 2005.

U.S. Congress, Medical Device Amendments, PL 94—295, 1976.

U.S. Congress, Safe Medical Devices, PL 101–629, 1990.

U.S. Congress, Safe Medical Devices, PL 102–300, 1992.

U.S. Congress, FDA Modernization Act, PL 105–15, 1997.

Bibliography

Black, J. and Hastings, G., *Handbook of Biomaterial Properties*, Chapman & Hall, London, 1998.

Cangelosi, R.J., Device standards: the view from the FDA, *Clin Eng.*, Jan–Mar, 5(1), 9, 1980.

Department of Health, Education, and Welfare, *Federal Food, Drug, and Cosmetic Act, as Amended*, Food and Drug Administration. U.S. Government Printing Office, Washington, D.C., 1972.

Food and Drug Administration, *Medical Devices Standardization Activities Report.* CDRH, FDA, HHS, Washington, D.C. FDA 94-4219. 1994.

Food and Drug Administration, *Standards Survey, National Edition*, Bureau of Medical Devices, Washington, D.C., 1979.

Health Industry Manufacturers Association, *Guidelines for the Development of Voluntary Device Law Standards, Report No. 79-6*, Health Industry Manufacturers Association, Washington, D.C., 1979.

Health Industry Manufacturers Association, *Guideline for Evaluating the Safety of Materials Used in Medical Devices, Report No. 78-7.* Health Industry Manufacturers Association, Washington, D.C., 1978.

Morton, W.A. and Veale, J.R., *Regulatory Issues in Artificial Organs: A Primer*, J.B. Lippincott, Philadelphia, 1987.

Ratner, B.D. et al., *Biomaterials Science: An Introduction to Materials in Medicine*, 1st ed., Academic Press, San Diego, 1996, 457.

21

Design and Selection of Implant Materials*

21.1 Introduction

21.1.1 What Is Design?

Design is what engineers do: they apply scientific knowledge and principles to the solution of practical problems. The object of their design may be a process, a new material, or a novel device. The process of design is artistic and creative, drawing from the same well at which the painter, sculptor, or writer does. What distinguishes the objects of engineering design from those of other artistic activities is the extent to which technological factors come into play in their realization (Asimow 1962).

As Cross (2000) points out, the separation between design and fabrication of man-made artifacts is a relatively recent event. When hand artisanship was the rule, design and fabrication were not separated: the maker designed as the final form of the artifact emerged. For the artist, there is still no separation in function: the design is the object. For the surgeon, the separation is incomplete: although surgical procedures are planned prospectively, detailed and complex decisions are made during the performance of the operation. However, for the engineer, the separation has become nearly total: today those who design rarely make and vice versa. This separation has led to vocational self-selection that produces significant problems for engineers involved in design. Engineering has become a linear analytical process, seeking the shortest distance to a solution. Engineers thus often have great difficulty in dealing with the creative, synthetic aspects of design that require attempts to devise as many alternative solutions as possible.

Even more than the creative aspects of design, the concept of a design process must be emphasized. Solutions to engineering design problems rarely, if ever, spring full blown from the mind of their creator. On the contrary, what is required is a systematic, dogged, iterative process stretching from exploration of initial requirements to evaluation of the preferred solution. In a sense, the design process and its necessary iterative design cycle

---

* Portions of this chapter appeared in an earlier form as Chapter 13 in Black (1988) and are reproduced by permission (Churchill–Livingstone Inc.).

represent attempts of engineering designers to deal with synthetic problems in an analytic fashion, rather in the manner of using digital computers to create analog models of systems. The use of a design process also has ethical implications: the iterative nature of design conducted in this fashion requires a continuous and repeated testing of goals and assumptions, thus introducing a system of checks and balances reflected as an inherent safety factor in the final product.

21.1.2   Introduction to the Orange

Engineers unfamiliar with design often have the same problem as a beginning art student: faced with a blank sheet of paper and an overall conception, they have no idea where to start. A useful exercise is a consideration of an orange in a process often referred to as reverse engineering. That is, given an object or finished artifact, one attempts to understand its rationale and determine details of the materials and processes of its construction retrospectively rather than design it prospectively. In this case, the use of an actual orange is a useful aid. The exercise proceeds in three steps:

1. *From observation and physical examination, make a list of all the things that it is possible to know about an orange.* In doing so, one usually begins with simple attributes, such as color, weight, size, etc., and moves to more complex ones, such as shape, number of seeds, amount of sugar contained, etc.

2. *For as many as possible of the quantitative attributes listed in step 1, estimate the value.* The benefit of this step is particularly seen when a number of individuals do the exercise separately or in groups and then compare their answers.

3. *For as many as possible of the attributes listed in step 1, propose as many methods as possible for finding their true or actual value.* This step provides clues to the later stages of design by requiring problem solving based upon estimates and other incomplete information.

The three steps of this exercise help to prime the creative pump. In form, they replicate steps 1, 2, and 4 of the design cycle, respectively (see Section 21.2.2). The first step teaches observation, the second estimation, and the third creation of alternatives.

This exercise also can be used to illustrate another point about design: it is better played as a team sport than as solitaire. This point may easily be demonstrated by setting the "orange exercise" for an individual and for a group to perform; the members of the group, no matter what its makeup, will always be more productive on average, let alone collectively, than the individual. Design can and often is performed by a single individual. However, it is far more productive if it is a group project; the resulting synergy increases in proportion to the variety of people involved.

21.2 The Design Process

21.2.1 The Phases of Design

Asimow (1962) defines design as a seven-phase process arising from a primitive need (Table 21.1). Materials design and selection, in the sense in which they are discussed in this chapter, fall within Asimow's phases I to III, depending upon the depth and detail required of the design process. In each instance, a structured design process or cycle (see the next section) is desirable. Device design is more likely to have to deal with all of Asimow's seven phases. In either case, a single phase may require a number of design cycles within its process. Design may be required for the development of manufacturing processes and design of devices, of surgical procedures and even of experiments. With suitable modifications, the same structured process may be utilized.

21.2.2 The Design Cycle

A structured design process consists of the consecutive execution of a repetitive design cycle. The design of a simple device, such as a tongue depressor and its dispensing container, may be achieved in as little as three or four such cycles; however, a complex design, such as a powered wheel chair, may require hundreds of such cycles, some in parallel and others in series.

The design of materials is a simpler problem, in general, than the design of devices. Materials design is rarely addressed directly because device designers tend to view themselves as expert in materials and to assume that materials design is merely a matter of selection from among the options available. This approach is illustrated by Lewis' (1990) otherwise excellent

TABLE 21.1

Seven Phases of Design

Primitive Need → Preliminary Phases

    I: Feasibility design
   II: Preliminary design
  III: Detailed design

Phases Related to Production/Consumption Cycle

   IV: Planning for production
    V: Planning for distribution
   VI: Planning for consumption
  VII: Planning for retirement

Source: Asimow, M., *Introduction to Design*, Prentice Hall, Englewood Cliffs, NJ, 1962, 1.

discussion of the design of a femoral medullary stem for a total hip replacement prosthesis.

(It is true that the selection of materials, with and without modification, has dominated biomaterials design until recently.) It is possible to use a formal design process for selection and/or modification of materials, but this may seem clumsy and unwarranted except for teaching purposes. However, today the advancing popularity of composite materials or, more properly, engineered materials makes necessary the use of a design process for the prospective selection of biomaterials properties for medical and surgical devices. The evolution of biomaterials as a field into the prospective design of interactive materials, such as resorbable ceramics and polymeric matrices subject to postimplantation cellular remodeling, further emphasizes this point.

The design of materials may require several cycles in series: first, selection of materials properties; then selection of processing methods and parameters, followed by consideration of the interaction of various biomaterials selected. These cycles cannot take place in isolation from the considerations involved in the design of the device (for which the biomaterials are designed/selected) because device requirements impose materials requirements and materials selections affect design choices.

A number of models may be utilized to develop a design cycle. The approach in this chapter is derived from that of Love (1986) and is shown in schematic form in Figure 21.1. The next section is devoted to a step-by-step discussion of this cycle.

21.2.3   Steps in Design

21.2.3.1   *Beginning the Design*

Design within a given cycle arises from a primitive need. This need may be an external statement (if the cycle is the first in the process) or may be the output of a previous cycle. The example in this chapter will take as the primitive need this possible statement by a product salesman for an orthopaedic implant company: "My customers are interested in a better total hip replacement (THR) system for younger patients." The engineering design group takes up the challenge and develops a concept for a novel femoral component. However, the group reports that none of the biomaterials in their handbooks and reference sources provide the appropriate combination of stiffness, strength, and fatigue life required to realize the preferred design approach. In Asimow's terminology, this finding, a result of a preliminary phase, becomes the input that begins the material design cycle to be examined here.

21.2.3.2   *Step 1: Analyzing Needs*

The first formal step in the design cycle is to examine the input statements, often in collaboration with those who made them, and to develop an

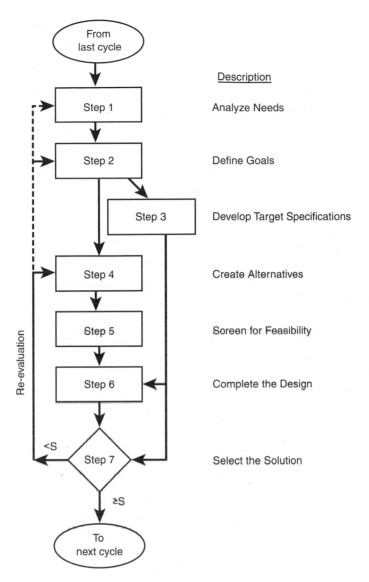

FIGURE 21.1

The design cycle. (Adapted from Love, S.F., *Planning and Creating Successful Engineering Designs: Managing the Design Process*, Los Angeles, Advanced Professional Development, Inc., 1986.)

objective summary statement that expresses the needs in an analytic way and represents a rational objective. For example, development of copper with a higher melting point is an irrational objective and seeking a higher strength-to-modulus ratio in the copper–silver binary alloy system is a rational one. In this case, after careful consultation and deliberation, the design objective is stated as: "The objective is the design of a new material suitable for use in fabrication of THR components that combines optimum stiffness (modulus) with greater strength and a higher endurance limit than that for presently available materials."

Note that the act of stating the objective limits the inquiry: a new material will be designed rather than a present one modified. It also completes the translation of the primitive need to a defined materials need, with three attributes: optimum (to be defined) modulus, increased strength, and higher fatigue endurance. In the same way that an experimental question (and its hypotheses) can be tested, this statement can be tested at the end of the cycle to see whether the objective has been realized.*

21.2.3.3   Step 2: Defining Goals

Design is not a simple process that leads to a unique output. Thus, objectives must be refined to limit the number of choices at each step and to guide the design cycle. This is achieved by selecting goals whose attainment (1) is necessary to reach the desired objective; or (2) represents generally "good" attributes of engineering design or reflects the desires of the designers. The first type are called *specific* goals (*demands*; Cross 2000) and the second type are called *general* goals (*wishes*; Cross 2000). An initial list of specific and general goals that might follow from the previously stated summary objective statement is given under the heading "initial" in Table 21.2.

The initial list of goals arises from a discussion with the customer — in this case, the device design group — and represents the definitive starting point of the material design cycle. It embodies the customer's concepts of what is desired as an end product of the design process. The material design team must now put its talents to work to understand these desires and to satisfy them. Some of the initial goals may come from other sources: the engineering manager is always worried about manufacturing costs; the color was suggested by the marketing manager because yellow is widely used in the company's packaging and has come to be identified positively with its products in the mind of the retail customer, the surgeon.

The material design team must actually go through two substeps to produce the refined set of goals shown in the lower part of Table 21.2. The first of these, the production of an initial set of goals, is the first creative act in the design cycle. The question posed at this point is, "What should a new material for a THR component look like?" As previously noted, the creation of ideas is not an easy process for engineers. The tendency is to "freeze": to be unable to produce ideas or, more commonly, to have an initial thought and then to proceed to develop it without consideration of further alternatives. The general solution for the individual designer is to produce a situation that is stimulatory and nonself-critical.**

---

* Discussion of the design and conduct of experiments is outside the scope of this work. However, the reader should note that this phase is identical to the statement of an experimental question.
** In this section, I refer to a single designer. In Section 21.2.3.5, the situation of creative effort by a group will be considered.

TABLE 21.2

Design Goals: New THR Material

Initial

Specific
  Modulus < 0.5 × Ti6Al4V
  Strength as high as possible
  Endurance limit as high as possible
  Corrosion/release rate "low"
  No wear against UHMWPE[a]
  Color: yellow
General
  Minimum cost
  No limit on source of supply
  Simplicity of fabrication

Refined

Specific
  Modulus < 0.5 × Ti6Al4V (H)
  Strength as high as possible (M)
  Endurance limit as high as possible (H)
  Corrosion/release rate as low as possible (H)
  Wear rate (against UHMWPE) as low as possible (M)
  Color: yellow (L)
  Formability in the operating room (M)
  Release of wear particles > 25 μm in size only (H)
General
  Minimum cost per kilogram (L)
  No limit on source of supply (M)
  Simplicity of fabrication (M)

[a] Ultrahigh molecular weight polyethylene

In this case, the designer may decide that "I'm going to set the problem aside, go for a 5-km run, and when I come in, write down the first ten things that come into my head." Such a procedure, with variants, has been adopted frequently by many if not most creative persons and is sometimes referred to as creative avoidance of the problem: undertaking other activities to distract the conscious mind (probably the analytic left brain function) and using the products of subconscious deliberation (probably the synthetic right brain function), without self-criticism or censoring.

The initial list is then reviewed for reasonableness and duplication and perhaps the process is repeated or extended until the sense is that all of the immediately possible options — in this case, design goals — have been acquired. Often the review triggers new ideas not previously considered. The designer in this example has added two specific goals and no general goal to previously cited desires. Note that this is an abbreviated example; step 2 of an actual design cycle might produce dozens of specific and general goals.

The second substep is the assignment of a priority to each of these initial goals to produce a set of refined goals. This is necessary because, in an actual design case, the number of goals very rapidly grows to a point at which it is obvious, *a priori*, that all cannot be met simultaneously. Thus, a ranking of relative importance is necessary. In this case, the designer employed a common practice and selected three levels of priority:

- High (H): must be met for successful design
- Medium (M): would like to meet during design cycle
- Low (L): desirable to meet but may be sacrificed

Therefore, the material's modulus is identified as a much more important attribute than its color, although the desire to satisfy the marketing manager is still considered as part of the later steps in the cycle. In a more subtle distinction, it is recognized that in the intended application, the endurance limit is a more important material attribute than the tensile strength, although both are important. During this substep, the sets of goals are also screened to eliminate absolute statements; statements of goals should not include the terms "never," "always," "none," etc.

21.2.3.4 Step 3: Developing Target Specifications

Setting specific and general goals and then refining the list and assigning priorities produce considerable clarification of the problem in hand but do not provide details necessary for later steps in the design cycle. To achieve this, it is necessary to translate the refined goals of step 2 into measurable quantities.

These measurable quantities are called specifications. They must be necessary, thus not setting limits unrelated to performance. They must also be sufficient: taken as a group, their satisfaction must be sufficient to produce a successful design and to assure that the formal requirements of the Medical Device Amendments (U.S. Congress 1976) of safety and efficacy are met.* Finally, they must be conservative: setting too high values or too stringent criteria will elevate cost unacceptably or possibly make the design unrealizable.

Consider the refined goal (Table 21.2):

- "Corrosion/release rate as low as possible (H)"

  This might be translated into these specifications:

  - Corrosion rate *in vivo* shall not exceed 0.1 mg/cm^2/year.
  - Release rate *in vivo* shall not produce a concentration of products ≥ 5 ppb at a distance of 1 cm from the implant–tissue interface.

---

* Note that materials used in medical devices are not explicitly regulated but are subject to this requirement indirectly because they perform in a device. See Section 20.5 for a further discussion of this point.

The attainment of minimum corrosion/release was judged to be of high importance; this is reflected in the use of design margins, multipliers of minimum values. In practice, these may vary between 10 (for extremely critical attributes) and 1.1 (for low importance or optional attributes). In this case, the actual allowable values might have been 1 mg/cm^2/year and 50 ppb, respectively, but were reduced by application of a 10× design margin. There are no objective criteria for deriving design margins: they reflect current practice in similar designs.

This is a good time to conduct a design conference to review the project because completion of phase 3 marks the boundary between defining the problem and, in a strict sense, solving it. It is worthwhile determining whether the team is on the right track before the really hard, time-consuming and costly parts of the cycle are undertaken.

21.2.3.5 Step 4: Creating Alternatives

Development of design concepts or alternative possible solutions is the heart of the design process and the point at which most fatal mistakes are made. It requires, again, a suspension of self-criticism and a source of external stimulation. For most people, concepts and alternatives evolve more readily in a group situation in which one person's ideas trigger another's imagination. This is the time in the design process when the prior formation of a multidisciplinary design team really pays dividends. The goal is the same as in step 2: to develop as many independent approaches to realization of the design goals as possible.

As an introduction to this step, the material's designer begins to gather supporting information on past and present materials used in THR prostheses components as well as on current progress in materials design and processing. Information acquired at this time serves the subconscious as a source of ideas and, if a design team is in existence, all members should have access to this resource information. This information will also be needed for the next step.

The primary tool in creating alternatives is the brainstorming or "blue sky" meeting. Cross (2000) lists the following essential rules for such a session:

- Offer no criticism during the session.
- A large number of ideas is wanted.
- Seemingly crazy ideas are welcome.
- Keep all ideas short and snappy.
- Try to combine and improve on the ideas of others.

Citing William J. Osborne, Love (1986) provides many practical suggestions on how to organize and run a successful session to create alternatives.

Table 21.3 presents a list of ideas that might arise from such a step 4 exercise. The initial list was developed in two creative sessions: a break was

TABLE 21.3

Design Alternatives: New THR Material

Initial List

Animal tusk
Modified wood
Cloned tree with new properties
Petrified wood
Coral
Metal impregnated coral
Woven ceramic fiber/resin impregnated
Carbon fiber/graphite
Carbon/silicon carbide powder composite
Carbon/polyethylene powder composite
Hydroxyapatite/polyethylene powder composite

Break Taken at this Point

Metal-fiber-reinforced silicon nitride
Alumina/polymer composite
Woven sapphire fiber/metal impregnated
Sapphire beads with spring connectors
Whisker-reinforced polymer
New titanium alloy
Titanium/polymer powder composite

Final List

Modified natural material
Fiber-reinforced composite
Powder composite
New titanium alloy

taken between the sessions, and the first part of the list was reviewed by the group to initiate the second session. The final list was developed some days later by review and analysis of the initial list.

In this hypothetical case, the creative sessions produced an initial list of 18 ideas that was then reduced to four concepts. The last of these was eliminated by reference to the objective summary statement (it was not judged to be able to lead to a new material) and the other three, which focus primarily on processing leading to new materials, could each be continued in parallel through later stages of the process. Trouble arises at this point or at a later point in the process when alternatives are not fully constrained and/or decisions are made that circumscribe the later steps too narrowly. Reduction in scope can occur later; what is needed at this point is to have created a maximum range of possibilities.

21.2.3.6 Step 5: Screening for Feasibility

It is now necessary to examine the alternatives created in the preceding step (Table 21.3) and select those with which to continue the process. In the example given, after analysis of the possibilities proposed, only three alternative approaches emerged; it might be reasonable to continue with all three. However, each would need to be screened for feasibility. If more than three approaches had resulted from the previous step, feasibility screening could be used to select the two or three most likely to lead to success.

Feasibility is the process of applying rational criticism, which was suspended in the previous step, to enable estimates to be made of the relative chance for success of each proposed approach. The primary aspects of each idea to be examined are: technical, economic, supply, and parsimony. These are justified as follows:

- Technical: the designer must avoid attempting to violate laws of nature.
- Economic: cost and resulting price are powerful considerations, even in materials design. This may refer to the final cost of the material and of its design and qualification.
- Supply: there should be no reasonable intrinsic or imposed barrier (through protection of intellectual property, etc.) to provision of sufficient material for the intended application.
- Parsimony: the simple is preferred over the complex.

Secondary attributes, including the designer's intuition, and political, legal, and/or perceptual issues (which may be unrelated to technical function) may also come into play. The specifications may be used to drive the screening process by attempting to estimate values for each of the material's physical attributes (identified in step 4) and using the apparent ease of achieving the specified values as an index of feasibility. The screening process may be qualitative — each alternative is ranked with respect to each aspect — or it may be made quantitative, with values assigned to rank and an overall score derived for each approach.*

21.2.3.7   Step 6: Completing the Design

Completing the design of the alternatives created in step 4 that survive feasibility screening in step 5 is the final pure design step of the design cycle. Not much needs to be said in that it involves traditional engineering processes of analysis, calculation, and simulation and may even require some pilot experiments to verify design and manufacturing concepts. Parametric studies, in which the effects of varying controllable independent variables are tested, are of great value in later considerations. The specifications must explicitly drive design choices because they will be the basis for testing the final design in the next step.

When alternative approaches were selected (step 5), design completion usually results in a definitive ranking in order of preference or in the elim-

---

* Ranking the three approaches selected in the last step is left as an exercise for the reader.

ination of one or more owing to an inability to realize a complete design. However, cost and time considerations may result in a decision to complete the design for only the most promising (most feasible) alternative.

21.2.3.8   Step 7: Selecting the Solution

Design selection (or evaluation) is a simple process of comparing the attributes of the final design to the specified values developed in step 3 and determining how well have been met. If no design conferences have been held (with the "customers") since the one at the end of step 3, now is the ideal time to do so. The customers (and outside reviewers, if possible) may serve as a board of review to complete this step. Ideally, all high- and medium-priority goals should be met, through satisfaction of their dependent specifications ($\geq$S, Figure 21.1), for the design to be said to be acceptable and for it to advance to the next cycle of the overall (device, etc.) design process.

If, in the opinion of the reviewers, the design is unacceptable (fails to meet one or more key specifications, <S, Figure 21.1), several options are open. These include reviewing design concepts to see whether additional ones can be developed, reviewing the specifications to see whether they (or their design margins) can be relaxed, and reviewing the goals to see whether they are all necessary and have appropriate priorities. If changes can be made retrospectively at any of these three steps, the cycle can be resumed at that point to determine whether a satisfactory design results.

21.3   The Value of Prospective Design

21.3.1   Why Have a Design Process Anyway?

The design process or even a single design cycle will not always yield a satisfactory result. Objectives may be unrealistic or even forbidden by basic physical principles or the goals selected may not be technologically achievable or financially feasible at the time. However, it is clear that, in the majority of cases, a structured design process does produce satisfactory results with well-articulated foundations and justification. In most cases, within the boundaries of assumptions and choices made at various steps, the resulting designs will represent optimum solutions. Thus, prospective design is to be preferred to inspired guesses in designing biomaterials, as in other areas of engineering.

21.3.2 Design in the Real World

The process elaborated here, based upon ideas put forward by Asimow (1962), Love (1986), and Cross (2000) as well as my experience in academic and industrial settings, reflects the ideal. The names of the seven steps encapsulate the central ideas: analysis of need, proposals for solution, elaboration of proposals, and testing of results against the original need. This cyclic, iterative approach is critical, whether it exists within a fully articulated process as described here or merely guides more informal considerations.

In the biomedical context, useful new materials and devices can result neither from pure analytical considerations of engineers and developers nor from pure synthetic suggestions of physicians and surgeons. What actually happens is that there is a continuing, interactive collaboration, made difficult at times by the necessary conflict between analysis and synthesis. Groups and companies that have been successful in bringing novel materials and devices incorporating them into clinical use have managed to preserve balanced collaboration. Robertson and Hyatt (1998) illustrate this interaction in the idealized development of spinal instrumentation hardware.

However, developments dominated by either party have been seen, in particular cases, to lead to unfortunate consequences. Engineers often express frustration in working with medical personnel who generally have difficulty in providing quantitative measures of their clinical observations. Clinicians tend to be overly impressed by engineering rigor, as exemplified by finite element analysis, and then disappointed when performance, which may have been based on inadequate inputs, fails to meet expectations.

As bioengineering matures professionally and clinical experience with existing materials now extends to periods of decades in some applications, additional barriers to successful design of materials have emerged. Although extensive testing protocols have been devised in the laboratory and in animal models (Chapter 17 and Chapter 18), it is still extremely difficult to predict biological performance of materials in the long term. Furthermore, the existence of an increasing range of materials with known host and materials responses in highly successful devices raises real ethical and practical issues concerning substitution of novel materials in such applications.

Success in design of materials or of devices requires an understanding of history as well as cultural and professional differences and all parties' willingness to be flexible and remain focused on the real goal: a better outcome for present and future patients.

References

Asimow, M., *Introduction to Design*, Prentice Hall, Englewood Cliffs, NJ, 1962, 1.
Black, J., *Orthopaedic Biomaterials in Research and Practice*, Churchill Livingstone, New York, 1988, 303.

Cross, N., *Engineering Design Methods: Strategies for Product Design*, 3rd ed., John Wiley & Sons, Chichester, U.K., 2000.

Lewis, G., *Selection of Engineering Materials*, Prentice Hall, Englewood Cliffs, NJ, 1990, 179.

Love, S.F., *Planning and Creating Successful Engineering Designs: Managing the Design Process*, Los Angeles, Advanced Professional Development, Inc., 1986.

Robertson, J.T. and Hyatt, D., Concepts and issues of spine device development and regulation, in Capen, D.A. and Haye, W. (Eds.), *Comprehensive Management of Spinal Trauma*, St. Louis, C.V. Mosby, 1988, 414.

U.S. Congress, *Medical Device Amendments*. PL 94-295, 21 USC 301, 1976.

Bibliography

Ashby, M.F., *Materials Selection in Mechanical Design*, 2nd ed., New York, Butterworth Heinemann (Elsevier), 1999.

Bronikowski, R.J., *Managing the Engineering Design Function*, Van Nostrand Reinhold, New York, 1986.

Collins, J.A., *Failure of Materials in Mechanical Design: Analysis, Prediction, and Prevention*, 2nd. ed., John Wiley & Sons, New York, 1993.

Norman, D.A., *The Design of Everyday Things*, Basic, New York, 2002.

Petroski, H., *The Evolution of Useful Things*, Vintage, New York, 1994.

Shackelford, J.F., Alexander, W. and Park, J., *CRC Practical Handbook of Materials Selection*, CRC Press, Boca Raton, FL, 1995.

22

Clinical Performance of Biomaterials*

22.1 Historical Aspects

Implants used for the alleviation and treatment of human disability and disease are derived from natural (biological donor) sources or are manufactured from organic and/or inorganic materials. The failure and success of live cell, tissue, and organ transplantation have been studied extensively. However, the study of the consequences of the use of manufactured biomaterials in implants, in their actual service setting, has been spotty at best and based primarily upon complications seen in reported clinical series or on local, intermittent study of devices retrieved at surgical revision (replacement) or at autopsy.

The use of manufactured implants in medicine has its roots in antiquity; however, the practice has only become prevalent in the last century and has gained widespread success only since World War II. Early efforts were distinguished by high rates of complications and failures and thus the use of nonbiological implants was long regarded as experimental. Historically, improved biomaterials and devices emerged from short-term animal studies and clinical observations that eliminate undesirable material and/or design-related performance on a case-by-case or small-group-study basis.

The result is that now a small group of biomaterials is, by and large, highly successful when used in a broad variety of designs; its use for many indications has become routine (see Interpart 1 for typical examples).** Heart valve replacements, heart pacemakers, and total hip and knee replacements are examples of devices incorporating such materials for which clinical experience of more than 10 years allows prediction of a high likelihood of success (>90 to 95%) for individual patients who meet appropriate indications. It is hard to estimate how many chronic (intended to remain *in situ* for more than 30 days) implants are in use today in the U.S., but national data (Moss 1991)

---

* Many of the ideas in this chapter were developed and elaborated during contractual studies for the USFDA, CDRH, whose support is gratefully acknowledged.
** However, there is no list of "generally recognized as safe" biomaterials, due to the modern, and correct, emphasis on biocompatibility being related to specific application requirements and to the resulting risk/benefit ratio.

suggest that the number was at least 11 million by 1988 with annual increases since then most probably of about 10%. Non-U.S. experience probably equals or slightly exceeds these figures; the 2005 worldwide total of chronic implants probably now exceeds 75 million.

However, success has produced a new set of problems, which can be summarized as follows:

- Large-scale, routine clinical use of implants, even with low failure rates, produces significant numbers of patients whose procedures fail to meet expectations.
- Clinical confidence in implants results in pragmatic extension of the indications for their use, especially to more difficult medical problems and to earlier intervention in disease processes.
- Routine use and earlier intervention produce an increasing mismatch between typically short development and evaluation cycles and longer intended (and actual) service periods.

Together, these factors have produced needs for certain types of data concerning the biomaterials from which implants are manufactured:

- Long-term effects of *in vivo* environments on biomaterials properties
- Chronic (including systemic and remote site) effects of manufactured biomaterials on human physiological processes
- Comparative service experience of different biomaterials in similar or different device designs used for the same clinical application/ indication

The response to these needs has been an effort, led primarily by bioengineers, to study implants and explants (retrieved devices) in a field that has come to be termed device retrieval and analysis (DRA). Early DRA efforts tended to focus on the disease state and view the device generically (medical or clinical pathology model) or to study the device closely, with little attention given to the generic disease or to individual patient conditions and use (engineering failure analysis model).

Since 1976, at least six major U.S. technical conferences* on DRA have had a primary, if unstated, goal to bring these two models together and thus produce a unified approach (using a single analytical model) to the study of biological performance (host and implant response) of devices (and the biomaterials from which they are fabricated) in human clinical use. Numerous professional societies, commercial concerns, and U.S. government

---

* Retrieval and Analysis of Orthopedic Implants, Bethesda, MD, 3/5/76; Corrosion and Degradation of Implant Materials, Kansas City, MO, 5/22-23/78; Implant Retrieval and Biological Analysis, Bethesda, MD, 5/1-3/80; Corrosion and Degradation of Implant Materials: Second Symposium, Louisville, KY, 5/9-10/83; Symposium on Implant Retrieval, Snowbird, UT, 8/12-14/88 and Implant Retrieval Symposium, St. Charles, IL, 9/17-20/92.

agencies have been involved in the sponsorship of these conferences and in support of numerous smaller symposia and workshops as portions of larger engineering and medical professional meetings.

Of outstanding note have been the efforts of the ASTM F-4 Committee on Medical and Surgical Materials and Devices, which, since 1972, has been codifying procedures and practices for the physical retrieval and analysis of individual implants. Although not believed to be widely used exactly as written, these procedures, such as F-561-05,* provide important and useful guidance to DRA activities. The American National Standards Institute (ANSI) and the International Standards Organization (ISO) have more recently begun to develop standard procedures for DRA. Of note is the work of Working Group 5 of ISO Technical Committee 150 that is developing standards for retrieval and analysis of implantable devices.**

However, despite early and continuing perceptions that the data and the knowledge that can be gained from study of retrieved devices are of vital importance, most of these efforts continue to focus on the implant and on the implications of its physical condition (engineering failure analysis model). The seven major parties to DRA (patient, physician, manufacturer, treating institution, insurer, regulatory agency, and society at large) recognize a shared common interest in DRA and its outcomes; however, individual benefit/risk calculations by each concerned party are in constant conflict (Black and Fielder 1992) and have stood in the way of emergence of a unified analytical model or of comprehensive and/or multi-institutional DRA programs. Table 22.1 briefly highlights the benefits and risks perceived by each party involved in DRA.

Notwithstanding this continued conflict, it is important for the advancement of the field of biomaterials and the practice of medicine that DRA efforts continue to advance and mature. The following sections outline some applicable methodology.

22.2 Procedures for Device Retrieval and Analysis

DRA today is of necessity a "team sport" brought about by the complexities of medical practice and of the social and legal setting of the early 21st century. Before one undertakes such activities, it is necessary to establish a supporting organization and for the parties involved to agree on a number of assumptions. The issues to be dealt with include goals, responsibility, methodology, and reporting.

---

* F-561-05 Practice for Retrieval and Analysis of Implanted Medical Devices, in *2005 Annual Book of ASTM Standards*, Vol. 13.01: Medical Devices; Emergency Medical Services, ASTM International, West Conshohocken, PA, 2005.
** ISO/DIS 12891-1: Retrieval and analysis of surgical implants — part 1: retrieval and handling.

TABLE 22.1

Benefits and Risks in Device Retrieval and Analysis

Party	Benefit	Risk
Patient	Improved medical care	Increased cost
		Increased concern related to device performance
Physician	Improved service to patient	Possible malpractice liability
Manufacturer	Increased knowledge of device performance	Increased administrative burden
		Possible increased cost
		Possible tort liability
Treating institution	Improved service to patient	Increased cost
		Possible liability
Insurer	Increased knowledge of device performance	Possible increased cost
	Reduced cost through use of "better" devices	
Regulatory agency	Increased knowledge of device performance	Increased administrative burden
Society at large	Increased knowledge of device performance	Possible alarm about device malfunction
	Reduced cost through use of "better" devices	
	Improved health care	

22.2.1 Goals

DRA is a general term that can cover a wide variety of activities, each of which has specific goals, such as:

- Premarket approval clinical evaluation: goals may include determining normal and abnormal device and/or material performance, meeting regulatory requirements for reporting adverse outcomes, and providing feedback for device and/or surgical technique modification.

- Routine clinical use of a device: goals may include monitoring of appropriateness of device/patient matching, determining specific device-related "failure" rates as part of survivorship calculations, establishing mechanisms underlying survivorship estimates, and planning future treatment for individual patients.

- Autopsy retrieval: goals may include investigation of local and systemic host response, long-term material property changes, and distribution and storage of implant degradation products.

In any of these or other activities, there should be formal written statement of and agreement to goals because such goals strongly affect the design and conduct of DRA studies.

22.2.2   Responsibility

Any DRA study should be conducted under the direction of a group of interested, appropriately trained, and committed individuals. The issues raised by DRA are such that careless or unplanned activities can produce extremely adverse outcomes for many of the parties involved. There should be a written, agreed upon set of procedures and methods. One individual, preferably a Ph.D.-trained person with experience in DRA, should have final responsibility for the program and should be designated as the custodian for the devices between their surgical recovery and their discharge from DRA study.

22.2.3   Methodology

In its most general form, DRA is an example of discovery science. Thus, it is inappropriate, except in very small, tightly focused studies, for all recovered devices to undergo a fixed set of procedures. Such an approach, especially in the usual setting of routine clinical practice, would produce insupportable costs without returning commensurably valuable information. Thus, it is good practice to classify devices prospectively before study. Three generic classes can be easily recognized. These are briefly described next, with examples of each type of device and of possible response within a DRA study:

- Class 3: no frank evidence of physical damage to the device pre- and postexplantation and no implication of involvement of device malfunction in clinical outcome
  - Example: routine (nonsymptomatic) removal of fracture fixation hardware
  - Response: positive identification of device, cataloging, discharge from recovery system*
- Class 2: frank evidence of physical damage to the device post- and possibly pre-explantation but no implication of involvement of device malfunction in clinical outcome
  - Example: component of total hip replacement, showing surface defects, recovered from site of early postoperative infection

---

* It is assumed in this chapter that any institution in which a DRA study is planned already has a working device recovery system in place. Most simply stated, a device recovery system is a set of procedures, parallel to those used for clinical pathology specimens, that dictate how a device is collected from the surgical field or clinic, handled postrecovery, examined for routine identification and evaluation purposes and then "discharged" (given to patient, retained for research, discarded, etc.) (see Section 22.3.4). It is difficult and ill advised to conduct DRA studies in the absence of such a recovery system; one of the first steps in designing and implementing a DRA program may have to be working with the host institution to install or improve a device recovery system.

TABLE 22.2

Conduct of DRA Studies

Steps	Removal Class		
Recovery Procedure			
Retrieve			
Package			
Identify			
Sterilize[a]			
Classify			
	Class 1	**Class 2**	**Class 3**
Evaluate			
Photographs	X	X	X
Culture reports	X	X	
Histology	X	X	
Metallography	X		
Mechanical analysis	X		
Chemical analysis	X		
Special tests	X	X	
Mechanical testing (device portions)	X		
Hardness	X		
Specific histologic stains	X		
Metal analysis (AAS) (fluids, tissues)	X		
Case disposition	X	X	X
Prepare report	X	X	X
Store/dispose of device	X	X	X

[a] Specific studies may require devices to be studied in unsterilized conditions; this may require deviations from routine recovery practice.

- Response: as for class 3 with additional procedures to examine and document noted device defects (see Table 22.2)

- Class 1: frank evidence of physical damage to the device pre- and postexplantation and implication of involvement of device malfunction in clinical outcome

  - Example: cardiac pacer lead with broken conductor

  - Response: as for class 2 with additional procedures to determine origin and/or cause of noted effects* (see Table 22.2)

22.2.4   Reporting

Timely reporting of results is the key to sustained and useful DRA studies. Reporting should take the following forms:

- Rapid reports should be made to the treating physicians, on a time schedule parallel to that in the treating institution for clinical

---

* Note: Clinical institutions frequently elect to deal with class 1 cases in a different manner than class 2 and 3 cases because the former involve devices that may become physical evidence in malpractice and/or product liability proceedings.

pathology studies. In addition to a personal report to the primary physician, a note should be placed in the hospital chart, over the signature of the DRA supervising professional. Although it is unusual for such individual studies to have an impact on the further treatment of the patient in question, such reporting is simply good manners and helps to maintain the professional relationships needed for DRA studies.

- In the case of class 1 and 2 devices, reports should be made directly to the manufacturer. This is especially necessary if more than one set of similar findings occurs during a study. Sensitivity should be shown to studies of class 1 devices: because of the possibility of litigation in such cases, reports should focus on physical findings and descriptions but omit theories of causation, unless they are supportable by peer-reviewed, published studies.

- Depending upon the nature of the findings and, in the case of a class 1 device, the degree of patient involvement, timely reports may need to be filed with a regulatory agency, such as the FDA in the U.S. Because this is a legal requirement, the treating institution should have already established an approved procedure for submitting such reports as a part of its device recovery system. DRA personnel should be aware of such a system and provide rapid access to their findings for the individuals responsible for making the report.

- Finally, there is a responsibility to make results of studies of groups of retrieved devices available to the scientific and engineering community. Such reports might include publication, presentation at professional meetings, and participation in workshops and instructional courses.

It cannot be too strongly emphasized that, except in reports to physicians within the treating institution, great care must be taken to preserve the privacy and identity of the patients involved. This is an ethical and legal requirement (Black and Fiedler 1992).

22.3 Common Concerns about Device Retrieval and Analysis

22.3.1 Cost

Costs for study and analysis of implants are extremely difficult to identify due to the varied nature of individual implants and the present indications for analysis. Survey results and anecdotal experience suggest ranges of direct costs as follows:

- Class 3: $5 to 25
- Class 2: $25 to $250
- Class 1: $250 to $10,000

These costs certainly are subject to economy-of-scale effects and can be expected to be nearer the lower ends of each range in large-scale and/or routine clinical retrieval and analysis studies.

22.3.2   Device Ownership

Central to any functioning DRA program is the concept of rapid availability of enrolled (recovered) devices, when selected, for nondestructive and destructive studies. It is good practice that all custodial and other procedures for handling implants and other medical devices satisfy minimum legal "chain of evidence" standards; however, the assumption* that patients may "own" devices removed from their bodies continues. It is suggested that concern for property rights may be satisfied in one of three ways:

- Institutions that conduct DRA studies beyond routine logging and discharge of recovered devices should probably alter their standard permission for treatment forms to include permission to study devices, including destructive testing. Possible language, as previously proposed,* is:

  I understand that part of my treatment may require removal of an artificial implant. If an implant is removed, I give permission for any studies of it related to my treatment. I understand that I and my doctor will be informed of the results of these studies in a timely fashion and that I will be consulted before the implant is discarded or if the implant is desired for other studies.

- In the case of individual (authorized by IRB) prospective studies, an additional approved permission form may be developed that explains the study's goals and conduct and asks for the patient's permission for any necessary destructive testing.
- Alternatively, because devices may already be in institutional custody at the time that they are selected for a study, treating institutions may elect to obtain permission for study retrospectively, using a form such as that described in the previous option (second bullet). This option is less desirable than the first (routine permission) because it may raise the patient's concern over possible device malfunction.

---

* Black 1996.

22.3.3 Patient Confidentiality

There is a clear need to retain a defined linkage between DRA data, which are devoid of patient identification, and medical records of each patient. This linkage is required because studies of device function and biomaterials properties may require correlation with disease state, mechanical environment, etc. encountered by the device during service. A possible linkage, as proposed in Section 22.4, is a coded identification number generated at the time of recovery of the device. The manual or electronic ways of generating such unique codes will not be discussed here. However, the key to the coding system will be deemed to be confidential and related to the patient, thus not accessible under Freedom of Information Act inquiry. The keys would be disclosed only to DRA study supervisors and then only after suitable assurances concerning maintenance of patient confidentiality were obtained and the "need-to-know" established on a patient-by-patient basis.

22.3.4 Recovery System

Repeated recommendations from many sources make it clear that all clinical facilities in which devices are explanted should possess and maintain recovery systems to deal with removed devices. The need for recovery systems has been frequently noted in individual hospital accreditation committee reports and exists independently of DRA studies or of the proposed implementation of a NIDRA structure (see Section 22.4).

A recovery system should, at a minimum, provide for the following documented steps:

1. Collection of the device from the surgical field
2. Entry into the patient's clinical record of a minimum data set
3. Handling and transport of the device to (1) minimize postexplantation damage to the device; and (2) minimize health risk* to support personnel
4. Examination and identification of the retrieved device
5. Discharge of the device from institutional care (adequate decontamination, disposal, or discharge to physician, patient, or third party)

---

* It is routine practice in DRA studies to assume that all explanted devices are contaminated with human pathogens unless positively sterilized. Because postexplantation sterilization procedures may affect materials' properties, routine sterilization is often not performed, during recovery or retrieval, and devices may need to be handled through some steps of the recovery process in an unsterilized state.

22.4   Proposed National Implant Data Retrieval and Analysis Program (NIDRA)

A 1981 conference* attempted to focus on data and knowledge resulting from DRA rather than on material and design aspects of implants. However, it primarily dealt with codification and standardization processes without addressing the need for an overall knowledge structure with defined internal data flows.

Notwithstanding this pioneering effort, little progress has been made in generalizing and unifying the intellectual product of DRA efforts and in making it accessible in real time. Contemporary DRA programs are still scarce and tend to be based in hospitals and academic research groups. Strongly influenced by liability considerations, the medical device industry, by and large, has elected to react to individual cases of apparent device malfunction rather than to study the general successful or unsuccessful performance of its products. Data interchange reflecting case or selected group studies performed largely without controls continues to be primarily by podium presentation and paper publication. Two further defects of many of these studies are that:

- They are performed in large centers that provide secondary or tertiary care and thus have nonrepresentative patient populations.
- They frequently involve or are directed by surgeons and engineers involved in development of the devices or device classes under study, without adequate third-party supervision, oversight, or quality control.

It was apparent by 1992 that a new effort needed to be made to gain necessary data from the vast human experience of routine clinical use of implants. The U.S. Food and Drug Administration commissioned me to develop a design specification for a national data management system. A questionnaire was developed, widely distributed and the results codified. The results of that survey clearly supported the need for development of a national knowledge structure and contain a number of recommendations that were drawn upon in preparation of this specification. Five guiding principles were proposed and, validated by the survey, can now be stated as system requirements for a national effort to study clinical performance of biomaterials:

- The emphasis should be on understanding biomaterial performance *in vivo* as it relates to biomaterials' composition and processing, individual patient variables, and device design classes.

* Medical devices: measurements, quality assurance, and standards, Gaithersburg, MD, 9/24-25/81.

- The program should be structured to provide early and continuing publicly utilizable data on device survival and biomaterial performance.

- The system design should embody low-level uniform data retrieval (for statistical results) combined with focused case studies related to perceived or possible clinical problems (for biomaterials' properties).

- The resulting database should be prospectively linked, in an interactive way, with existing and planned engineering, biological, and clinical databases.

- The system should be decentralized and extramural (nongovernmental) insofar as possible, with central intramural activities involving only planning, direction, data analysis, and audit functions.

The final design specification described the database and its associated device- and data-acquisition and management systems (termed collectively the "NIDRA structure") needed for low-cost, reliable production of bioengineering data from current clinical implant experience to meet the needs of expanding use of implants.

22.5 Elements of a NIDRA System

The aim of the NIDRA proposal is to describe a system capable of generating, in a timely fashion, a number of minimum data sets. The driving idea of this approach is to make the implantation and removal of chronic (>30 days) implants statistical events much as births and deaths or, for that matter, purchase and scrapping of automobile tires are. A secondary goal is to make recovered implants available for larger scale DRA studies than are now possible within single institutions.

22.5.1 Data Sets

Three data sets are proposed:

- A minimum explantation data (EDATA) set containing no more than six items:
  - Date of removal
  - Identification number (ID number) of medical facility where explantation occurred (per HSS FDA 92-4247*)

---

* HSS FDA 92-4247: Medical device reporting for user facilities, December 1991.

- Coded ID number creating link to patient hospital records (may include previous two items)
- Device identity (per HSS FDA 91-4246*)
- Retrieval grade: recommended codes (referring to device rather than to clinical outcome)**:
  - RG1: no pre- (diagnostic imaging, functional test result, etc.) or postremoval (naked eye, functional test result, etc.) defects
  - RG2: preremoval defects; no postremoval defects
  - RG3: pre- and postremoval defects
  - RG4: no preremoval defects; postremoval defects
- Device serial/model number (when available) (optional)
- An expanded explantation data set (expanded EDATA): this data set would include the EDATA set as well as information on implantation (e.g., original anatomical location), service (e.g., implantation duration), and analysis (e.g., lipid content of silicone rubber) as well as the minimum IDATA set (when available). Although it is clear that the use of standardized analytical procedures would simplify comparison of expanded EDATA sets, the careful definition of test methods and the use of control (reference) materials would permit full data merger in the envisioned data base.
- A minimum implantation data (IDATA) set containing no more than six items:
  - Date of implantation
  - ID number of medical facility where implantation occurred (per HSS FDA 92-4247)
  - Coded ID number creating link to patient hospital records (may included previous two items)
  - Device identity (per HSS FDA 91-4246)
  - Indication for use (per DRG)
  - Device serial/model number (when available) and/or coded ID number creating link to manufacturing records

22.5.2 Organizational Elements

The proposed NIDRA structure designed to generate, collate, and analyze these data sets has four principal elements:

---

* HSS FDA 91-4246: Classification names for medical devices and *in vitro* diagnostic products. August 1991.
** These correspond, respectively, to DRA classes (section 22.2): RG1: class 3, RG2: class 2, RG3: class 1 (possibly class 2), RG4: class 2.

- Clinical institutions
- Study centers
- Data analysis and device management center (DADMC)
- Steering committee

The proposed responsibilities of each element and their manner of interaction are briefly outlined next.

22.5.2.1 Clinical Institutions

Any participating clinical institution would be expected to modify its (informed) "consent for treatment" procedure to enable off-site analysis of devices, to operate a recovery system, and to enroll each device by informing the DADMC (see later section) by FAX transmission of a minimum EDATA set on the day of explantation of each device. The clinical institution would then hold the device for a set period (2 to 10 days; recommendation: 3 working days) and subsequently:

- If informed affirmatively (during the holding period) of a need for the device for an approved DRA study in another center and, upon receipt of a prepaid shipping container, ship the device to a specified study center, *or*
- If not informed affirmatively, dispose of the device in accordance with recovery system routine practice

The costs for a clinical institution to participate in this program would be minimal and deviation from conventional recovery practice would in many cases not be necessary beyond NIDRA case enrollment (FAX preparation and transmission).

22.5.2.2 Study Centers

The principal public need is for an accessible flow of uniform, high-quality data concerning properties and clinical performance of implants. It is proposed to support present analysis programs and, if needed, to encourage the establishment of new ones in academic, medical, or industrial settings, by defining and funding a set of prospective studies. Support would be provided from traditional public funding sources as well as from a fund to be established in relation to the DADMC.

Briefly, experimental questions would be proposed by the NIDRA Steering Committee and advertised through traditional RFP/RFC channels for response by interested groups. Examples of such areas of study are *in vivo* degradation of silicone elastomers and fatigue processes in spinal fixation devices. A study center with a funded NIDRA study would have real-time access to the device enrollment data flowing into the DADMC so that devices meeting the criteria defined for each experimental program could be retrieved rapidly in large numbers. The study center would, as part of its responsibilities, design and fabricate appropriate shipping containers. It would identify devices that met the criteria of its study, cause DADMC to make an affirmative selection of these devices on its behalf, and dispatch appropriate prepaid shipping containers to the clinical institutions that enrolled the selected devices. The study center would also bear the responsibility (and cost) of directly contacting the clinical institutions from which it received selected devices to obtain supplementary data, laboratory test results, etc. as needed for the specific study. As the study progresses, the study center would transmit results in real time to the DADMC.

Although many highly capable interdisciplinary research groups are currently active in the analysis of device materials and performance, as mentioned previously, it may sometimes prove necessary to establish dedicated study centers focusing on a particular perceived device related clinical problem, on a class of devices in a particular medical/surgical field, or on a particular biomaterial class. The need for such centers would be defined by the NIDRA Steering Committee and conventional center support funds would be sought from NIH, NSF, and other public sources as well as funds provided from the central fund.

22.5.2.3   *Data Analysis and Device Management Center (DADMC)*

The DADMC would be the only new permanent federal element of the proposed NIDRA data management system. Its principal responsibility would be the creation of the software and hardware to host a publicly accessible relational database to house the minimum EDATA sets and the integrated results of focused studies by the study centers, on a grouped basis as well as through generation of an expanded EDATA set for each specific device studied. This relational database would be provided with functional linkages to present databases, such as the MDR system, and proposed bases such as the proposed FDA-based Biomaterials Compendium.* The DADMC's secondary roles would include management and oversight of clinical institutions' recovery and enrollment systems, recruitment of new clinical institutions to the program, performance of statistical analyses on the database, and design and provision of products for electronic access and hard-copy publication.

22.5.2.4   *Steering Committee*

It is intended that the NIDRA Data Management System be coordinated and directed by a nationally organized steering committee. This committee would be responsible for further design of NIDRA, for field test and

---

* At the time of the original NIDRA study (1992), the FDA (CDRH) was compiling data base of clinically used biomaterials, including properties and relevant standards, from various forms of pre-approval applications. This effort has apparently been abandoned.

implementation, and for scientific oversight and management in the steady state. Initially, this committee should be staffed by invitation; however, it might be reasonable for a definitive committee to have identified seats to be filled by representatives from various professional, scientific, and industrial organizations. As of today, NIDRA remains a proposal, although limited efforts are under way in the U.S. and elsewhere to develop and test various elements of such a national system.

22.6 Autopsy Retrieval Studies

Conventional DRA programs, however well conceived and executed, will continue to be studies of "failure"; that is, they focus on the few devices for which the outcome has been unexpectedly less than desired and/or frank damage is noted on retrieved implants. For a long time, researchers have recognized this problem and have attempted to compensate for this by *in situ* studies and recovery of successful implants after death.

In situ studies have so far been largely limited to the use of conventional imaging techniques, such as x-ray, CT, and MRI, and occasional sampling and analysis of fluids and tissues. However, ethical and practical considerations have severely limited the scope and utility of these studies. This is a still primitive field of effort when compared to the *in situ* study of natural systems, but it can be expected to develop in the future.

A number of investigators, such as Sir John Charnley, have recognized the need to study success and have asked patients prospectively to "return" their devices when they are no longer needed — that is, after death. The success of the studies of such devices and the important insights that they have provided have encouraged a wider approach to autopsy retrievals of successfully functioning devices and associated tissues, as well as tissues and fluids from systemic and remote locations.

Involvement in one such program since 1990 (Jacobs et al. 1999) has highlighted the benefits and the inherent difficulties of its operation. Several comments can be made about such programs in general:

- Patients and their close relations are generally interested in their medical condition and have an inherent willingness to take part in studies, if they have a fairly low impact on their day-to-day lives, in order to benefit others. However, individuals have social, religious, and ethical standards and principles that must always be honored. Thus, programs must be flexible enough to accommodate a wide variety of individual concerns.
- Permitting study of one's body after death for scientific purposes is a personal decision, much like agreeing to donate organs. As a result,

successful autopsy retrieval programs depend to a great extent on continuing, repeated contact with the prospective subjects and their families by caring, concerned personnel with minimum interference after death.

- Death rarely arrives on schedule or at a convenient time and the window of opportunity for satisfactory, uncontaminated retrieval of device components and tissue specimens is usually quite brief. Therefore, successful programs require well defined and established protocols, previously prepared instrument and sample recovery kits, trained one- to three-person retrieval teams on 24-hour standby (with adequate coverage for sick leave, vacations, holidays, etc.), and a reliable communication system to alert all parties as quickly as possible after death occurs.

In general, autopsy retrieval programs function much as more conventional DRA studies do. However, as the previous comments suggest, costs are considerably higher. On balance, the scientific results from the few in operation today have more than repaid the effort required. and they represent one of the frontiers of biomaterials research.

22.7 Concluding Remarks

It should be a truism that one can only really learn about the clinical performance of biomaterials by actually examining that clinical performance. A vast human experiment is under way; significant numbers of patients now have had chronic devices *in situ* for more than 20 years. The time when important new discoveries about the biological performance of biomaterials can be made in the laboratory or in limited animal studies without primary reference to this clinical experience has probably passed. Device retrieval and analysis studies, national data systems, and autopsy retrieval programs will come to play important roles in obtaining data and insight to benefit future generations of patients.

It is clear that the failure of such systems to emerge, for whatever reasons, has profound impacts on the quality and cost of health care. In 2000, a U.S.–NIH-sponsored national consensus development conference* concluded in part that:

- "Implant retrieval and analysis is of critical importance in the process of improving care of patients…"

---

* Improving medical implant performance through retrieval information: challenges and opportunities, Bethesda, MD, January 10–12, 2000.

- "The [continuing] failure to appreciate the value of…retrieval and analysis is a serious impediment to medical device research… [R]etrieval will lead to the acquisition of information necessary to improve the quality of future devices."

In other words, better understanding of biological performance of devices (and their materials of construction) in actual clinical settings is and remains important and necessary.

References

Black, J. and Fielder, J.H., Ethical aspects in device retrieval, *Proc. Implant Retrieval Symposium*, Society for Biomaterials, St. Charles, LA, 9/17–20/92, 14–1.

Jacobs, J.J. et al., Postmortem retrieval of total joint replacement components, *J. Biomed. Mater. Res. (Appl. Biomat.)*, 48(3), 385, 1999.

Moss, A.J., *Advance Data from Vital and Health Statistics, No. 191*, National Center for Health Statistics, 1991, 1.

Bibliography

Anderson, J.M., Procedures in the retrieval and evaluation of vascular grafts, in Kambic, H.E., Kantrowitz, A. and Sung, P. (Eds.), *Vascular Graft Update: Safety and Performance, STP 898*, American Society for Testing and Materials, Philadelphia, 1986, 156.

Anderson, J.M., Cardiovascular device retrieval and evaluation, *Cardiovasc. Pathol.*, 2(3)(suppl.), 199S, 1993.

Black, J., An overview of goals and perspectives of implant retrieval, *Int. J. Risk Safety Med.*, 8, 99, 1996.

Brooks, C.R. and Choudury, S.A., *Metallurgical Failure Analysis*, McGraw–Hill, New York, 1992.

Collins, J.A., *Failure of Materials in Mechanical Design*, 2nd ed., John Wiley & Sons, New York, 1993.

Das, A.K., *Metallurgy of Failure Analysis*, McGraw–Hill, New York, 1997.

Engel, L. et al., *An Atlas of Polymer Damage: Surface Examination by Scanning Electron Microscope*, Prentice Hall, Englewood Cliffs, NJ, 1981.

Fraker, A.C. and Griffin, C.D. (Eds.), *Corrosion and Degradation of Implant Materials: Second Symposium, STP 859*, American Society for Testing and Materials, Philadelphia, 1985.

Scheirs, J., *Compositional and Failure Analysis of Polymers: A Practical Approach*, John Wiley & Sons, New York, 2000.

Syrett, B.C. and Acharya, A. (Eds.), *Corrosion and Degradation of Implant Materials, STP 684*. American Society for Testing and Materials, Philadelphia, 1979.

Weinstein, A., Horowitz, E. and Ruff, A.W. (Eds.), *Retrieval and Analysis of Orthopaedic Implants*, NBS Special Publication 472, U.S. Government Printing Office, Washington, D.C., 1977.

Glossary

G.1 Introduction

From its beginning, the intellectual field of biomaterials science and engineering has been hampered by having grown up from a group of supporting basic and applied endeavors (Chapter 1). As a result, its vocabulary has been drawn from a number of varied historical sources. The practice in the discipline has been, in some cases, to give new meanings to old terms. In addition, practitioners in the field have had to invent or adopt terminology to describe their insights. The resulting vocabulary is so far a piecemeal assemblage and, except for efforts by various authors, does not appear in any one place. Perhaps the most noteworthy attempt to solve this problem has been *The Williams Dictionary of Biomaterials* (1999). An earlier effort by Szycher (1992) is of little practical use because it is simply a compilation of U.S. legal medical device definitions as required under the Medical Device Amendments (1976) (Chapter 20) and later legislation, previously published in Title 21 of the *Code of Federal Regulations (CFR)* (FDA91-4246).

At international consensus conferences in 1987 (Williams 1987) and 1991 (Williams et al. 1992), attempts were made to develop a standard core nomenclature for biomaterials. All of the definitions considered at these two meetings are included in the following two sections. Adopted ones are identified as follows:

* * = 1987 conference consensus definition
* *p = 1987 conference provisional definition
* ** = 1991 conference consensus definition

Beyond these specialized terms, the vocabulary of biomaterials is still drawn from a broad base in the engineering and scientific disciplines. Many of the terms used have common language meanings, so a popular dictionary can be used. For medical terms, a more specialized source is required. Many medical dictionaries are available; *Dorland's Illustrated Medical Dictionary*, 30th edition (2003) in the pocket edition is recommended. Its small size makes it convenient to keep on the desk and to carry to the library, leaving no excuse for misunderstanding.

G.2 Glossary

Note: When two definitions are provided, the first is the more common usage.

Acute   Duration of less than 30 days; however, durations associated with clinical treatment (such as use of instruments, dialysis equipment, etc.) are usually termed short term or intraoperative. See also: chronic.

Adaptation   The ability of tissues to adapt to local requirements, including reaction to the chemical, physical, or electrical properties of implants.

Allograft   See: graft, allo-.

Artificial organ*   A medical device that replaces, in part or in whole, the function of one of the organs of the body.

Autograft   See: graft, auto-.

Bioactive   The ability of a biomaterial surface or coating to adhere directly to soft or hard tissue without an intermediate layer of modified tissue.

Bioactive material

> 1.** A biomaterial designed to elicit or modulate biological activity.
>
> 2.* One designed to induce specific biological activity.

Bioadhesion*   The adhesion of cells and/or tissue to the surface of a material.

Bioattachment*   The fastening of cells and/or tissue to the surface of a material, including mechanical interlocking (see: ingrowth; ongrowth).

Bioceramic   Strictly, any ceramic biomaterial. Usually used as equivalent to bioactive material, although bioactive polymers also exist.

Biocompatible material   One having acceptable host and material response in a specific application (see: host response; material response; first definition of biocompatibility).

Biocompatibility

> 1.* The ability of a material to perform with an appropriate host response in a specific application.
>
> 2. Biological performance in a specific application that is judged suitable to that situation. Note: the implication that biocompatibility implies little or only beneficial host response is to be avoided by context.

Biodegradation

1.** The breakdown of a material mediated by a biological system.

2.*ᴾ The gradual breakdown of a material mediated by specific biological activity.

Biological environment See: environment, biological.

Biological performance The interaction between materials and living systems (see: host response; material response).

Biomaterial

1.** A material intended to interface with biological systems to evaluate, treat, augment, or replace any tissue, organ, or function of the body (most general; see below; see also bioactive material).

2.* A nonviable material used in a medical device, intended to interact with biological systems.

3. A material of natural or manmade origin that is used to direct, supplement, or replace the functions of living tissues.

Also compound forms may be used: ceramic biomaterial, composite biomaterial, metallic biomaterial, polymeric biomaterial.

Biomaterial, inert One that elicits little or no host response. Also termed: type 1 biomaterial.

Biomaterial, interactive One designed to elicit, promote, or modulate a specific host response, such as hard tissue adhesion. Also termed: type 2 biomaterial.

Biomaterial, manmade (or manufactured) One that is significantly processed from raw materials of inorganic or organic origin.

Biomaterial, native (or natural) One obtained from natural organic sources and implanted essentially unprocessed.

Biomaterial, replant One consisting of live native cells or tissue, cultured *in vitro* from cells obtained previously from specific patients. Also termed: type 4 biomaterial.

Biomaterial, viable One that incorporates host tissue and/or live cells and/or active DNA plasmids and is capable of being remodeled and/or is resorbable and/or bioresorbable. Also termed: type 3 biomaterial.

Biomaterials The organized study of the materials properties of the tissues and organs of living organisms; the development and characterization of pharmacologically inert materials to measure, restore, and improve function in such organisms; and the interaction between viable and nonviable materials.

Biomaterials engineering   The application of the principles of biomaterials science and its foundation sciences to the solution of practical problems of human health, disability, and disease.

Biomaterials science   The study and knowledge of the interaction between living and nonliving materials.

Biomaterials science and engineering   Compound form; modern descriptor for the intellectual, academic, and industrial field previously referred to as biomaterials (see: biomaterials engineering; biomaterials science).

Biophysiological environment   See: environment, biophysiological.

Bioprosthesis*   An implantable prosthesis that consists totally or substantially of nonviable, treated donor tissue.

Bioresorbable   The ability of a biomaterial to be digested by or as a consequence of cellular activity and thus disappear in part or in whole after implantation. Should be used to imply specific action of cells or tissues (see: resorbable).

Bioresorption*P   The process of removal by cellular activity and/or dissolution of a material in a biological environment.

Bone bonding**   The establishment by physicochemical processes of continuity between implant and bone matrix.

Calor   Local tissue temperature rise; one of the four classic signs of inflammation (see also: dolor; rubor; tumor).

Cancer   A disease of multicellular organisms characterized by uncontrolled multiplication and spread of abnormal forms of host cells.

Capsule   Tissue surrounding an implant produced by local host response (see also: incapsulization; host response, local).

Carcinogen   An agent capable of causing cancer.

Carcinogenesis   Malignant, inheritable change in mammalian cells.

Carcinogenesis, chemical (attribute of an implant)   Carcinogenesis induced by the chemical composition of an implant or its degradation products.

Carcinogenesis, foreign body (attribute of an implant)   Carcinogenesis induced by the physical form of an implant, independent of its chemical composition.

Chelation   A type of interaction between an organic compound (having two or more points at which it may coordinate with a metal) and the metal to form a ring-type structure.

Chemotaxis   Orientation or movement of cells towards a chemical source.

Chronic   Duration of 30 days or longer (see also: acute).

Coagulation Sequential process in blood leading to thrombus formation (see also: thrombus).

Colony-forming unit The minimum number of bacteria required to grow a cell cluster or colony on a suitable solid culture medium. Abbreviated: cfu.

Control material See: reference material.

Coordination The joining of an ion or molecule to a metal ion by a nonionic valence bond to form a complex ion or molecule.

Cytokine Chemical species used for intercellular signaling.

Cytotoxic Having a deleterious or adverse effect on cells. Note: does not necessarily imply cell death.

Device matching Selecting an implant suited to the expected implant life history of a particular patient. (See also implant life history.)

Device, medical* An instrument, apparatus, implement, machine, contrivance, *in vitro* reagent, or other similar or related article, including any component, part, or accessory, that is intended for use in the diagnosis of disease or other conditions, or in the cure, mitigation, treatment, or prevention of disease in man. (Note: in modern usage, for "man" read "humans." Such a definition may be equally well used in veterinary medicine; however, there the preferred term would be veterinary medical device.)

Device, percutaneous*ᴾ A medical device that passes through the skin, remaining in position for a significant length of time (may be equivalent to implant [acute; chronic], permucosal).

Device, permucosal*ᴾ A medical device that passes through a mucosal layer and remains in position for a significant length of time (may be equivalent to implant [acute; chronic], percutaneous).

Diapedesis The outward passage of blood cells through intact vessel (arterial or venous) walls.

Dilantant Property of a lubricant; increasing shear viscosity with increasing shear rate (see also: thixotropic).

Dolor Local pain; one of the four classic signs of inflammation (see also: calor; rubor; tumor).

Environment, biological Conditions encountered within an animal or human body.

Environment, biophysiological Controlled chemical (inorganic) and thermal conditions, with addition of appropriate cell products, simulating a portion of a biological or pericellular environment.

Environment, pericellular Conditions encountered immediately adjacent to living cells *in vitro* or, more generally, within an animal or human body.

Environment, physiological   Controlled chemical (inorganic) and thermal conditions simulating a portion of a biological, biophysiological, or pericellular environment.

Extrusion   Resolution in which implants in contact with epithelial tissue (skin and the lining of natural internal body cavities) are surrounded by a down-growing extension of such tissue, directed towards extruding the implant from the body. This is termed marsupialization, due to the resemblance of the newly formed tissue to a kangaroo's pouch.

Factor XII   Initial factor in intrinsic pathway for blood coagulation; also called Hageman factor.

Foreign body reaction   A variation in normal tissue behavior caused by the presence of a foreign material (see also: host response, local).

Glycocalyx   A protective enveloping film formed on the surface of implants by some types of bacteria.

Graft*ᴾ   A piece of viable tissue or collection of viable cells transferred from a donor site to a recipient site for the purpose of reconstruction of the recipient site (most general; see following).

Graft, allo-*ᴾ   A graft taken from another individual of the same species as the recipient. (Note: all humans are members of a single species.)

Graft, auto-*ᴾ   A graft taken from a source in the individual who receives it; that is, the donor and the recipient are the same person (see also: replant).

Graft, xeno-*ᴾ   A graft taken from an individual of a different species from the recipient's. (Note: the source is explicitly nonhuman.)

Granuloma   Actively growing provision soft tissue that precedes remodeling phase of inflammatory response; may become chronic in the absence of resolution.

Hageman factor   See factor XII.

Hemolysis   Release of hemoglobin due to damage to red blood cells.

Heterograft   Old term for autograft (see: graft, auto-).

Homeostasis   The maintenance of conditions necessary for mammalian life.

Homograft   Old term for allograft (see: graft, allo-).

Host response

1.   The local and systemic response, other than the intended therapeutic response, of living systems to the material; a component of biological performance (most general, see below).

2.*   The reaction of a living system to the presence of a material.

Host response, level of The nature of the host response in a standard test with respect to the response obtained with a reference material.

Host response, local The response, other than the intended therapeutic response, of tissue and organs contacting a biomaterial.

Host response, remote The response, other than the intended therapeutic response, of remote tissue and organs in an individual with one or more implants.

Host response, systemic The distributed or disseminated response, other than the intended therapeutic response, of tissue and organs in an individual with one or more implants.

Hybrid artificial organ* An artificial organ that is a combination of viable cells and one or more biomaterials (see: biomaterial, viable; hybrid device).

Hybrid device One utilizing cells from patient or donor sources cultured *in vitro* and combined with resorbable or metabolizable supports and matrices (may be equivalent to hybrid artificial organ; see also: biomaterial, viable).

Implant

1. A device placed within an animal or human body by the act of implantation (see: implantation).

2.* A medical device made from one or more biomaterials that is intentionally placed within the body, totally or partially buried beneath an epithelial surface (most general, see following).

Implant, acute A device that remains *in situ* for less than 30 days.

Implant, chronic (or permanent) A device that remains *in situ* for 30 or more days.

Implant, intraoperative A device removed within hours to days at the termination of the surgical or therapeutic procedure.

Implant, percutaneous A device that, after placement, penetrates the skin (see also: device, percutaneous).

Implant, permucosal A device that, after placement, penetrates the mucosa (see also: device, permucosal).

Implant life history Lifetime performance requirements for an implant.

Implantation Placement of a device or material within the body of an animal or human by a medical or surgical professional, in such a way as to breach one or more epithelial layers and to leave materials and/or components in place after the initial procedure is completed.

Incapsulization Resolution in which the implant is surrounded and walled off from normal tissue by a collagenous, relatively acellular tissue termed capsule that much resembles scar tissue. In a bony location, the capsule may be mineralized and is called a sequestrum.

Inflammation   See: inflammatory response.

Ingrowth   Formation of tissue within pores, etc. in the body of an implant (see also: ongrowth).

Integration   Resolution for a very limited number of materials, such as "bioactive" glasses of selected compositions and some metals, such as pure titanium for which direct "bonding" or apparent adhesion to normal tissue may take place.

Iontopheresis   Facilitation of diffusion by imposing an electrical gradient on a charged diffusing species.

Ligand   Any ion or molecule that, by donating one or more pairs of electrons to a central metal ion, is coordinated with it to form a complex ion or molecule.

Marsupialization   See: extrusion.

Material response   The response of a material to living systems; a component of biological performance.

Material response, level of   The nature of the material response in a standard test with respect to the response obtained with a reference material.

Mutagenesis   Induction of a permanent (inheritable) genetic change.

Ongrowth   Formation of tissue directly on the surface of an implant (see also: ingrowth). Does not imply adhesion.

Oppenheimer effect   Induction of primarily subcutaneous tumors in rodents through a foreign body mechanism; named after its discoverers, E. and B.S. Oppenheimer.

Opsonization   Coating of bacteria or biomaterial particles with native proteins, such as complement factors, rendering them dectable as "foreign" by phagocytic cells.

Orthosis   A device applied externally to the body to provide stability and to control motion. May or may not replace a portion of a limb (see also: prosthesis).

Osseointegration

1.   Clinical stability of an implant anchored in bone; often taken to refer to implants with bioactive coatings.

2.**   A description of clinical performance of devices; not applicable to the description of biomaterial–bone interactions. (Note: sometimes spelled osteointegration; however, osseintegration is preferred.)

Osteoconductive   Property of a biomaterial that encourages bone, already being formed, to lie close to or adhere to its surface.

Osteogenic   Property of a biomaterial that stimulates bone growth in the implant site.

Osteoinductive   Property of a biomaterial that encourages bone to form close to or adhering to its surface. Note: the term should be used to apply to the material (matrix) in the absence of specific osteoinductive signaling molecules or ligands.

Osteointegration   See osseointegration.

Osteolysis   Cellularly mediated bone loss (also called small particle disease) secondary to debris production and/or release by implants in or near to bone. Notes: previously, also incorrectly called "cement disease." Do not confuse with stress shielding.

Pericellular environment   See: environment, pericellular.

Phagocytosis   The process of internalizing small particles by mammalian cells.

Phagocytosis, frustrated   The failure of mammalian cells to phagocytose particles due primarily to their size, resulting in release of cytokines.

Physiological elements   Elements (calcium, phosphorus, potassium, sulfur, sodium, chlorine, and iron) — other than oxygen, hydrogen, nitrogen, and carbon — required for mammalian homeostasis.

Physiological environment   See: environment, physiological.

Prosthesis*   A device that replaces a limb, organ, or tissue of the body. Note: externally worn prostheses, especially ones not permanently attached to the body, are more properly termed orthoses; see: orthosis.

Pseudointima   Tissue consisting of a firm fibrin clot, with occasional islands of endothelial cells, formed by resolution on interior (blood-contacting surfaces) of cardiovascular implants.

Pseudoneointima   Pseudointima in which cells form a continuous layer.

Pyrogen   A substance producing fever (heat) *in vivo.*

Reference material   A material that, by standard test, has been determined to elicit a reproducible, quantifiable host or material response.

Replant   An autograft produced *in vitro* from DNA, cells and/or tissues obtained from the donor, utilizing one or more techniques of tissue engineering.

Resolution   The stable end state of the inflammation or inflammatory response associated with an implant.

Resorbable   The ability of a biomaterial to be dissolved or digested and thus disappear after implantation. Note: does not imply specific action of cells or tissues; see: bioresorbable.

Resorption   Resolution associated with resorbable or bioresorbable implants in which the tissue site condenses to a collapsed scar or, in the case of bone, completely remodels to normal (regenerated) tissue.

Response, acute   Host response or material response in less than 30 days after implantation.

Response, chronic   Host response or material response in 30 days or more after implantation.

Response, host   See host response.

Response, immune   Host response involving humoral or cellular specific immune mechanisms.

Response, inflammatory   The cell-mediated local and regional response directed towards stabilizing injured tissue, restoring physiological status quo ante, removing dead or damaged tissue elements and foreign material, and correcting the structural and functional loss due to the initial insult. The four classical signs of inflammation are: redness (rubor), swelling (tumor), pain (dolor), and heat (calor).

Response, material   See: material response.

Rubor   Local tissue reddening; one of the four classic signs of inflammation (see also: calor; dolor; tumor).

Sequestrum   Mineralized capsule, generally in or on bone. In the absence of bone, more properly referred to as ectopic calcification.

Small particle disease   See osteolysis.

Sonopheresis   Facilitation of diffusion, particularly transdermally, by inducing reversible ultrasonic microcavitation.

Standard test   A well-defined, repeatable test of host or material response, generally involving the use of one or more reference materials.

Stress shielding   Effect resulting in a decreased density of bone as a consequence of load sharing between an implant and tissue.

Thixotropic   Property of a lubricant; decreasing shear viscosity with increasing shear rate (see also: dilantant).

Three-phase junction   Referring to percutaneous implants; the point at which tissue, implant, and air meet.

Thrombogenicity*   The property of a material that induces and/or promotes the formation of a thrombus (most general, see below).

Thrombogenicity, general*P   Thrombogenicity of a blood–material system.

Thrombogenicity, inherent

  1.** Thrombus formation controlled by the material surface.

  2.*P Reaction-controlled thrombogenicity at the surface of a material.

Thrombogenicity, non-*P   The characteristic of a material that leads to minimal thrombogenicity.

Thrombus   A solid mass formed from the molecular and cellular constituent of blood (see also: thrombogenicity).

Tissue engineering (provisional definition)   Elaboration of cells and tissues outside a living organism, intended for use as components of a viable biomaterial or replant by use of engineering methods and techniques.

Tumor   Local tissue swelling; one of the four classic signs of inflammation (see also: calor; dolor; rubor).

Vroman effect   The temporal succession of molecular species adherent to surfaces of implants, named after its discoverer, Leo Vroman.

Wolff's law   "The form being given, tissue adapts to best fulfill its mechanical function" (after Wolff 1892 in Maquet and Furlong 1986).

Xenograft   See graft, xeno-.

G.3 Deprecated Terms

Williams (1987) also lists the following terms, which the attendees to the first consensus conference considered redundant or inappropriate under certain conditions; it is suggested that these should be deprecated:

Antithrombogenic

Bioceramic   To be consistent with the advice on biopolymer and biometal (see following), this term should also be deprecated. However, see ceramic biomaterial and bioceramic (Section G.2), notwithstanding the advice of the 1991 conference to deprecate the latter.

Biocompatible   When used as an adjective.

Bioinert

Biological performance   Preferred term is biocompatibility.

Biometal   Preferred term is metallic biomaterial.

Biopolymer   Term has an agreed meaning in molecular biology; the preferred term is polymeric biomaterial.

Biostability

Blood compatibility

Material rejection

Material response

Thromboresistant   The preferred term is nonthrombogenic (see: non-thrombogenicity, Section G.2).

Tissue response   Preferred term is host response, local.

References

FDA 91-4246: *Classification Names for Medical Devices and in Vitro Diagnostic Products.* U.S. Government Printing Office, Washington, D.C., 1991.

Maquet, P. and Furlong, R., *The Law of Bone Remodeling, Wolff, H. (1892)*, Springer–Verlag, Berlin, (transl.), 1986.

Newman Dorland, W.A., *Dorland's Illustrated Medical Dictionary*, 30th ed., W.B. Saunders, Philadelphia, 2003.

Szycher, M., *Szycher's Dictionary of Biomaterials and Medical Devices*, Technomic Publishing Co., Lancaster, PA, 1992.

Williams, D.F. (Ed.), *The Williams Dictionary of Biomaterials*, Liverpool University Press, Liverpool, U.K., 1999.

Williams, D.F. (Ed.), *Definitions in Biomaterials: Proceedings of a Consensus Conference of the European Society for Biomaterials*, Chester, England, March 3–5, 1986. Elsevier, Amsterdam, 1987.

Williams, D.F., Black, J. and Doherty, P.J., Definitions in biomaterials, Second Consensus Conference on Definitions in Biomaterials, in Doherty, P.J., Williams, R.L., Williams, D.F. and Lee, A.J.C. (Eds.), *Biomaterial–Tissue Interfaces. Advances in Biomaterials* Vol. 10, Elsevier, Amsterdam, 1992, 525.

Index

A

Ablative surfaces, thromboresistant materials development, 170
Abrasion, 116, 117
Absorbable materials, fracture strength, 101
Absorption, 36–38
    drug release devices, 46
    mechanical properties
        elastic modulus, 92
        environment effects, 91
        fracture strength, 103
    mineral metabolism
        chromium, 283–295
        iron, 276–277
    undesirable, examples of, 38–41
    and wear debris, 121
Acellular fibrous capsule, 146
Acid treatment, passivation, 54
Activation, surface/interface interactions, 80–81
Acute response, inflammation, 148, 149
Adaptation, 183–199
    examples, implant applications, 186–197
        bone response, remodeling near implants, 191–196
        bone response, to electrified implants, 196–197
        tendon replacement, 189–191
        vascular prosthesis, 186–189
    factors in local host response, 198–199
    interdependency of effects, 198–199
    systemic/remote site response mechanisms, 322
    tissue growth strategies, 183–185
    utility of active tissue response, 197–198
Adhesion
    adaptation, physical induction factors, 199
    surface/interface interactions, 78–86
Adhesive wear, size of debris particles, 119
Adsorption
    hypersensitivity reactions, implant-associated, 230–231

surface/interface interactions, 77, 78–79
Age, and inflammatory response, 148
Aggregation, surface/interface interactions, 74
Albumin, surface/interface interactions, 77, 81'
Alkaline/basic conditions, corrosion, 50
Allergic foreign body response, 225–241
    clinical performance of biomaterials, 331
    hypersensitivity reactions, classes of, 230
    hypersensitivity reactions, implant-associated, 230–240
        metals, 231–240
        polymers, 230–231
    immune response, mechanisms of, 226–229
    specific versus nonspecific response, 225, 226
    systemic/remote site response mechanisms, 323
Allo-, defined, 210
Allobiopsy cells, *in vitro* tissue growth and replantation, 211, 214
Allografts
    cell sources, 211, 212
    vascular, 174
Alloys
    carcinogenicity, 253, 255
    corrosion, 65–66
        leaching, 62
        pitting, 61
        uniform attack, 59
    corrosion product distribution, 299
    electrochemical series, 54, 55, 56
    inflammation, phagocytosis, 156–157
    systemic distribution and excretion
        dissolved species, distribution and excretion of, 303
        multicompartment distribution models, 306–309
        one compartment distribution models, 304, 305
    test methods, *in vivo*, 369
    wear, size of debris particles, 119, 120